Endoscopy

Editors

STEPHEN J. DIVERS
LAILA M. PROENÇA

VETERINARY CLINICS OF NORTH AMERICA: EXOTIC ANIMAL PRACTICE

www.vetexotic.theclinics.com

Consulting Editor
AGNES E. RUPLEY

September 2015 • Volume 18 • Number 3

ELSEVIER

1600 John F. Kennedy Boulevard • Suite 1800 • Philadelphia, Pennsylvania, 19103-2899
http://www.vetexotic.theclinics.com

VETERINARY CLINICS OF NORTH AMERICA: EXOTIC ANIMAL PRACTICE Volume 18, Number 3
September 2015 ISSN 1094-9194, ISBN-13: 978-0-323-39589-2

Editor: Patrick Manley
Developmental Editor: Meredith Clinton

Veterinary Clinics of North America: Exotic Animal Practice (ISSN 1094-9194) is published in January, May, and September by Elsevier, Inc., 360 Park Avenue South, New York, NY 10010-1710. Subscription prices are $255.00 per year for US individuals, $399.00 per year for US institutions, $130.00 per year for US students and residents, $305.00 per year for Canadian individuals, $482.00 per year for Canadian institutions, $340.00 per year for international individuals, $482.00 per year for international institutions and $165.00 per year for Canadian and foreign students/ residents. To receive student/resident rate, orders must be accompanied by name of affiliated institution, date of term, and the *signature* of program/residency coordinator on institution letterhead. Orders will be billed at individual rate until proof of status is received. Foreign air speed delivery is included in all *Clinics* subscription prices. All prices are subject to change without notice. **POSTMASTER:** Send address changes to *Veterinary Clinics of North America: Exotic Animal Practice*, Elsevier Health Sciences Division, Subscription Customer Service, 3251 Riverport Lane, Maryland Heights, MO 63043. **Customer Service: Telephone: 1-800-654-2452** (U.S. and Canada); **1-314-447-8871** (outside U.S. and Canada). **Fax: 1-314-447-8029. E-mail: journalscustomerservice-usa@elsevier.com (for print support); journalsonlinesupport-usa@elsevier.com (for online support).**

Reprints. For copies of 100 or more of articles in this publication, please contact the Commercial Reprints Department, Elsevier Inc., 360 Park Avenue South, New York, New York 10010-1710. Tel.: 212-633-3874; Fax: 212-633-3820; E-mail: reprints@elsevier.com.

Veterinary Clinics of North America: Exotic Animal Practice is covered in *MEDLINE/PubMed (Index Medicus).*

Contributors

CONSULTING EDITOR

AGNES E. RUPLEY, DVM
Diplomate, American Board of Veterinary Practitioners (Avian Practice); Director and Chief Veterinarian, All Pets Medical and Laser Surgical Center, College Station, Texas

EDITORS

STEPHEN J. DIVERS, BSc(Hons), BVetMed, DZooMed, DipECZM (Herpetology, Zoo Health Management), DACZM, FRCVS
RCVS Recognized Specialist in Zoo and Wildlife Medicine; European Veterinary Specialist in Zoological Medicine (Zoo Health Management); Professor of Zoological Medicine, Department of Small Animal Medicine and Surgery, College of Veterinary Medicine, University of Georgia, Athens, Georgia

LAILA M. PROENÇA, MV, DVM, MS, PhD
Director of the Exotic Animal Medicine Service, VCA Animal Hospitals, Los Angeles, California

AUTHORS

FERRAN BARGALLÓ, DVM
Zoologic Badalona Veterinary Clinics, Badalona, Spain

NORIN CHAI, DVM, MSc, PhD
Ménagerie du Jardin des Plantes, Muséum national d'Histoire naturelle, Paris, France

MARION R. DESMARCHELIER, DVM, IPSAV, DES, MSc
Diplomate of the American College of Zoological Medicine; Zoological Medicine Service, Faculté de médecine vétérinaire, Université de Montréal, Saint-Hyacinthe, Quebec, Canada

NICOLA DI GIROLAMO, DMV, MSc (EBHC)
Clinica per Animali Esotici, Centro Veterinario Specialistico, Roma, Italy

STEPHEN J. DIVERS, BSc(Hons), BVetMed, DZooMed, DipECZM (Herpetology, Zoo Health Management), DACZM, FRCVS
RCVS Recognized Specialist in Zoo and Wildlife Medicine; European Veterinary Specialist in Zoological Medicine (Zoo Health Management); Professor of Zoological Medicine, Department of Small Animal Medicine and Surgery, College of Veterinary Medicine, University of Georgia, Athens, Georgia

SHANNON T. FERRELL, DVM
Diplomate of the American Board of Veterinary Practitioners (Avian); Diplomate of the American College of Zoological Medicine; Granby Zoo, Granby, Quebec, Canada

JORDI GRÍFOLS, DVM, MSc
Zoologic Badalona Veterinary Clinics, Badalona, Spain

JEAN-MICHEL HATT, Prof Dr med vet, MSc
Diplomate of the European College of Zoological Medicine (Avian); Diplomate of the American College of Zoological Medicine; Department of Small Animals, Clinic for Zoo Animals, Exotic Pets and Wildlife, Vetsuisse Faculty, University of Zurich, Zurich, Switzerland

KAREL HAUPTMAN, DVM, PhD
Avian and Exotic Animal Clinic, Faculty of Veterinary Medicine, University of Veterinary and Pharmaceutical Sciences Brno, Brno, Czech Republic

ROMAN HUSNIK, DVM, PhD
Department of Veterinary Clinical Sciences, School of Veterinary Medicine, Louisiana State University, Baton Rouge, Louisiana; International Clinical Research Center (ICRC), St. Anne's University Hospital Brno, Brno, Czech Republic

MINH HUYNH, DVM
Diplomate of the European College of Zoological Medicine (Avian); Exotics Medicine Service, Centre Hospitalier Vétérinaire Frégis, Arcueil, France

VLADIMIR JEKL, DVM, PhD
Diplomate of the European College of Zoological Medicine (Small Mammal); European Recognised Veterinary Specialist in Zoological Medicine (Small Mammal), Avian and Exotic Animal Clinic, Faculty of Veterinary Medicine, University of Veterinary and Pharmaceutical Sciences Brno, Brno, Czech Republic

ZDENEK KNOTEK, DVM, PhD
Professor, Diplomate of the European College of Zoological Medicine (Herpetology); European Recognised Veterinary Specialist in Zoological Medicine (Herpetology), Avian and Exotic Animal Clinic, Faculty of Veterinary Medicine, University of Veterinary and Pharmaceutical Sciences Brno, Brno, Czech Republic

ALBERT MARTÍNEZ-SILVESTRE, DVM, MSc, PhD, Acred AVEPA (Exotic Animals)
Diplomate European College Zoo Medicine (Especiality Herpetology); Scientific Director, CRARC (Catalonian Reptile and Amphiobian Rescue Center), Masquefa, Spain

CHARLY PIGNON, DVM
Diplomate of the European College of Zoological Medicine (Small Mammal); Exotics Medicine Service, Alfort National Veterinary School, Maisons-Alfort, France

LAILA M. PROENÇA, MV, DVM, MS, PhD
Director of the Exotic Animal Medicine Service, VCA Animal Hospitals, Los Angeles, California

PAOLO SELLERI, DMV, PhD
Diplomate of the European College of Zoological Medicine (Herpetology and Small Mammals); Clinica per Animali Esotici, Centro Veterinario Specialistico, Roma, Italy

SANDRA WENGER, Dr med vet, MSc
DECVAA; Diplomate of the European College of Zoological Medicine; Department of Small Animals, Clinic for Zoo Animals, Exotic Pets and Wildlife, Vetsuisse Faculty, University of Zurich, Zurich, Switzerland

Contents

> The definitive diagnosis has often been elusive in exotic pet medicine, and its absence has been, and continues to be, the source of much client anguish and practitioner frustration. To reach a definitive diagnosis, demonstration of a pathologic response and the etiologic agent are required. This article demonstrates why such an approach is necessary and how it can be readily achieved in practice using endoscopy.

> Urinary diseases are commonly found in guinea pigs. Diagnostic workup includes clinical examination, blood testing, imaging studies, urine culture, and urinalysis. This article describes the use of transurethral cystoscopy in female guinea pigs as an ancillary tool to diagnose abnormalities within the bladder and urethra. In addition, the transurethral cystoscopic removal of uroliths measuring up to 5 mm and situated within the urinary bladder is described.

> Gastrointestinal disease is a common complaint in ferrets (*Mustela putorius furo*). Their relatively simple and short gastrointestinal tract makes them good candidates for flexible endoscopy. However, apart from a few references in biomedical research articles, there is little information on the use of flexible endoscopy in ferrets. This review describes patient preparation, equipment, and select gastrointestinal endoscopy techniques in ferrets, including esophagoscopy, gastroscopy, duodenoscopy, percutaneous endoscopic gastrostomy, jejunoileoscopy, colonoscopy, and biopsy.

> Laparoscopic ovariectomy has been advocated as the preferred sterilization method for dogs for some time. The same arguments and benefits can be extended for many zoologic mammals, including carnivores, suids, primates, lagomorphs, and large rodents. This article summarizes the benefits, equipment options, surgical technique, recovery, and complications associated with this sterilization procedure.

Ophthalmic diseases are common in rabbits and rodents. Fast and definitive diagnosis is imperative for successful treatment of ocular diseases. Ophthalmic examination in rabbits and rodents can be challenging. Oculoscopy offers great magnification for the examination of the ocular structures in such animals, including the evaluation of cornea, anterior eye chamber, limbus, iris, lens, and retina. To date, oculoscopy has been described only sporadically and/or under experimental conditions. This article describes the oculoscopy technique, normal and abnormal ocular findings, and the most common eye disorders diagnosed with the aid of endoscopy in rabbits and rodents.

Ear disease is a common disorder seen in exotic companion mammals, especially in ferrets, rabbits, and rats. This article describes patient preparation, equipment, and video otoscopy technique in exotic companion mammals. This noninvasive technique facilitates accurate diagnosis of diseases affecting the external ear canal or middle ear. Moreover, therapeutic otoscopic evaluation of the external ear facilitates foreign body removal, external ear canal flushing, intralesional drug administration, myringotomy, and middle ear cavity flushing.

Endoscopy in nonhuman primates (NHPs) has resulted in improvements in research and clinical care for more than 4 decades. The indications and procedures are the same as in humans and the approach is similar to that in dogs, cats, and humans. Selected procedures are discussed including rhinoscopy, tracheobronchoscopy, upper gastrointestinal endoscopy, laparoscopy, and endoscopic salpingectomy. This short overview provides practitioners with pragmatic elements for safe and effective endoscopy in NHPs.

Although endoscopy is part of the basic standard of care in most avian practices, many wildlife rehabilitation centers do not have access to the equipment or do not use it on a regular basis. Endoscopic equipment is easily available at a lower cost on the used market or can be acquired through donations from local human hospitals. Several medical conditions encountered in wild raptors have an improved prognosis if they are diagnosed or treated early with the aid of endoscopy. In many cases, endoscopy provides a noninvasive alternative to exploratory surgery, saving cost and time and decreasing postoperative pain.

Despite advances in exotic animal endoscopy, descriptions involving amphibians are scarce. Amphibian endoscopy shares some similarities with reptiles, especially in lizards. Selected procedures are discussed, including stomatoscopy, gastroscopy, coelioscopy, and biopsy of coelomic organs and lesions. This short overview provides the practitioner with pragmatic advice on how to conduct safe and effective endoscopic examinations in amphibians.

Pulmonoscopy is a practical diagnostic tool for investigating respiratory diseases in snakes. Two different approaches exist for pulmonoscopy, tracheal and transcutaneous. The access to the proximal or distal lung is limited by the length and diameter of the endoscope when using the tracheal approach. The transcutaneous approach allows direct evaluation of the lung and distal trachea through the air sac. Both of the methods are safe, and specific contraindications for pulmonoscopy in snakes are not known except for any anesthesia contraindication.

The medical approach to chelonians can be challenging. Cystoscopy may be useful to evaluate morphologic changes in the viscera without the need of celiotomy, and is a valuable diagnostic tool. The size and transparency of the urinary bladder in chelonians allows visualization of most coelomic organs. Through cystoscopy the external aspect of stomach, intestine, heart, lungs, liver, pancreas, spleen, kidneys, testes, and ovaries may be visualized. Although a definitive diagnosis cannot be achieved, rapid identification of the diseased system through cystoscopy may be possible. Furthermore, cystoscopy is fundamental for diagnosis and treatment of lower urogenital disorders.

 Videos of endoscopic evaluation and cystoscopy evaluation accompany this article

Cloacoscopy and cystoscopy are simple, noninvasive to minimally invasive techniques that provide excellent visualization, and result in fast recovery. General or intrathecal anesthesia is sufficient. They can be performed in free-ranging turtles under field conditions. Cloacoscopic gender identification of external genitalia is not reliable because of the high degree of misinterpretation between phallus and clitoris, especially in juveniles. However, saline-infusion or air insufflation cystoscopy through the urinary bladder (or accessory vesicles/bladders) is often effective for the visualization of gonads and to identify the sex. Visualization of gonads is feasible through the urinary bladder or accessory vesicle wall in many species.

A video of a two-portal access laparoscopic ovariectomy accompanies this article

Laparoscopic sterilization techniques are becoming accepted in veterinary medicine, and there has been interest in reducing the number and size of portals. Computer-controlled bipolar electrocoagulation devices facilitate sealing and dividing ovarian pedicles, reducing operative time. The 2-portal laparoscopic ovariectomy has been proved to be safe, feasible, and effective in dogs and cats, but has not yet been described in exotic companion mammals. Based on the author's experience, the 2-portal laparoscopic ovariectomy seems to be safe and feasible in rabbits, but complications such as emergency conversion to laparotomy and severe postoperative ileus have occurred in pigs.

VETERINARY CLINICS OF NORTH AMERICA: EXOTIC ANIMAL PRACTICE

RELATED INTEREST

Veterinary Clinics of North America: Small Animal Practice
July 2015 (Vol. 45, No. 4)
Urology
Joseph W. Bartges, *Editor*

THE CLINICS ARE NOW AVAILABLE ONLINE!
Access your subscription at:
www.theclinics.com

Preface

Endoscopic Research and Practice Development Marches Forward

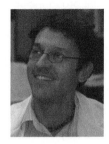
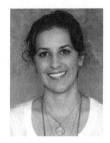

Stephen J. Divers, BSc(Hons), BVetMed, DZooMed, DipECZM (Herpetology, Zoo Health Management), DACZM, FRCVS

Laila M. Proença, MV, DVM, MS, PhD

Editors

Inquisitive thinking, the popular "curiosity," is timeless. It occurred to Philipp Bozzini in 1806 when developing the first rudimental endoscope, and so on to many veterinarians hungry to use this novel technique. It was no different with the innovative group of veterinarians that came up with the great *Veterinary Clinics of North America: Exotic Animal Practice* 2010 Endoscopy issue. The issue covered the basics of diagnostic endoscopy and some endosurgery, and it is still considered a contemporary publication.

Fortunately, curiosity has not stopped since, and many novel techniques have been developed in zoological medicine. Grouping all of them together and sharing all this knowledge was the perfect way to keep stimulating minds and more inquisitive thinking. This current Exotic Endoscopy issue comes to complement, not substitute, the previous publication.

Information is only useful when shared and practiced. To be practiced, it needs to be relevant. To be relevant, it needs to relate to our everyday work, to our needs. With that in mind, and with the help of all the authors, we chose the articles you will find in this issue. The information presented here originated out of curiosity, by simply trying to answer questions raised by our daily activities.

It has been 5 years since the last issue of *Veterinary Clinics of North America: Exotic Animal Practice* was dedicated to Endoscopy. That previous publication attempted to bring the basics of exotic animal endoscopy to the forefront. If it failed to convince you in 2010, we hope that the first article will convince you today. This issue, however, is different for several reasons. First and foremost, and despite some initial resistance

Vet Clin Exot Anim 18 (2015) xi–xii
http://dx.doi.org/10.1016/j.cvex.2015.06.001
1094-9194/15/$ – see front matter © 2015 Published by Elsevier Inc.

vetexotic.theclinics.com

from the publishers, I was able to have my then resident, Dr Laila Proença, assist as a guest editor. It is unusual for the *Veterinary Clinics of North America: Exotic Animal Practice* to permit a nonspecialist to edit an issue, but during her residency, Dr Proença was consistently excited about endoscopic techniques and benefited from the unique training possibilities at University of Georgia (UGA). Although I was disappointed that she left UGA prematurely, I have no doubt that her singular focus and drive for personal success will continue. I am grateful for the dedication and professionalism that she has shown throughout this process.

This issue also sees a departure from the usual broad inclusive taxa-based reviews. We both felt that it was important to showcase the great advances that are occurring not just in North America but also throughout Europe. To that end, we are delighted with the international flavor of this issue with contributions from Canada, Switzerland, France, Czech Republic, Italy, Spain, and the United States. We gave colleagues, whom we know to be active in the field, freedom to create an article on something that they find exciting, and the issue offers real practical benefits in zoological medicine. They delivered quality articles on time, and even more amazingly, generally not in their primary language. That deserves huge credit all by itself. In addition to describing endoscopy procedures that vary from basic to advanced, we also tried to tackle some problem practice management areas such as fee structures. The diversity of topics covered here is considerable, and we trust that there is something for everyone whether you work with exotic pets, zoo collections, or wildlife. There is no better way to finish this preface than with a quote by James Cameron: "Curiosity is the most powerful thing you own." So grab yours, along with a cup of coffee, and enjoy this issue.

Stephen J. Divers, BSc(Hons), BVetMed, DZooMed, DipECZM (Herpetology,
Zoo Health Management), DACZM, FRCVS
RCVS Recognized Specialist in Zoo and Wildlife Medicine;
European Veterinary Specialist in Zoological Medicine (Zoo Health Management)
Department of Small Animal
Medicine and Surgery
College of Veterinary Medicine
University of Georgia
2200 College Station Road
Athens, GA 30602, USA

Laila M. Proença, MV, DVM, MS, PhD
Exotic Animal Medicine Service
VCA Animal Hospitals
12401 West Olympic Boulevard
Los Angeles, CA 90064, USA

E-mail addresses:
sdivers@uga.edu (S.J. Divers)
laila.proenca@vca.com (L.M. Proença)

Making the Difference in Exotic Animal Practice

The Value of Endoscopy

Stephen J. Divers, BSc(Hons), BVetMed, DZooMed,
DipECZM (Herpetology, Zoo Health Management), DACZM, FRCVS

KEYWORDS

- Definitive diagnosis • Endoscopy • Biopsy

KEY POINTS

- A definitive diagnosis requires demonstration of a pathologic change and identification of the causative agent.
- Endoscopic biopsy represents a noninvasive to minimally invasive technique that facilitates internal evaluation and biopsy.
- Training is required, but basic clinical competency is quickly achieved.

INTRODUCTION

Zoologic medicine has been plagued with numerous problems, many of which our domestic animal counterparts do not have to face. As exotic animal veterinarians, we have to deal with a variety of diverse species, general lack of pathognomonic clinical signs, limited serologic tests, and few tried and tested therapeutic modalities. I myself used to be frequently frustrated with many of my reptile, avian, and small mammal cases. My inability to reach a definitive diagnosis often adversely affected the accuracy of my prognoses, and the effectiveness of my treatments. In 1994, I took the Harris and Taylor avian endoscopy laboratory at the North American Veterinary Conference, and that forever changed the way I practiced zoological medicine. During the last two decades, my research and clinical experiences have only strengthened my belief that endoscopy is a diagnostic cornerstone of zoological medicine, and offers major benefits to exotic pet practitioners. From the outset it is important to state that my interests in endoscopy are solely clinical. I am not a paid consultant for any endoscopy company, and all equipment used in my clinical service (**Table 1**) at the Veterinary Teaching Hospital, University of Georgia, has been purchased (not

The author has nothing to disclose.
Department of Small Animal Medicine and Surgery, College of Veterinary Medicine, University of Georgia, 2200 College Station Road, Athens, GA 30602, USA
E-mail address: sdivers@uga.edu

Table 1
Endoscopy equipment frequently used in exotic animal procedures

Equipment Description	Primary Indications
Telescopes and Endoscopes	
1 mm × 20 cm semirigid miniscope, 0°	Stomatoscopy, otoscopy, rhinoscopy, tracheoscopy in animals up to 1 kg
1.9 mm × 18.5 cm telescope, 30° oblique, with integrated 3.3-mm operating sheath	Stomatoscopy, otoscopy, rhinoscopy, tracheoscopy, gastroscopy, colonoscopy, cloacoscopy, and coelioscopy in animals up to 3–4 kg
2.7 mm × 18 cm telescope, 30° oblique (wide angle) 4.8-mm operating sheath	Stomatoscopy, otoscopy, rhinoscopy, tracheoscopy, gastroscopy, colonoscopy, cloacoscopy, and coelioscopy in animals between 100 g and 10 kg
5 mm × 8.5 cm otoendoscope, 0°, with integrated operating sheath	Stomatoscopy and otoscopy in animals between 1 and 100 kg
Mechanical holding arm (VITOM)	Enables the telescope to be held in place by a table-clamped mechanical arm
3-mm, 100-cm fiberoptic bronchoscope with 1.2-mm channel	Two-way deflection and biopsy channel for flexible gastrointestinal and respiratory endoscopy
2.8-mm, 60-cm video bronchoscope with 1.2-mm channel	Two-way deflection and biopsy channel for flexible gastrointestinal and respiratory endoscopy
5.9-mm, 110-cm videogastroscope with 2-mm channel	Four-way deflection, irrigation, suction, and biopsy channel for flexible gastrointestinal
Visualization and Documentation	
Endovideo camera and monitor Xenon light source and light guide cable Digital capture device (eg, AIDA-DVD)	Required for all endoscopy procedures
Flexible Instruments for Use with Operating Sheaths	
1-mm biopsy forceps 1-mm grasping forceps	For use with 1.9-mm telescope and integrated sheath
1.7-mm biopsy forceps 1.7-mm single-action scissors 1.7-mm remote injection needle 1.7-mm grasping/retrieval forceps 1.7-mm wire basket retrieval 1.7-mm needle end radiosurgery electrode 1.7-mm polypectomy snare	For use with 2.7-mm telescope and 4.8-mm operating sheath, and 5-mm otoendoscope
Insufflation	
CO_2 insufflator with silicone tubing	Used for insufflation during reptile coelioscopy
Sterile saline suspended above endoscopy table with intravenous drip line to a port on the operating sheath	Used for sterile saline infusion for otoscopy, rhinoscopy, cystoscopy, cloacoscopy, reptile (especially of small and/or aquatic species), or fish coelioscopy

(continued on next page)

Table 1 (continued)	
Equipment Description	**Primary Indications**
Rigid instruments, Handles, and Cannulae for Multiple-Entry Coelioscopy	
2.5-mm graphite and plastic cannula 2-mm Reddick-Olsen dissecting forceps, plastic handle without racket 2-mm Metzenbaum scissors, plastic handle without racket 2-mm Babcock forceps, plastic handle with racket	Used with the 1.9-mm telescope for coelioscopy in animals <1 kg
3.9-mm graphite and plastic cannula (accommodates 2.7-mm telescope and 3.5-mm protection sheath) 3.5-mm graphite and plastic cannula (accommodates 3-mm instruments) 3-mm fenestrated grasping forceps 3-mm Reddick-Olsen dissecting and grasping forceps 3-mm short curved Kelly dissecting and grasping forceps 3-mm atraumatic dissecting and grasping forceps 3-mm Babcock forceps 3-mm Blakesley dissecting and biopsy forceps 3-mm scissors with serrated curved double-action jaws 3-mm micro hook scissors, single-action jaws 3-mm Mahnes bipolar coagulation forceps 3-mm irrigation and suction cannula 3-mm palpation probe with cm markings 3-mm distendable palpation probe 3-mm ultramicro needle holder 3-mm knot tier for extracorporeal suturing 2 plastic handles without rackets 1 plastic handle with Mahnes style racket 1 plastic handle with hemostat style racket	Used with the 2.7-mm telescope for coelioscopy in animals <10 kg. These same instruments are also available in 5 mm for use with 5 mm scopes and 6 mm cannulae.
Radiosurgery Equipment	
3.8- or 4.0-MHz dual radiofrequency unit with foot pedal Monopolar lead to connect to plastic instrument handles Bipolar lead to connect to 3-mm Mahnes bipolar coagulation forceps	Enables endoscopic instruments to be used as monopolar devices and facilitates bipolar coagulation
5-mm Ligasure laparoscopic seal and cut instrument connected to electrosurgical unit	This unit facilitates sealing and cutting with a single instrument but is only available in 5 mm, and not smaller sizes

donated). The purpose of this article is to convince those that do not use endoscopy regularly to start; you will never look back!

THE DEFINITIVE DIAGNOSIS

Much of what we do as veterinarians is governed by accurate diagnosis. It informs the client of the likely prognosis, which is often their primary concern. An accurate diagnosis also tends to dictate appropriate therapeutic approaches, and removes the flawed guesswork associated with antibiotic choice, or whether surgery or medical treatment may be more appropriate.

It is concerning that many exotic animal diagnoses are made merely to the organ level with a presumed, generic cause (eg, parrots with respiratory disease, iguanas with renal disease, and rabbits with cystitis). What is required is a definitive diagnosis to a histologic and etiologic level. A definitive diagnosis relies on the demonstration of a patient's pathologic response, and identification of the causative agent. Essentially, the pathologic response can be demonstrated through histopathology, cytology, or paired rising serologic titers. There are few serologic tests available for most exotic pets, and those that are available typically require several weeks between sample collection (the patient may well be better or dead by the time results are obtained). Consequently, they are typically used for retrospective confirmation. Cytology is most rapid, but suffers from a lack of tissue architecture, and therefore histopathology is often considered the gold standard. Demonstration of the causative agent relies on microbiologic culture or polymerase chain reaction for bacteria, fungi, viruses (and some parasites), sensitive assays to identify toxins, and a variety of other techniques for parasite identification.

It is well appreciated that the collection of samples from lesions and tissues for histopathology, microbiology, parasitology, and/or toxicology remains the best hope of reaching a specific diagnosis. Samples can be easily collected postmortem; however, diagnosis in the live animal requires an antemortem biopsy.

As an example to illustrate these points, take an iguana with renal disease. An iguana with chronic weight loss and reversed calcium to phosphorus plasma biochemistry ratio most likely has renal disease, but this is not a definitive diagnosis, and does not indicate specific therapy. Radiology and ultrasonography may confirm renomegaly and again the likelihood of renal disease, but that still does not provide a definitive diagnosis. An iohexol excretion study can demonstrate decreases in glomerular filtration rate and renal function, and although accurate is still is not a definitive diagnosis. Biopsy of the kidney with the histologic demonstration of interstitial nephritis with calcification, and culture of *Klebsiella* bacteria with antimicrobial sensitivity testing is a definitive diagnosis, from which more targeted and specific therapy can be prescribed.

THE ENDOSCOPIC SOLUTION

There are a variety of ways that antemortem biopsies can be collected, including surgical excision, guided imagery (eg, computed tomography, ultrasonography), or endoscopy. Surgical access to a lesion or diseased tissue, unless part of the integument, typically requires an invasive approach that may involve extensive laparotomy or coeliotomy. Computed tomography and ultrasound-guided biopsies are certainly possible, and techniques have been reported in the exotic animal literature. However, iatrogenic trauma is certainly more likely than when compared with direct endoscopic visualization.[1] There are multiple examples in the domestic and human literature to indicate the superior diagnostic capability of biopsy over ultrasound-guided aspirate cytology.[2–4] There are also many examples of how endoscopy, being less invasive, is less traumatic and less painful than traditional surgical approaches. In human medicine, faster recovery, reduced hospital stay, and decreased pain scores have been attributed to endoscopic procedures.[5–7]

The endoscopic approach is typically noninvasive to minimally invasive. Endoscopic evaluation of the gastrointestinal (via the mouth, anus, or cloaca) and respiratory tracts (via the glottis) requires no surgical incision, and yet the endoscopist can access deep, internal structures (**Fig. 1**). Coelioscopy and laparoscopy enable internal visceral evaluation and biopsy through a much smaller incision than would be required for traditional laparotomy and biopsy (**Fig. 2**). The benefits of endoscopy and endoscopic biopsy have been well demonstrated in human and domestic animal medicine. However, an increasing number of studies and reports in the exotic pet literature have also demonstrated the safety and effectiveness of these techniques in birds, reptiles, mammals, and fish.[8-16] Once competency has been achieved, endoscopic techniques tend to percolate into other areas of veterinary practice. For example, at the University of Georgia we now recommend laparoscopic ovariectomies for exotic mammals and offer gender identification of juvenile turtles.[11,12,17]

Diagnostic and surgical endoscopy are not innate skills, and appropriate training is required. However, the learning curve is rapid (especially for diagnostic procedures) and clinicians can quickly become competent in the basic techniques. The reptile and avian diagnostic endoscopy course of the University of Georgia takes novices to basic clinical competency in 2 days (http://www.vet.uga.edu/ce/calendar.php). Shorter, more introductory courses, are frequently available at conferences of the

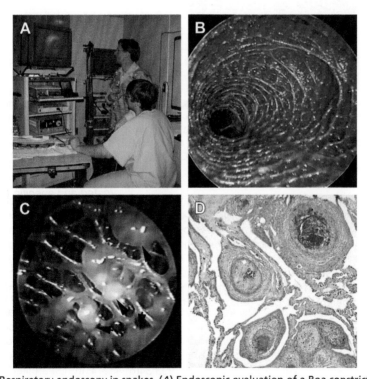

Fig. 1. Respiratory endoscopy in snakes. (*A*) Endoscopic evaluation of a Boa constrictor (*Boa constrictor*) using a fine flexible bronchoscope. (*B*) Endoscopic view of the lung of a healthy Ball python (*Python regius*). (*C*) Endoscopic view of the lung of a Ball python with chronic respiratory disease. Note the granulomata (*arrows*). (*D*) Histopathologic view of a biopsy taken from the same Ball python in C. The granulomas were caused by *Mycobacterium haemophilum*, which were only identified by endoscopic biopsy, and 9 months later by culture. Multiple lung lavage procedures, cytology, and aerobic cultures failed to diagnose this disease.

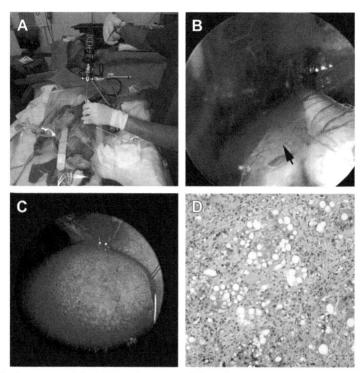

Fig. 2. Coelioscopy and liver biopsy in parrots. (*A*) Coelioscopic liver evaluation and biopsy in a macaw via the left caudal thoracic air sac. (*B*) Endoscopic view of a normal avian liver (*arrow*). (*C*) Endoscopic view of the liver in an Amazon parrot without elevation of liver enzymes or bile acids. Note the pinpoint paler across the surface. (*D*) Hepatic histopathology from the same Amazon parrot as shown in C. Note the fibrotic changes characteristic of hepatic cirrhosis.

Association of Reptilian and Amphibian Veterinarians (www.arav.org), Association of Avian Veterinarians (www.aav.org), Association of Exotic Mammal Veterinarians (www.aemv.org), and the American Association of Zoo Veterinarians (www.aazv. org). I started this discussion with reference to the first endoscopy training course that I attended in 1994, and at that time I clearly remember Dr Don Harris saying "you can't be an avian veterinarian without endoscopy." After 20 years I can offer no argument against his sentiment, and would only expand on it by stating that "you can't be an exotic pet veterinarian without endoscopy."

REFERENCES

1. Ramiro I, Ackerman N, Schumacher J. Ultrasound-guided percutaneous liver biopsy in snakes. Vet Radiol Ultrasound 1993;34(6):452–4.
2. Roth L. Comparison of liver cytology and biopsy diagnoses in dogs and cats: 56 cases. Vet Clin Pathol 2001;30(1):35–8.
3. Falcone RE, Wanamaker SR, Barnes F, et al. Laparoscopic vs. open wedge biopsy of the liver. J Laparoendosc Surg 1993;3(4):325–9.
4. Rawlings CA, Diamond H, Howerth EW, et al. Diagnostic quality of percutaneous kidney biopsy specimens obtained with laparoscopy versus ultrasound guidance in dogs. J Am Vet Med Assoc 2003;223(3):317–21.

5. Rau B, Hunerbein M. Diagnostic laparoscopy: indications and benefits. Langenbecks Arch Surg 2005;390(3):187–96.
6. Parker WH, Cooper JM, Olive DL. Benefits of laparoscopy. Am J Obstet Gynecol 2001;184(6):1309–10.
7. Yu SY, Chiu JH, Loong CC, et al. Diagnostic laparoscopy: indication and benefit. Zhonghua Yi Xue Za Zhi (Taipei) 1997;59(3):158–63.
8. Divers SJ. Diagnostic endoscopy. In: Mader DR, Divers SJ, editors. Current therapy in reptile medicine and surgery. St Louis (MO): Elsevier; 2014. p. 154–78.
9. Divers SJ, Boone SS, Berliner A, et al. Nonlethal acquisition of large liver samples from free-ranging river sturgeon (Scaphirhynchus) using single-entry endoscopic biopsy forceps. J Wildl Dis 2013;49(2):321–31.
10. Mejia-Fava J, Divers SJ, Jimenez DA, et al. Diagnosis and treatment of proventricular nematodiasis in an umbrella cockatoo (Cacatua alba). J Am Vet Med Assoc 2013;242(8):1122–6.
11. Divers SJ. Exotic mammal diagnostic and surgical endoscopy. In: Quesenberry KE, Carpenter JW, editors. Rabbits, ferrets and rodents – clinical medicine and surgery. 3rd edition. Philadelphia: Elsevier; 2012. p. 485–501.
12. Hernandez-Divers SJ, Stahl SJ, Farrell R. An endoscopic method for identifying sex of hatchling Chinese box turtles and comparison of general versus local anesthesia for coelioscopy. J Am Vet Med Assoc 2009;234(6):800–4.
13. Stahl SJ, Hernandez-Divers SJ, Cooper TL, et al. Evaluation of transcutaneous pulmonoscopy for examination and biopsy of the lungs of ball pythons and determination of preferred biopsy specimen handling and fixation procedures. J Am Vet Med Assoc 2008;233(3):440–5.
14. Hernandez-Divers SJ, Stahl SJ, McBride M, et al. Evaluation of an endoscopic liver biopsy technique in green iguanas. J Am Vet Med Assoc 2007;230(12): 1849–53.
15. Hernandez-Divers SJ, Stahl S, Hernandez-Divers SM, et al. Coelomic endoscopy of the green iguana (Iguana iguana). J Herp Med Surg 2004;14:10–8.
16. Hernandez-Divers SJ. Endoscopic renal evaluation and biopsy of Chelonia. Vet Rec 2004;154(3):73–80.
17. Divers SJ. Clinical technique: endoscopic oophorectomy in the rabbit (oryctolagus cuniculus): the future of preventative sterilizations. J Exot Pet Med 2010; 19(3):231–9.

Transurethral Cystoscopy and Endoscopic Urolith Removal in Female Guinea Pigs (*Cavia porcellus*)

CrossMark

Sandra Wenger, Dr med vet, DECVAA, DACZM, MSc*,
Jean-Michel Hatt, Prof Dr med vet, DECZM (avian), DACZM, MSc

KEYWORDS

- Guinea pig • *Cavia porcellus* • Female • Transurethral • Cystoscopy
- Urolith removal • Endoscopy

KEY POINTS

- Micturition abnormalities are common in guinea pigs with urolithiasis.
- Transurethral cystoscopy can be a useful additional diagnostic tool for the evaluation of the lower urinary tract of female guinea pigs.
- Cystoscopy provides a magnified view of the lumen of the urethra and urinary bladder.
- Transurethral cystoscopic removal of small calculi is a simple, minimally invasive treatment method in female guinea pigs with urolithiasis.
- Transurethral cystoscopic removal of uroliths in female guinea pigs is less invasive and more rapid than cystotomy.

INTRODUCTION

Guinea pigs (*Cavia porcellus*) are commonly presented to veterinary clinics with micturition abnormalities, such as hematuria, stranguria, dysuria, or polyuria.[1] There are numerous possible causes, including cystitis, urolithiasis, tumors of the bladder wall, as well as renal and uterine disease, which can cause the aforementioned abnormalities.[1,2] Diagnostic workup includes clinical examination, blood testing, imaging studies, urine culture, and urinalysis. In some cases, it can be difficult to determine the origin and cause of the urogenital abnormality in the female guinea pig and cystoscopy can be an ancillary tool for further diagnostics. Cystoscopy allows the direct

The authors have nothing to disclose.
Department of Small Animals, Clinic for Zoo Animals, Exotic Pets and Wildlife, Vetsuisse Faculty, University of Zurich, Winterthurerstrasse 260, Zurich 8057, Switzerland
* Corresponding author.
E-mail address: swenger@vetclinics.uzh.ch

visualization of the mucosal surface of the urethra and urinary bladder, and biopsy of mucosal lesions.[3]

Urolithiasis is a common problem in both female and male guinea pigs older than 2 years.[4] Clinical signs, such as micturition problems, lethargy, anorexia, and abdominal pain, are commonly seen in guinea pigs with uroliths.[2] In guinea pigs, urinary calculi are usually composed of calcium carbonate, generally radio-opaque, and easily seen on radiographs.[1,4] Uroliths can cause discomfort and obstruction and are a potential source for cystitis. Medical treatment is unrewarding, and surgical removal of the stone is often required.[1] Uroliths can recur despite dietary modification in guinea pigs.[1,2]

Transurethral cystoscopic removal of a urolith situated within the urinary bladder has been described in an adult pet female guinea pig.[5] Cystoscopic urolith removal is a rapid and less invasive alternative to surgical cystotomy in female guinea pigs with urolithiasis. The anesthesia time required for cystoscopy is shorter than for laparotomy, and the patients are usually discharged earlier. Clients are likely more willing to permit cystoscopic examination of the urinary bladder for urolith removal from their female guinea pigs if cystotomy can be avoided.

Female guinea pigs lack a vaginal vestibulum, and the urethra opens outside the vagina. The urethral papilla is located ventrally to the vaginal orifice.[6] The separate urethral opening present in female guinea pigs makes introduction of the cystoscope into the bladder simpler than in dogs and cats.[5] The urethral mucosa is longitudinally folded. The urinary bladder is relatively large and triangular in shape. The urinary bladder is thin-walled and lined with transitional epithelium.[6]

This article describes the use of transurethral cystoscopy in female guinea pigs to diagnose abnormalities within the bladder and urethra. In addition, the cystoscopic removal of uroliths measuring up to 5 mm and situated within the urinary bladder is described.

INDICATIONS/CONTRAINDICATIONS

Indications for transurethral cystoscopy in veterinary medicine include lower urinary tract inflammation of unknown origin, urolithiasis, recurrent urinary tract infections, urinary incontinence, bladder and urethral masses, and anatomic abnormalities.[7–9]

Transurethral cystoscopic urolith removal of the female guinea pig is feasible only if the calculi are smaller than the diameter of the urethra. In the authors' opinion, uroliths measuring more than 5 to 6 mm in diameter cannot be removed via transurethral cystoscopy because of excessive trauma caused to the urethra. Alternatively, larger calculi can be broken into smaller pieces within the bladder during cystoscopy using flexible grasping forceps before retrieval.

Transurethral cystoscopy is limited to female guinea pigs with a urethra that is large enough to pass an endoscope; the authors do not recommend the procedure in subadult guinea pigs. In male guinea pigs, cystoscopy and urethroscopy are difficult, if not impossible, due to the small size of the urethra and the presence of an os penis.[2,10] Other contraindications include factors leading to an increased anesthetic risk, such as anemia, azotemia, electrolyte imbalance, and increased liver enzymes.[11] Such conditions need to be corrected before performing the procedure.

PATIENT PREPARATION AND POSITIONING

Routine general anesthesia is necessary to perform cystoscopy to ensure adequate immobilization and muscle relaxation and to avoid iatrogenic injury.[7,8,10] The authors typically use a combination of midazolam-opioid or medetomidine-ketamine as premedication before induction and maintenance of anesthesia with isoflurane using a face mask. Additional analgesia can be provided with a nonsteroidal anti-inflammatory drug such as meloxicam in animals without kidney compromise. In animals with moderate to severe inflammation of the urethra, it might be necessary to administer meloxicam for several days before performing the cystoscopy to reduce the inflammation and allow the introduction of the telescope. In cats and dogs, it has been recommended that acute inflammatory processes, such as cystitis, be resolved before cystoscopy is attempted. Theoretically, instillation of fluids into the bladder may induce a vesicoureteral reflex and thus promote pyelonephritis in an animal with cystitis.[8]

The guinea pig is placed in the dorsal recumbency position with the perineum close to the table edge (**Fig. 1**). The perineal region is given a standard surgical scrub using a disinfectant such as dilute chlorhexidine. The endoscopist should wear sterile gloves and minimize any contamination of the urinary tract.

ENDOSCOPIC EQUIPMENT

The basic equipment for cystoscopy includes the following materials:

- 1.9-mm × 18.5-cm telescope, forward 0° view with a 4-mm operating sheath
- 2.7-mm diameter × 18-cm telescope, 30° forward–oblique with a 4.8-mm operating sheath
- 1.7-mm flexible grasping forceps
- 1.7-mm flexible biopsy forceps with double-action jaws
- 1.7-mm wire basket retrieval
- Fluids (eg, 0.9% sterile saline solution bag with infusion set)
- Xenon light source and light cable
- Endovideo camera and monitor
- Alternatively, the mobile endoscopic imaging system (Tele Pack System, Karl Storz, Tuttlingen, Germany) can be used, replacing the need of light source and monitor.

The authors typically use the 1.9-mm telescope (**Fig. 2**) with a xenon light source to evaluate the urethra and urinary bladder. For the actual removal of the urolith, the authors typically use the 2.7-mm telescope with the operating sheath (**Fig. 3**) because it allows the introduction of the instruments (eg, wire basket and grasping forceps).

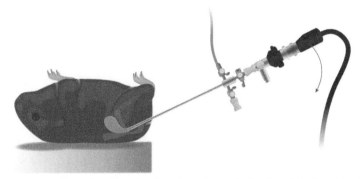

Fig. 1. For cystoscopic evaluation, the female guinea pig is placed in the dorsal recumbency position with the perineum close to the table edge. The endoscope is initially inserted in angle pointing toward the spine (toward the table) and then redirected horizontally.

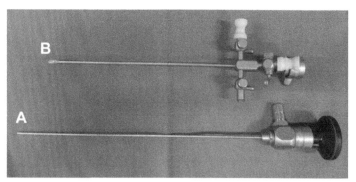

Fig. 2. Rigid cystoscopy equipment that can be used to evaluate the urethra and urinary bladder in female guinea pigs. (*A*) 1.9-mm × 18.5-cm telescope, forward 0° view; (*B*) 4-mm operating sheath.

The larger system produces images of better quality, and it has been used successfully in guinea pigs weighing 800 g and more. An operating sheath is used with both telescope systems to allow introduction of instruments and instillation of fluids.

PROCEDURE

The lubricated endoscope is inserted gently via the urethral orifice using warm 0.9% saline infusion. The endoscope is initially inserted in a 35° to 40° angle toward to spine (toward the table) and then redirected horizontally (see **Fig. 1**). The saline infusion should be adjusted to a rate preventing the mucosa from collapsing around the endoscope and therefore hindering visualization (approximately 1 drop per second using a macro fluid line). The rate of the saline infusion should not be excessive to prevent disproportionate dilation and possible rupture of the bladder wall. Once the bladder is entered, instillation of saline can typically be discontinued or reduced, while keeping the port of the operating sheath closed. Regular palpation of the caudal abdomen during the procedure is recommended to prevent overdistension of the bladder. Excess fluids can quickly be removed through the operating sheath.

Endoscopic retrieval devices, such as grasping forceps, snares, or baskets, are necessary for retrieval of uroliths situated within the urinary bladder or urethra. The urolith can be grasped with the 1.7-mm flexible grasping forceps (**Fig. 4**) via the

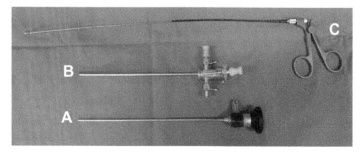

Fig. 3. Equipment for transurethral cystoscopy and endoscopic urolith removal in female guinea pigs. (*A*) 2.7-mm diameter × 18-cm telescope, 30° forward–oblique; (*B*) 4.8-mm operating sheath; (*C*) 1.7-mm flexible grasping forceps, which can be introduced through the operating sheath.

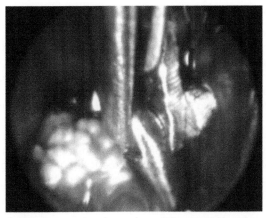

Fig. 4. Transurethral cystoscopy and endoscopic urolith removal in a female guinea pig. The urolith is grasped with a 1.7-mm flexible grasping forceps and removed through the urethra.

4.8-mm operating sheath. The operating sheath is then removed together with the forceps and the urolith through the urethra. When using the grasping forceps, it can be difficult to maintain a grip on the urolith during retrograde passage through the urethra, therefore necessitating several attempts. Brittle stones might break into smaller pieces during retrieval, requiring several attempts. The risk of inadvertently damaging the mucosa when grasping the urolith must also be taken into consideration.

Another option for retrieval of uroliths includes endoscopic baskets and nets, which need to be inserted cranially to the stone and then opened. Retrieval baskets and nets (**Fig. 5**) are constructed from a soft, flexible mesh material attached to the noose of a snare. When the snare loop is opened, the mesh forms a concave compartment capable of capturing the urolith. Closure of the snare captures the retrieval target in this compartment. Again, the operating sheath is removed together with the basket/net and the urolith through the urethra. The flexible baskets are available in small sizes in the range of 1 mm to 1.7 mm and can therefore be used with the smaller endoscopes measuring 1.9 mm or 2.7 mm in diameter, respectively.

Bladder tumors are reported in guinea pigs and can lead to intermittent hematuria. Biopsy or grasping forceps can be used to obtain tissue specimens via cystoscopy.[2] The forceps are advanced through the operating sheath, and tissue samples are obtained under direct visualization.[9]

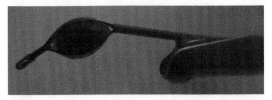

Fig. 5. Retrieval net (Urotech basket; UROTECH, Achenmühle, Germany) used for transurethral endoscopic urolith removal in a female guinea pig. Transurethral endoscopy was performed using the 1mm-diameter telescope. (*Courtesy of* Anklin AG, Binningen, Switzerland).

ENDOSCOPIC FINDINGS

The normal urethra is smooth with an even, pale pinkish color. The urethral mucosa contracts into longitudinal folds (**Fig. 6**). The normal urinary bladder is thin-walled with a smooth surface and pale pinkish mucosa. The submucosal vascular pattern can be easily identified (**Fig. 7**). Some sediment is often found in the urinary bladder and can obscure visualization (**Fig. 8**). To increase visibility, the bladder can be flushed by repeatedly instilling saline solution and removing it through the operating sheath.

Abnormal findings of the mucosa include irregular mucosal surface, hyperemic mucosa, ecchymosis, and abrasions. Evidence of hemorrhage can appear as clots adhered to the bladder mucosa or floating free in the urine.[10] Other abnormalities include nodules, polyps, and thickened bladder wall. Uroliths can be readily identified and often have an irregular whitish to yellowish surface (**Fig. 9**).

Cystoscopy can also be used to evaluate anatomic abnormalities, such as strictures and diverticula. In cats and dogs, cystoscopy is considered the gold standard for diagnosis of ectopic ureters.[7]

BENEFITS OF CYSTOSCOPY

The benefits of cystoscopy for female guinea pigs include the direct visualization of the mucosal surface of the urethra and bladder, the possibility of taking biopsies of nodules or altered bladder wall, and allowing the removal of smaller uroliths. The endoscopic retrieval of uroliths is more rapid and less invasive than surgical removal via cystotomy. With endoscopic retrieval of uroliths, there is a limitation regarding the size of the urolith that can pass the urethra. In the authors' experience, it is not possible to remove uroliths larger than 5 to 6 mm in diameter in one piece through the urethra. Cystotomy is associated with more risks, such as postoperative suture dehiscence. The suture material used to close the bladder wall is a possible site for infection or nidus for future urolith formation.[12]

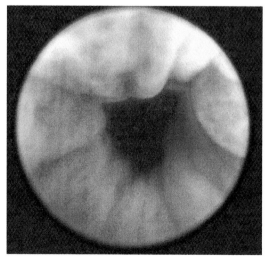

Fig. 6. Cystoscopic appearance of a normal urethra in a healthy female guinea pig showing even pink color and mucosal folds. In the center, the entrance to the urinary bladder can be seen.

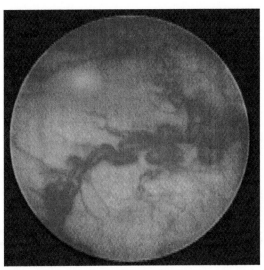

Fig. 7. Cystoscopic appearance of the normal urinary bladder of a female guinea pig. The wall of the urinary bladder is thin, and the blood vessels can be readily identified. The abdominal fat can be seen shimmering through the wall.

COMPLICATIONS OF TRANSURETHRAL CYSTOSCOPY

Published complications in guinea pigs include iatrogenic abrasions of the bladder wall and urethra caused by the tip of the endoscope.[10] Bladder rupture due to overinfusion is a possibility.[10] Perforation of the urethra or urinary bladder is described as possible complications in dogs when using inappropriate-sized equipment.[11] Another potential risk of cystoscopy is retrograde infection. Several authors recommend the administration of antibiotics for 3 to 5 days after the procedure in cats and dogs to avoid urinary

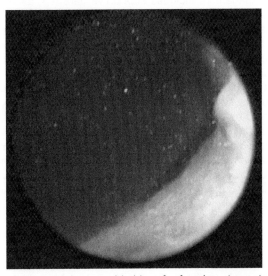

Fig. 8. Cystoscopy of the normal urinary bladder of a female guinea pig. Sediment (white dots) can often be found in the urine of the guinea pig and might reduce visibility.

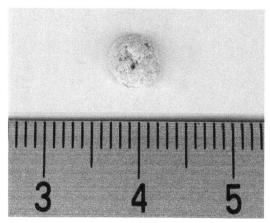

Fig. 9. Bladder calculus measuring 5.5 mm in diameter that was removed endoscopically from the urinary bladder of a female guinea pig using a retrieval basket. The urolith has an irregular whitish surface.

tract infection.[7,9] The authors routinely administer prophylactic antibiotics (eg, trimethoprim/sulfonamide or enrofloxacin) after performing cystoscopy, especially after urolith removal, to avoid urinary tract infections secondary to iatrogenic lesions. If possible, antibiotic choice should be based on urine culture and sensitivity.

In contrast to other diagnostic modalities such as radiography or sonography, general anesthesia is necessary to perform cystoscopy. General anesthesia in guinea pigs is associated with a higher risk than in dogs and cats.[13] The overall risk of anesthetic-related death needs to be taken into consideration and communicated to the owner.

PATIENT MANAGEMENT

Postcystoscopy management includes supportive care (eg, assisted feedings and fluid therapy), analgesics, and antibiotics (based on culture and sensitivity).[1] The authors routinely administer meloxicam for 3 to 5 days after performing cystoscopy. Additional analgesia can be provided by administering oral opioids (eg, buprenorphine) and local anesthetic, for example, lidocaine 1% (diluted 1:1 in saline), instilled topically into the urethra and bladder at the end of the procedure.

Calculi analysis should be performed and specific methodologies are needed to differentiate calcium carbonate crystals from calcium oxalate monohydrate; therefore, the laboratory should be chosen accordingly.

In guinea pigs with urolithiasis, important preventative measures are to increase water intake and reduce dietary calcium intake. Reducing dietary calcium has been advocated for the prevention of the disease. Diets containing a high percentage of timothy, oat, or grass hays, a lower overall percentage of pellets, and a wide variety of vegetables and fruits decrease the risk of urolith development in pet guinea pigs. Despite treatment and prevention, recurrence of the disease is common.[1]

SUMMARY

Cystoscopy is a useful diagnostic tool to assess the urethra and bladder in female guinea pigs. Cystoscopic urolith removal is a rapid and less invasive alternative to surgical cystotomy in female guinea pigs with urolithiasis.

REFERENCES

1. Hawkins MG, Bishop CR. Disease problems of guinea pigs. In: Quesenberry KE, Carpenter JW, editors. Ferrets, rabbits and rodents: clinical medicine and surgery. 3rd edition. Philadelphia: WB Saunders; 2012. p. 295–310.
2. Ewringmann A, Glöckner B. Urinveränderungen. In: Ewringmann A, Glöckner B, editors. Leitsymptome bei Meerschweinchen, Chinchilla und Degu. Enke Verlag Stuttgart; 2005. p. 167–84.
3. Divers SJ. Exotic mammal diagnostic and surgical endoscopy. In: Quesenberry KE, Carpenter JW, editors. Ferrets, rabbits and rodents: clinical medicine and surgery. 3rd edition. Philadelphia: WB Saunders; 2012. p. 485–501.
4. Hawkins MG, Ruby AL, Drazenovich TL, et al. Composition and characteristics of urinary calculi from guinea pigs. J Am Vet Med Assoc 2009;234:214–22.
5. Pizzi R. Cystoscopic removal of a urolith from a pet guinea pig. Vet Rec 2009;165: 148–9.
6. Breazile JC, Brown EM. Anatomy. In: Wagner JE, Manning PJ, editors. The biology of the guinea pig. New York: Academic Press; 1976. p. 53–62.
7. Chew DJ, DiBartola SP, Schenck PA. Clinical evaluation of the urinary tract. In: Chew DJ, DiBartola SP, Schenck PA, editors. Canine and feline urology. 2nd edition. St Louis (MO): Elsevier Saunders; 2011. p. 54–5.
8. Pressler B, Bartges JW. Urinary tract infections. In: Ettinger SJ, Feldmann EC, editors. Textbook of veterinary internal medicine. 7th edition. St Louis (MO): Saunders Elsevier; 2010. p. 2036–47.
9. Senior DF. Endoscopy. In: Osborne CA, Finco DR, editors. Canine and feline nephrology and urology. Philadelphia: Williams and Wilkins; 1995. p. 303–15.
10. Lennox AM. Endoscopy of the distal urogenital tract as an aid in differentiating causes of urogenital bleeding in small mammals. Exot DVM 2005;7(2):43–7.
11. Grzegory M, Kubiak K, Jankowski M, et al. Endoscopic examination of the urethra and the urinary bladder in dogs – indications, contraindications and performance technique. Pol J Vet Sci 2013;16:797–801.
12. Fossum T. Surgery of the bladder and urethra. In: Fossum T, editor. Small animal surgery. 3rd edition. St Louis (MO): Mosby Elsevier; 2007. p. 663–701.
13. Brodbelt DC, Blissitt KJ, Hammond RA, et al. The risk of death: the confidential enquiry into perioperative small animal fatalities. Vet Anaesth Analg 2008;35: 365–73.

Flexible Gastrointestinal Endoscopy in Ferrets (*Mustela putorius furo*)

Charly Pignon, DVM, DECZM (Small Mammal)[a,*],
Minh Huynh, DVM, DECZM (Avian)[b], Roman Husnik, DVM, PhD[c,d],
Vladimir Jekl, DVM, PhD, DECZM (Small Mammal)[e]

KEYWORDS

- Ferret • Endoscope • Esophagoscopy • Gastroscopy • Colonoscopy
- Percutaneous endoscopic gastrostomy • *Mustela putorius furo*

KEY POINTS

- Gastrointestinal diseases are common complaints in ferrets. However, apart from a few references in biomedical research articles, there is little information on the use of flexible endoscopy.
- The anatomy of the ferret gastrointestinal tract is relatively simple and short. The small intestine distal to the duodenum forms coiled tubes suspended by a mesentery; the large intestine is a straight dilated tube that is differentiated into ascending, transverse, and descending colon.
- Because of the small lumen size of the ferret gastrointestinal tract, small-diameter bronchoscopes have been traditionally used.
- Gastroscopes can be used in ferrets weighing more than 1 kg, while the new generation of smaller videoscopes is likely to make this practical in smaller ferrets.
- Percutaneous endoscopic gastrostomy is a promising and useful technique for anorectic or dysphagic ferrets.

INTRODUCTION

Gastrointestinal diseases are common complaints in ferrets (*Mustela putorius furo*). Causes include infection (*Helicobacter* gastritis, campylobacteriosis, salmonellosis,

The authors have nothing to disclose.
[a] Exotics Medicine Service, Alfort National Veterinary School, 7 Avenue du Général de Gaulle, Maisons-Alfort 94700, France; [b] Exotics Medicine Service, Centre Hospitalier Vétérinaire Frégis, Rue Aristide Briand, Arcueil 94110, France; [c] Department of Veterinary Clinical Sciences, School of Veterinary Medicine, Louisiana State University, Skip Bertman Drive, Baton Rouge, LA 70803, USA; [d] International Clinical Research Center (ICRC), St. Anne's University Hospital Brno, Pekarska 53, Brno 656 91, Czech Republic; [e] Avian and Exotic Animal Clinic, University of Veterinary and Pharmaceutical Sciences Brno, Brno 65691, Czech Republic
* Corresponding author.
E-mail address: cpignon@vet-alfort.fr

epizootic catarrhal enteritis, rotavirus infection, mycobacteriosis, proliferative enteropathy), neoplasia (gastrointestinal lymphoma and adenocarcinoma, stromal tumor adenomatous polyp), but also other conditions (foreign body, eosinophilic gastroenteritis, lymphoplasmacytic enteritis, inflammatory bowel disease).[1,2] The relatively simple and short gastrointestinal tract of ferrets makes them ideal candidates for flexible endoscopy.[3] Although routinely used in cats and dogs,[4] little information is available about flexible endoscopy in ferrets, apart from a few references in biomedical research articles.[5,6] Recent technical advances, especially in smaller videoendoscopy, have both decreased the diameter and purchase price of flexible endoscopes. General practitioners now have affordable access to suitably sized endoscopes for ferrets that provide high-quality images.

CLINICAL ANATOMY OF THE FERRET GASTROINTESTINAL TRACT

The anatomy of the ferret gastrointestinal tract is comparable to cats and dogs. However, differences include dental formula, small length of the intestine, lack of differentiation between jejunum and ileum, absence of a cecum, and small lumen size of the colon. The relatively simple anatomy results in a short gastrointestinal transit time of 4 to 8 hours, whereas in cats the rate of food passage is 24–37 hours.[7]

Esophagus

The esophagus starts at the pharynx, just above the laryngeal cricoid cartilage, extends to the cardia, and measures 17 to 19 cm.[3] It is divided into cervical, thoracic, and abdominal segments. The cervical segment is dorsal to the trachea, but at the thoracic inlet veers to left. The esophageal lumen decreases in size when it crosses the left bronchi and passes through the diaphragm. As a strong gastroesophageal sphincter does not exist, ferrets can vomit easily. The musculature is composed only of striated fibers like the dog, making the esophagus thin and fragile.[8] Characteristic of animals that are able to ingest food rapidly, the mucosa is covered with a layer of squamous, keratinized epithelium.[8]

Stomach

The stomach is simple, J-shaped, and similar to the dog. It consists of a cardia, fundus, body, antrum, and pylorus.[8] The stomach is located in the cranial abdomen, under the hypochondrium, and positioned transversally, left of the median plane. It is in contact cranially with the left liver lobe and diaphragm, dorsally with the ascending colon, and caudally with the spleen and left pancreatic lobe. The greater curvature of the stomach is in communication with the visceral side of the spleen, the 2 organs being linked by the gastrosplenic ligament that contains nerves and blood vessels.

The lesser curvature of the stomach is oriented craniodorsally and is separated from the papillary process of the caudate liver lobe by the lesser omentum. The pylorus is well developed and in contact with the abdominal wall. The capacity of the stomach is large in ferrets relative to their size and can easily hold 50 mL/kg or more.[9] The fullness of the stomach determines its shape, size, and position. When it is full, the stomach occupies all of the subcostal area and pushes the intestines to the right. The cranial border of the stomach is located under the 11th thoracic vertebra and the caudal border is located under the first or second lumbar vertebra. The fundus can also move caudoventrally. The musculature is composed of 2 layers: a smooth longitudinal external muscular layer and a smooth circular muscular layer.[8]

Small Intestine

The small intestine is relatively short in comparison with other carnivores, possibly explaining the fast (4–8 h) gastrointestinal transit time of the ferret.[9] The small intestine measures 182 to 198 cm, with a ratio of 5:1 for intestine length to body length (in dogs it is 4–5:1).[3] The lumen of the small intestine is narrow, and foreign bodies greater than 1 cm diameter are unlikely to pass without the need for intervention.

Duodenum

The duodenum is 10 cm in length and divided into 3 segments.[8] The cranial duodenum is the shortest (2 cm) and has a sigmoid shape. It is in contact with the liver, pancreas, stomach, and greater omentum. The descending duodenum (5 cm) is caudally in contact with the right abdominal wall, liver, right kidney, and ascending colon. The ascending duodenum (3 cm) lies cranially in the medial plane and is in contact with the jejunoileum, descending colon, aorta, caudal vena cava, and left ureter. The biliary and pancreatic ducts enter the duodenum via the major duodenal papilla, which is 3 cm from the pylorus. The minor duodenal papilla is often absent.[8]

Jejunoileum

There is no anatomic distinction between the jejunum and the ileum in ferrets, and hence the term jejunoileum is used.[8] It is 140 cm in length and in contact with the duodenum, colon, liver, pancreas, spleen, and urogenital organs.[8] As the ferret does not have a cecum or ileocecal valve, the junction between the jejunoileum and the colon is not distinct. It is identified by the anastomosis between the ileojejunal and colic arteries. Intraluminally, it is characterized by a change in the mucosal surface. The jejunoileal mucosa is flat, whereas the colonic mucosa forms longitudinal folds. At the jejunoileal-colic junction, a band of connective tissue that prevents propagation of small intestinal electrical activity (migrating myoelectric complexes) to the colon interrupts the muscular layers. Electrical activity changes suddenly to characteristic colonic short and long spike burst activity.[10]

Large Intestine

The large intestine is approximately 10 cm and comprises the colon, rectum, and anus.[9] Ferrets do not have cecum.

Colon

The diameter of the large intestine is 0.6 cm.[3] The length of the colon is 7 cm, and it is divided into 3 segments. The ascending colon lies cranially to the jejunoileal-colic junction and is in contact with the pancreatic right lobe dorsally and the right kidney. The transverse colon is located cranially in the abdomen where it extends from the right side to the left side. It is in contact with the stomach cranioventrally and the left lobe of the pancreas craniodorsally. The descending colon runs along the left abdominal wall. It is in contact with the ventral surface of the left kidney, and dorsal surface of the uterus and urinary bladder.[11]

The colonic mucosa is devoid of villi, which cease abruptly at the ileocolic junction. Tubular glands are organized within the longitudinal folds of mucosa. The muscularis is composed of longitudinal and circular layers.[8]

Rectum and Anus

The border between the colon and the rectum is located at the entrance of the pelvis. The rectum is 2 cm in length and ends at the anus.[11]

The anus consists of 2 sphincters: the internal anal sphincter composed of smooth muscle and the external anal sphincter composed of striated muscle. The anal glands are present between these 2 sphincters. They measure 10×5 mm and their ducts open at 4 and 8 o'clock at the mucocutaneous junction.[11]

EQUIPMENT

The flexible endoscope, like the rigid endoscope system, is composed of a light source, light-transmitting cable, endoscope, camera, and monitor (**Fig. 1**). On many flexible endoscopes, the light-transmitting cable is permanently attached to the endoscope and has a connector that plugs directly into the light source. Additional accessories may include various instruments for biopsy, grasping, aspiration, fluid infusion, cytologic sampling, electrosurgery, laser surgery; pumps for suction, insufflation, and irrigation; and image management systems for recording, printing, and digital storage or transmission of still photographs and video (**Fig. 2**).

Flexible Endoscope

The 2 basic types of flexible endoscopes are the fiberscope and the video endoscope. The difference between the 2 is in their method of sensing and transmitting images. In a fiberscope, the image is carried from the distal tip of the endoscope to the eyepiece or camera by bundles of optical glass fibers. In a video endoscope, the image is

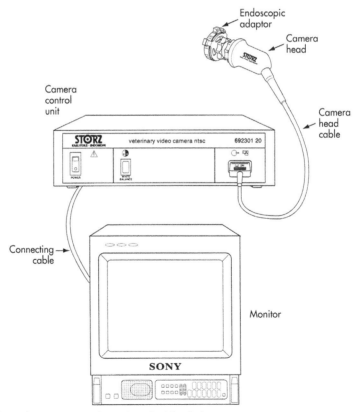

Fig. 1. An endoscope system is equipped with a light source, a camera, and a monitor. (*Courtesy of* Karl Storz Co, Tuttlingen, Germany.)

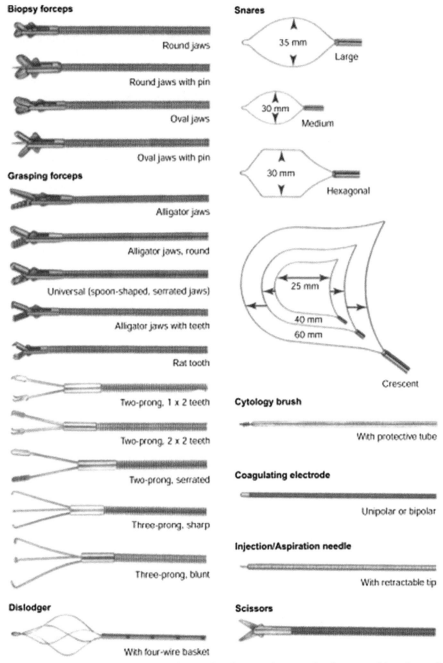

Fig. 2. Flexible instruments that can be used with an endoscope that has a working channel. (*Courtesy of* Karl Storz Co, Tuttlingen, Germany.)

transmitted electronically to a video monitor from the distal tip of the endoscope where it is sensed by a charge-coupled device chip.

True video endoscopes are preferred for their superior visualization in gastrointestinal endoscopy. Because the image produced by a video endoscope is not fiber-optic, it will never display the honeycomb pattern or broken fibers seen as black dots in a fiber-optic image. The smallest flexible video endoscope currently available for medical use has a 2.8-mm outer diameter (OD) (**Fig. 3**). However, endoscope size is dependent on chip technology and mechanical functions, such as channel size and deflection capability.

Fiberscopes are available in diameters ranging from 14 mm to less than 1 mm. Most flexible scopes greater than 2 mm in diameter are equipped with a working channel and a deflectable tip. The working channel is the section of the endoscope through which ancillary instruments like biopsy forceps are advanced into the patient. Because of their versatility, the most popular endoscopes in small animal practice are 4-way tip deflection (up, down, left, and right) gastro-fiberscopes and have a smallest OD of 8.6 mm (**Fig. 4**). This gastro-fiberscope can be used in ferrets weighing more than 1 kg.[6] The tip's 2-plane, 4-direction deflection capability (up, down, left, and right) is useful to navigate the gastrointestinal tract, especially the more challenging maneuver of advancing through the pylorus into the duodenum. However, because of the small lumen size of the ferret gastrointestinal tract, bronchofiberscopes are used most of the time, although continued advances are likely to result in smaller videoscopes in the future. Broncho-fiberscopes only have 2-way tip deflection in a single plane (up and down) and suitable models for the ferret gastrointestinal tract can range from 5.2 mm OD (operating channel 2.3 mm, 113 cm long) to 3 mm OD (operating channel 1.2 mm, 100 cm long) (**Fig. 5**).

Basic Construction and Handling

A flexible endoscope has 3 major sections: the insertion tube, the hand piece, and the umbilical cord (**Fig. 6**).

The insertion tube contains fiber-optic bundles (fiberscope) or electrical wiring (videoscope), channels for suction, irrigation, and insufflation, 2 to 4 deflection cables, and several layers of protective materials along the entire length of the tube. The last several centimeters of an endoscope with tip deflection capability is called the bending section. Controlled by the deflection knobs in the hand piece, this portion of the insertion tube may be deflected in one (eg, bronchoscopes and

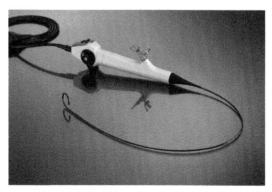

Fig. 3. Video endoscope (Flex XC, Karl Storz Co, Tuttlingen, Germany) with a 2.8-mm OD with an operating channel of 1.2 mm and 70 cm long. (*Courtesy of* Karl Storz Co, Tuttlingen, Germany.)

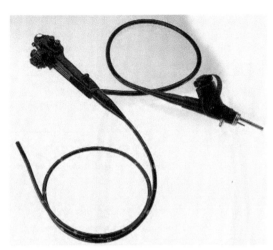

Fig. 4. Gastrofiber endoscope with an outside diameter of 8.6 mm, 2.8-mm working channel, 140 cm long. This flexible endoscope is suitable for a large ferret that is larger than 1 kg body weight. (*Courtesy of* Karl Storz Co, Tuttlingen, Germany.)

small-diameter endoscopes) or 2 planes (eg, gastroscopes). The degree of tip deflection varies among models, but complete retroflexion (180° or greater) in at least one direction is desirable.

The working channel is used for suction of air and fluids as well as the passage of flexible instruments into the patient. However, the effectiveness of suction is greatly reduced when an instrument is inside the channel. In a gastroscope, an additional irrigation and insufflation channel is available. The insufflation channel allows room air to be blown into the gastrointestinal tract, distending the viscous and enabling a clearer

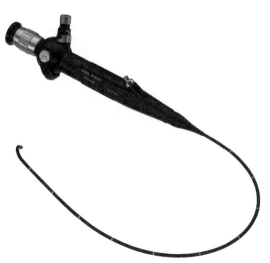

Fig. 5. Bronchofiber endoscope of 3 mm diameter, operating channel 1.2 mm, and 100 cm long. This is a commonly used flexible endoscope in ferrets. (*Courtesy of* Karl Storz Co, Tuttlingen, Germany.)

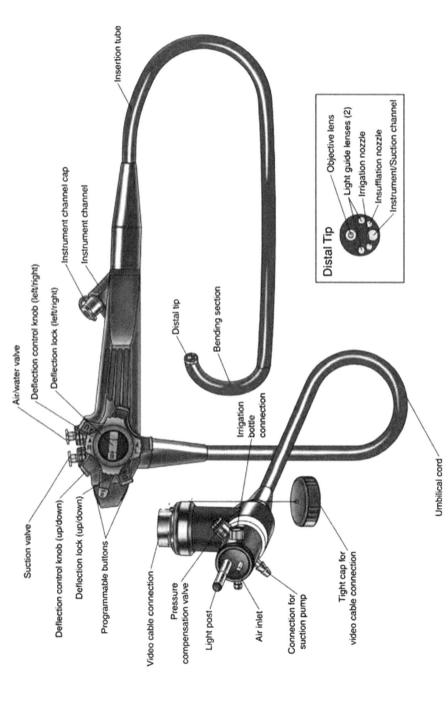

Fig. 6. The parts of a gastrovideo endoscope. (*Courtesy of Karl Storz Co, Tuttlingen, Germany.*)

and more thorough examination of the mucosa. The water jet exiting the irrigation nozzle is directed over the distal objective lens to remove debris and mucus when necessary. In a broncho-fiberscope, the operating channel can also be used for insufflation or irrigation.

The hand piece contains the deflection control knobs and locks, the opening to the working channel, and the suction valves for air or water in a gastro-fiberscope. The hand piece of a fiberscope also contains the eyepiece with its diopter adjustment ring, for direct viewing without video. The hand piece is designed to be held in the left hand. The index finger controls suction. The air/water valve can be controlled by the index or middle finger. The thumb of the left hand is used to control the up and down deflection knob. The right hand controls the left and right deflection knob, inserts channel accessories, and advances the insertion tube into the patient, applying rotational torque when necessary. The umbilical cord contains the portion of the fiberscope that connects to the light source and includes connectors for insufflation and irrigation in gastro-fiberscopes.

Flexible Instruments

A variety of flexible instruments are available for use with endoscopes that have a working channel (see **Fig. 2**). The most widely used instruments are biopsy forceps and grasping forceps for foreign body retrieval. Other useful flexible instruments include cytology brushes, aspiration tubing, injection/aspiration needles, polypectomy snares, and coagulating electrodes. A vast number of styles and sizes are available.

Pumps and Insufflators

Most endoscopic procedures require some combination of insufflation, irrigation, or suction so that a clearly visible space is created and maintained between the distal lens of the endoscope and the area under examination. For both upper and lower gastrointestinal endoscopy, the gaseous distension medium is simply room air. An air pump either may be included in the light source or may be separate and connected to the scope with an appropriate adapter and tubing (**Fig. 7**). In either case, the pressure of the air pump must be of suitable power to drive the insufflation and irrigation of the endoscope, without being so powerful that it causes damage to the instrument or

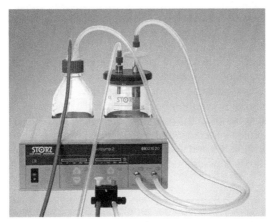

Fig. 7. An example of a pump (Vetpump 2; Karl Storz Co) that provides insufflation, irrigation, and suction during the endoscopic procedure. (*Courtesy of* Karl Storz Co, Tuttlingen, Germany.)

patient. If no pump is available, insufflation in ferrets can be performed with a 60-mL syringe attached to the working channel.

PATIENT PREPARATION AND POSITIONING
Evaluation of the Patient

Routine evaluation of the patient should include a complete physical examination and hematology and biochemistry panel before the procedure. Total protein and albumin are parameters of particular importance, because animals with gastrointestinal disease are at risk for hypoproteinemia. Anesthetic risk must be evaluated, and although it may result in a delay, the procedure should not be performed until the protein level is adequate.

Ultrasonography is a superior imaging method compared with endoscopy for diagnosing and differentiating between submucosal lesions in the gastrointestinal tract. Ultrasonography should be performed for first staging of submucosal lesions by lymph node visualization and checking for signs of neoplasia in the deeper layers. If performed before the endoscopic procedure, it allows checking for complete gastric emptying.

Preparation

Before endoscopic evaluation, anti-inflammatory and antibacterial drugs should be stopped for at least 2 weeks to collect proper histologic and microbiologic samples. It may be difficult to control vomiting in such patients, and the clinician must assess the risk and benefit of withholding treatment. Antiemetic drugs can help in controlling the disease periodically. Ideally, endoscopy and biopsy sampling should be performed before anti-inflammatory or antibiotic drugs are initiated. Hypoproteinemic patients may benefit from colloid administration. In cases of severe hypoalbuminemia, blood transfusion should be considered.

Good gastrointestinal luminal visualization is achieved by allowing the bowel to empty. In cats and dogs, the recommended food withholding time is 12 hours for esophagoscopy and 36 hours for colonoscopy.[12,13] In the ferret, gastrointestinal transit time is 4 to 8 hours, but in an animal with gastrointestinal disease, the time may be longer.[2,7] One way of dealing with potentially delayed gastrointestinal emptying is to hospitalize the ferret, starve it for 12 hours, and check the blood glucose level before anesthesia. Alternatively, provide carnivore formulas (eg, Carnivore Emeraid; Lafeber, Chicago, IL, USA) for 8 hours and then remove the food for the next 4 hours.

For colonoscopy, dog and cat bowel preparation recommendations include administering a high-volume colonic lavage solution orally 18 hours before the procedure and performing multiple enemas.[13] The authors have found that removal of feces from the descending colon and good mucosal colonic cleansing can be achieved in ferrets using only enemas, with the patient under sedation. A lubricated urinary catheter (2.6 mm × 50 cm) is inserted into the anus and advanced slowly to the middle of the abdominal cavity (**Fig. 8**), and warm saline (maximum 20 mL/kg) is flushed into the colon. This procedure is repeated until the fluid coming out of the anus is clear.

Anesthesia

For all flexible endoscopy procedures, ferrets must be anesthetized. Theoretically, avoid the use of drugs that can slow gastrointestinal motility; however, one study in cats showed premedication with hydromorphone, glycopyrrolate, medetomidine, or butorphanol did not affect the time and difficulty to perform gastroduodenoscopy.[14]

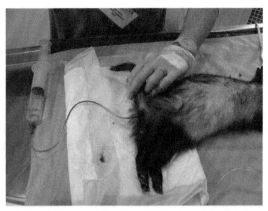

Fig. 8. Enema performed in a sedated ferret using warm saline (maximum 20 mL/kg) and a urinary catheter (2.6 mm × 50 cm). (*Courtesy of* Charly Pignon, Maisons-Alfort, France.)

Morphine and α_2-agonists can induce emesis and should be avoided. Morphine can also increase the pyloric tone. Atropine and glycopyrrolate may alter lower esophageal sphincter tone. Analgesics are essential as passage of a flexible endoscope into the gastrointestinal tract causes stretching of mesenteric attachments, and insufflation causes stretching of the intestines that results in discomfort. The authors prefer to premedicate using butorphanol (0.03 mg/kg intramuscularly) and midazolam (0.2 mg/kg intramuscularly), place an intravenous catheter, and induce with propofol to effect (1–5 mg/kg intravenously). After intubation, an inhalant anesthetic (isoflurane or sevoflurane) is administered.

Patients must be intubated as inflation of the stomach can depress respiratory function by pushing against the diaphragm and limiting the depth of inspiration.[15] Furthermore, endotracheal tube placement is important to avoid inadvertent aspiration of irrigation or gastric fluids during the procedure (**Fig. 9**).

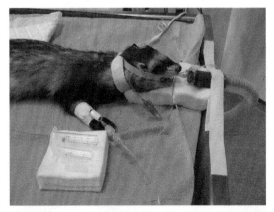

Fig. 9. Ferret anesthetized for a gastroscopy. Note the endotracheal tube placement, which is important to avoid inadvertent aspiration of fluids during the procedure. On the bottom left, the barrels of syringes have been prepared to be used to protect the endoscope. (*Courtesy of* Charly Pignon, Maisons-Alfort, France.)

Minimal monitoring during upper gastrointestinal endoscopy includes monitoring of heart rate, respiration, and oxygen saturation using pulse oximetry and ensuring that the degree of gastric distension does not hinder respiration. Insufflation of the stomach is critical for ensuring a complete gastric examination. However, prolonged insufflation can cause cardiovascular and respiratory compromise.

Positioning

The current accepted standard for gastroscopy in cats and dogs is to place the patient in left lateral recumbency position.[16] This position improves the endoscopist's ability to examine the stomach completely. When a dog or cat is in the right lateral recumbency position, it is more difficult to clearly identify and pass the endoscope around the incisura angularis and through the antrum to the pylorus.[16] One of the authors uses the sternal recumbency position in ferrets and does not encounter any difficulties. To protect the endoscope from being chewed or scratched, an appropriately sized mouth speculum should be used. A syringe body with the tip cut off is a suitable replacement for a mouth speculum (see **Figs. 9** and **10**).

For colonoscopy, cats and dogs can be placed in either the sternal or the right lateral recumbency position.[13] One of the authors uses the sternal recumbency position with good results (**Fig. 11**).

UPPER GASTROINTESTINAL TRACT ENDOSCOPY
Indications

Indications for upper gastrointestinal endoscopy include investigation of common problems such as salivation, bruxism, chronic vomiting, hematemesis, anorexia, weight loss, and melena. Foreign body retrieval is also another indication, especially if the owner sees the foreign body being ingested and the ferret is quickly presented. Evaluation of gastric hairballs in ferrets has also been reported.[17] Gastroscopy should always be performed whenever hematemesis is demonstrated. Acute vomiting, apart from foreign-body-ingestion–associated vomiting is not a common indicator for gastroscopy.

Limitations

Limitations of upper gastrointestinal endoscopic investigation in ferrets are similar to those seen with cats and dogs. Endoscopy allows the detection of morphologic

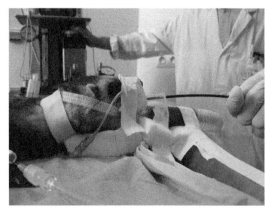

Fig. 10. Esophagoscopy in a ferret using a syringe body with the tip cut off placed in the mouth to protect the endoscope. (*Courtesy of* Charly Pignon, Maisons-Alfort, France.)

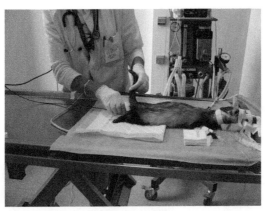

Fig. 11. Colonoscopy in a ferret positioned in sternal recumbency. (*Courtesy of* Charly Pignon, Maisons-Alfort, France.)

changes but, to a lesser extent, functional disease. Lesions located in the muscular and submucosal layers are more difficult to detect and prescreening with ultrasonography is recommended. Midintestinal exploration is limited by the size of the endoscope, even more so in ferrets because the distal duodenum and jejunum cannot be visualized. Laparotomy and laparoscopy are superior to oral endoscopy for diagnosing intestinal lymphoma in cats because the lymphomas are located more frequently in the jejunum and ileum, which are not accessible via an oral approach.[18] Finally, in contrast to exploratory laparotomy or laparoscopy, upper gastrointestinal tract endoscopy does not provide information about the health of other abdominal organs, such as mesenteric lymph nodes, liver, or pancreas.

Contraindications

Contraindications include high-risk anesthetic patients. When gastrointestinal perforation is suspected, insufflation of air with the endoscope may enhance bacterial contamination of the peritoneum. Endoscopy is also discouraged in animals with coagulation disorders.

Complications

Complications of upper gastrointestinal tract endoscopy in small mammals are rare.[16,19] The most common complication is associated with gastric inflation. Air should always be suctioned from the stomach after the procedure is completed. Overinflation of the stomach may cause hypotension and bradycardia, vasovagal stimulation, diaphragmatic compromise, and pain. Careful anesthetic monitoring during the procedure is critical. In cases of venous return compression due to gastric dilation, a suction pump is advantageous to deflate the stomach rapidly.[19]

The pylorus is particularly sensitive to potential gastrointestinal perforation by the endoscope.[16] Whenever perforation is suspected, immediately take abdominal radiographs. Visualization of free air in the abdominal cavity will confirm the diagnosis.[19]

Esophagoscopy

The tip of the endoscope is advanced to the distal esophagus (**Fig. 12**A). The position and configuration of the gastroesophageal junction are noted. The normal esophagus appears flaccid and drapes over the trachea; normal mucosa is pale and smooth (see

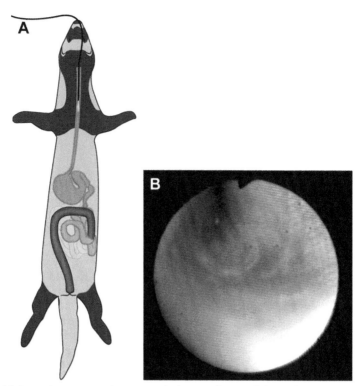

Fig. 12. (*A*) To perform an esophagoscopy in ferrets, the tip of the endoscope is advanced to the distal esophagus. (*B*) The normal mucosa of the esophagus is pale and smooth. (*Courtesy of* Charly Pignon, Maisons-Alfort, France; and Eric Pignon, Maisons-Alfort, France.)

Fig. 12B), and superficial vessels are sometimes visible. In cases of sucralfate administration, white deposits can be seen on sites of mucosal erosion. The cardia is visualized (**Fig. 13**), and any signs of gastric reflux can be noted.

Gastroscopy

To enter the gastroesophageal junction, the tip of the endoscope is deflected approximately 30° to the left of the ferret (**Fig. 14**A). Minimal or no upward deflection is needed. No resistance should be encountered. If the tip is advanced too far, the endoscope will become stuck in the esophagus. Should this occur, the tip of the endoscope must be retracted and repositioned. As the tip enters the stomach, the rugal folds on the greater curvature of the stomach are seen. At this point, insufflation should be performed. The amount of distension required should allow separation of the rugal folds. Satisfactory insufflation allows identification of an ulcer, mass, or foreign body. The gastric mucosa is usually smooth, bright pink to red (see **Fig. 14**B), and paler in the pylorus. Erythema is sometimes seen. In cases of mucosal thickening due to edema, reflection of the light is observed. Gastric ulcers have a raised thickened margin and the ulcer bed is usually dark brown because of accumulated blood.

During insufflation, care must be taken not to overdistend the stomach. The respiratory rate may increase. The rugal folds become flattened; superficial blood vessels can be observed, and the mucosa may appear blanched. When available, narrow band imaging endoscopy can be used to enhance visualization of the mucosa and vasculature, allowing early diagnosis of gastric lesions.[20,21]

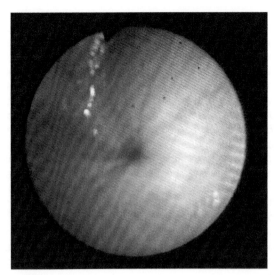

Fig. 13. Visualization of the normal ferret cardia during esophagoscopy. (*Courtesy of* Charly Pignon, Maisons-Alfort, France.)

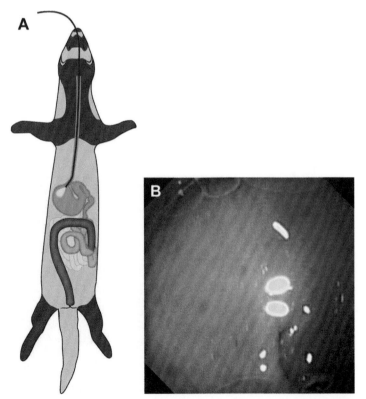

Fig. 14. (*A*) To enter the gastroesophageal junction in ferrets, the tip of the endoscope is deflected approximately 30° to the left. (*B*) The normal gastric mucosa is smooth, bright pink to red. (*Courtesy of* Charly Pignon, Maisons-Alfort, France; and Eric Pignon, Maisons-Alfort, France.)

The smooth lesser curvature is on the endoscopist's right and rugal folds are on the left. The endoscope is advanced along the greater curvature until the incisura angularis, a large fold extending from the lesser curvature, is identified. To perform a complete gastric evaluation, the endoscopist has to perform retroversion (**Fig. 15**A). The proximal stomach cannot be seen when the endoscope enters the stomach. The maneuver is started when the endoscope tip is midway into the body of the stomach. The tip is deflected upward as far as possible as the endoscope is advanced. The retroversion requires a 180° tip deflection and provides a face view of the incisura angularis (see **Fig. 15**B), cardia, and fundus. Two cavities appear on each side of the incisura angularis. The upper area is the gastric body; the lower area is the antrum. The gastric body is examined. Retroversion should be reversed gradually so the mucosa can be further inspected. The incisura angularis and entrance to the antrum usually appear as a circular orifice that is smaller than the distended body of the stomach. The endoscopist should advance the endoscope to the antrum, pylorus, and duodenum.

The pylorus is easily identified as the endoscope is advanced through the antrum (**Fig. 16**A). Sometimes the opening can be difficult to visualize because of an overlapping fold of the pyloric ring (see **Fig. 16**B) or because the opening is obscured by fluids.

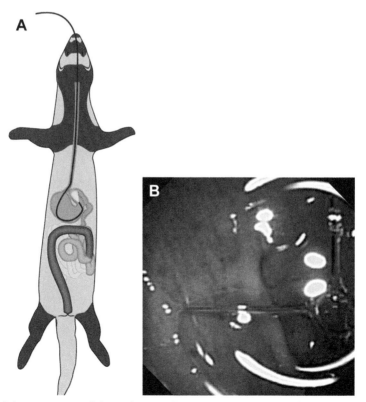

Fig. 15. (*A*) Retroversion of the endoscope during a gastroscopy in order to perform a complete gastric evaluation in a ferret. (*B*) This maneuver allows a face view of the incisura angularis. (*Courtesy of* Charly Pignon, Maisons-Alfort, France; and Eric Pignon, Maisons-Alfort, France.)

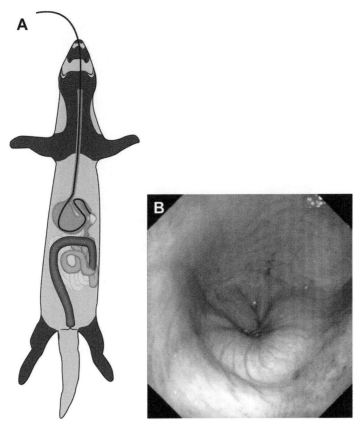

Fig. 16. (*A*) To identify the pylorus during a gastroscopy in a ferret, the endoscope is advanced through the antrum. (*B*) Overlapping fold of the pyloric ring can be visualized. (*Courtesy of* Charly Pignon, Maisons-Alfort, France; and Eric Pignon, Maisons-Alfort, France.)

Duodenoscopy

The pylorus must be kept in the center of the endoscopic field. The tip of the endoscope should be aligned properly with the pyloric canal. Because the position of the pylorus changes every time the patient breathes, minor adjustments are needed as the endoscope tip is gradually advanced toward the pylorus. In some cases, the pylorus may be closed and may offer resistance when the endoscope is advanced into the duodenum. A distinct sensation is felt as the pylorus relaxes and allows the endoscope to enter the duodenum (**Fig. 17**). An additional step to aid in passing the endoscope into the duodenum involves passing the biopsy instrument through the pylorus and then using it as a guidewire over which the endoscope can be passed.

Because of the sharp angle between the pylorus and duodenum, it is necessary to make a directional change as soon as the pylorus is passed so the endoscope tips falls into the duodenal canal. Care must be taken not to cause undue damage to the mucosa.

If considerable resistance is encountered and the endoscope tip can only be slightly advanced into the pylorus, it may not be possible to enter the duodenum. In those cases, a blind biopsy of the duodenum can be obtained. With the endoscopic tip positioned in the distal antrum and the pyloric orifice centered in the image, the biopsy forceps are guided through the pylorus.

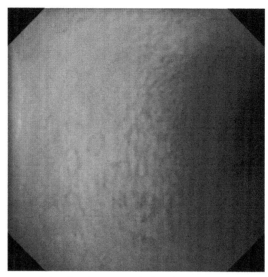

Fig. 17. View of a normal duodenal mucosa during ferret gastroenteroscopy. (*Courtesy of Charly Pignon, Maisons-Alfort, France.*)

Biopsy

Biopsies are performed after visualization of the stomach and duodenum. Biopsy samples should be obtained regardless of whether gross abnormalities are present. Many patients with histologic diagnosis of gastritis have no gross gastric mucosal lesions, whereas patients with gastric motility disorders may have mucosal erythema with no histologic abnormalities.

Gastric biopsies

Biopsy forceps with serrated edges or bayonet-type instruments usually obtain good-quality mucosal biopsy samples. The best area to take a biopsy specimen is the rugal fold of the gastric body. Several samples should be obtained from the body, fundus, and antrum. If it is difficult to obtain samples from the antrum, moderate deflation of the stomach helps in grasping the rugal folds.

When the biopsy instrument is close to the sampling site, the forceps are opened and advanced firmly into the tissue. Once resistance to movement is met, the forceps are closed firmly. As the forceps are withdrawn in a closed position, the mucosa that has been grasped is drawn up to the objective lens. A tissue sample is then torn off as the forces are withdrawn in the working channel. It is preferable to approach the mucosal fold at a 45° to 90° angle rather than parallel. The endoscopist must exercise caution when maneuvering around the pit of an ulcer to avoid perforation.

The biopsy instrument is opened and shake in sterile saline to free the biopsy, and then the biopsy specimen is decanted into a biopsy cassette or a microbiological receptacle. It is critical that the biopsy samples do not dry or adhere to the biopsy instrument. Biopsy specimens obtained from each area of the stomach and duodenum, or locations where dissimilar sampling areas are seen, should be placed in separate containers. A separate biopsy jar should be used for each lesion to correlate with the endoscopic findings.

Duodenal biopsies

Intestinal mucosa is generally not drawn up to the tip of the endoscope. Instead, samples are lifted off as the forceps cups are snapped shut. The forceps cups are opened as soon as they are passed beyond the endoscope and advanced until resistance is met. The forceps cups are usually beyond view. The forceps are generally retracted slightly so the cups can be reopened. They are then firmly readvanced into the mucosal wall. After closure, the forceps cups are withdrawn with minimal resistance.

Biopsy interpretation

Poor correlation has been reported between endoscopic, pathologic, and clinical findings in canine and feline gastroenterology.[22] A major hypothesis is that histologic findings may be inaccurate because of the lack of endoscopic and microscopic standardization for intestinal biopsy specimens. Histopathological standards have been developed by the World Small Animal Veterinary Association Gastrointestinal Standardization Group to allow comparison of different studies.[23,24] Although no standards have been developed for ferrets, the clinician and pathologist should refer to these guidelines when interpreting biopsy samples. Furthermore, as agreement between pathologists can be a source of misinterpretation, the authors recommend using the same pathologist to compare different biopsy samples.[25]

Percutaneous Endoscopic Gastrostomy

Ferrets respond to a diverse range of emetic stimuli. They are animal models of nausea and vomiting[26] and gastroesophageal reflux.[27] Pet ferrets may present for vomiting caused by gastric foreign body or *Helicobacter mustelae* chronic infection.[28,29] Less common causes include gastrointestinal neoplasia, toxin ingestion, and azotemia. Initial treatment includes administration of antiemetic drugs to prevent reflux esophagitis and force-feeding, because most animals are anorectic. However, ferrets can refuse to syringe feed, especially when anorectic. An alternative treatment is percutaneous endoscopic gastrostomy (PEG; **Fig. 18**), a method of placing a tube into the stomach percutaneously, aided by endoscopy. In ferrets and dogs, PEG tubes are

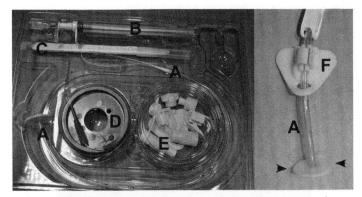

Fig. 18. Surgical set for percutaneous gastrostomy tube placement. In ferrets, a radio-opaque 9-Fr diameter gastric tube is preferred. The set consists of a polyurethane gastrotomy tube with an integral loop (A), puncture cannula (B), scalpel (C), introducer cone with double thread (D), quick release clamp and external silicone fixation plate (E), and luer lock adapter, funnel adapter (F). The funnel adapter is sutured to the skin, whereas the internal disc of the PEG tube (*arrowheads*) should be in light contact with the gastric mucosa, creating a wound seal and avoiding possible complications (eg, ischemic pressure necrosis) at the stoma site. The size of the internal disc (*arrowheads*) can be adjusted using scissors. Care should be taken not to create sharp margins because it could cause gastric wall damage. (*Courtesy of* Vladimir Jekl, Brno, Czech Republic.)

tolerated better than pharyngostomy or nasogastric tubes and can be easily managed at home by the owner.[19]

Indications for PEG tube placement in ferrets include regurgitation associated with chronic reflux esophagitis, anorexia nonresponsive to treatment, and surgery of the oral cavity, larynx, or esophagus that impede appropriate food intake. PEG tube placement is generally contraindicated in ferrets with gastrointestinal foreign bodies and high-anesthetic-risk patients. Ideally, the patient has been stabilized and a diagnosis established before performing the procedure.

Patient preparation and positioning

For PEG tube placement, intravenous access and endotracheal intubation are necessary. The ferret should be fasted for 3 hours before procedure. The ferret is anesthetized, placed in the right lateral recumbency, and a 5 cm × 5 cm area caudal to the last rib is surgically prepared (**Fig. 19**). Local anesthesia is infiltrated at the placement site.

Percutaneous endoscopic gastrostomy tube placement

A mouth speculum is placed and the lubricated endoscope introduced into the stomach. Endoscopic examination of the stomach prior to tube placement is vital as certain pathology, such as neoplasia, severe inflammation or ulceration, may hinder proper placement. Slowly inflate the stomach until moderately distended, but not tympanic, and transilluminate the abdominal wall using the endoscope light. The light is visible externally on the abdominal wall and is used to ensure that the spleen and other organs (eg, liver, and intestine) are not between the stomach and abdominal wall (see **Fig. 19**). The site of tube insertion is typically determined by a combination of endoscopic monitoring while intermittent digital pressure on the abdominal wall is applied by an assistant. An indentation of the gastric wall is visible endoscopically (**Fig. 20**A). Typically the tube is inserted approximately 1 cm caudal to the last rib and as dorsally as possible (approximately one third of the distance dorsally from the ventral abdominal wall). The site can be marked with a surgical pen.

The placement site is aseptically prepared and a small skin incision is made with a no. 15 scalpel blade. The endoscope is withdrawn into the cardia to avoid any

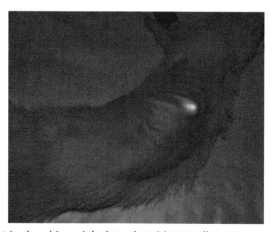

Fig. 19. The ferret is placed in a right lateral position to allow percutaneous gastrostomy tube placement in the left parasternal area. Endoscopic light is clearly visible through the skin and ensures that the spleen and other organs are not present between the stomach and abdominal wall. (*Courtesy of* Vladimir Jekl, Brno, Czech Republic.)

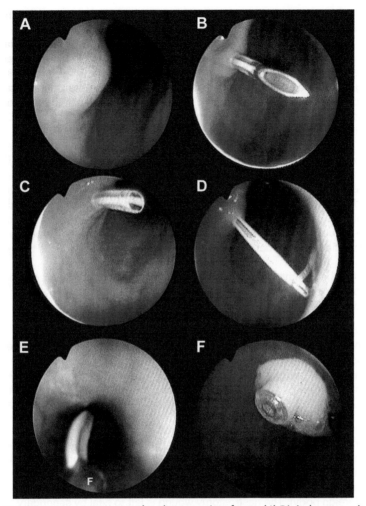

Fig. 20. Percutaneous gastrostomy tube placement in a ferret. (*A*) Digital pressure is applied on the abdominal wall by an assistant and can be seen on gastroscopy as an indentation. (*B*) An intravenous catheter is introduced through the body wall into the gastric lumen. (*C, D*) The stylet is removed and a retrieval suture is advanced through the catheter into the stomach. (*E*) The suture is grasped with an endoscopic forceps and the endoscope and instrument are carefully retracted through the esophagus and out of the mouth. (*F*) Proper placement of the internal disc against the gastric mucosa as verified by gastroscopy. (*Courtesy of* Roman Husnik, Baton Rouge, Louisiana.)

unintentional damage. An intravenous catheter is placed through the abdominal wall into the stomach and its position is confirmed by endoscopic visualization (see **Fig. 20**B). A nylon or polyester suture that serves as a guidewire is then passed through the catheter into the stomach (see **Fig. 20**C, D). The external portion of the suture is secured with a hemostat to prevent it from accidentally being pulled into the stomach during the next step. The suture material is grasped with the endoscopic biopsy forceps, and the endoscope and forceps are carefully pulled out of the mouth along with the endoscope (see **Fig. 20**E).

The suture is released from the endoscopic forceps and attached to the PEG tube. The internal disc at the distal end of the PEG tube is adjusted to the size of the ferret. Lubricant is applied to the PEG tube and the suture is pulled from the abdominal wall end so that the whole PEG tube goes through the mouth, down the esophagus, into the stomach, and emerges out of the incision site until the internal disc is seated snugly against the gastric mucosa. If not using a commercial kit, further steps are needed to attach the PEG tube. Suture is passed through the end of a pipette tip. The feeding tube is cut at an angle, removing the proximal end, and an 18 G needle is feed through perpendicularly. Then, the suture mentioned above is carefully threaded through the needle. The needle should be removed since the suture is now properly positioned. The suture should then be tied circumferentially around the tube, with the knot centered in the middle. The pipette tip, attached to the suture, should then by pushed down and over the tube's end. The PEG tube's descent can be monitored with the endoscope. The proper placement of the internal disc against the gastric mucosa is confirmed endoscopically (see **Fig. 20**F). The internal disc of the PEG tube should contact the gastric mucosa to create a seal. Once proper positioning has been verified, an external flange can be placed to fix the PEG tube to the skin using suture.

The PEG tube is trimmed to an appropriate length, and a catheter adapter can be placed on the opening of the PEG tube for ease of use (**Fig. 21**). The incision site is covered with gauze and the PEG tube secured to the ferret with a stockinette.

Complications and postoperative care

Ensure that excessive pressure of the PEG tube internal disc against the gastric mucosa is avoided to prevent ischemic necrosis. Thoroughly monitor the incision site for the first 2 days for any signs of gastric fluid leakage or infection. Flush the PEG tube with saline or water after each feeding to prevent obstruction. If complications should arise, a repeat endoscopic evaluation of the gastric mucosa is warranted.

Percutaneous endoscopic gastrostomy tube removal

In dogs and cats, tube feeding is generally required for 6 to 14 days.[19] In ferrets, tube feeding may be required for up to 14 to 42 days. The PEG tube should be left in place until full recovery, spontaneous food intake, and patient weight gain occur. To remove, the PEG tube is cut as close to the skin as possible, and removed endoscopically (like a gastric foreign body). The gastrostomy wound is left to heal by secondary intention.

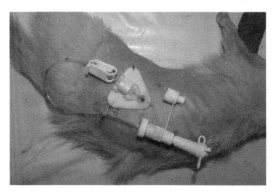

Fig. 21. Postoperative view of a ferret with a percutaneous gastrostomy tube in place. An external flange has been placed and sutured to the skin, securing the tube in place. A catheter adapter can be placed on the tube to facilitate tube manipulation and feeding. (*Courtesy of* Vladimir Jekl, Brno, Czech Republic.)

Percutaneous endoscopic gastrostomy feeding

Ferrets should be fed (based on patient body weight and caloric needs) through the PEG tube for 2 to 6 days using a commercial recovery diet for carnivores (eg, Convalescent Support Instant Diet Royal Canine, Emerald Exotic Carnivore, Oxbow Carnivore Care).[30] Feeding of a small amount of food (2–10 mL) several times a day is recommended. After 2 to 6 days, small amounts of an easily digestible diet are offered in a bowl, and the ferret's diet is slowly introduced until full patient recovery occurs.

Diseases of the Upper Gastrointestinal Tract

Esophageal disease

Ferrets seem prone to esophagitis and gastric reflux.[31] An affected esophagus shows erythema, multiple erosions (**Fig. 22**), irregularity (**Fig. 23**), and strictures. Another condition is megaesophagus, which has been well described in the ferret.[32] Assessing megaesophagus by endoscopy is difficult because the normal esophagus appears flaccid and is inflated for visualization; however, the presence of food and fluid within the esophagus is suggestive. Management of esophageal stricture has been described using endoscopic placement of self-expanding mesh stent and balloon dilation.[33,34] Esophageal foreign bodies have been described in ferrets but endoscopic retrieval has not been documented.[35] Circumferential thickening, erythema, and turgidity of the esophagus is described as pathognomonic for disseminated idiopathic myofasciitis but so far an endoscopic description has not been reported.[36]

Gastric disease

Chronic *H mustelae* infection results in chronic gastritis, duodenitis, and ulcer formation.[37] There is virtually 100% prevalence of infection from selected commercial US breeders. The prevalence in other countries is unknown. Ferrets are an animal model of *H pylori*-associated gastritis.[38] Gastroscopy has been used to demonstrate the role of hypergastrinemia in the pathogenesis of gastric ulcers and the control of helicobacter disease.[39–42] Surprisingly, very few descriptions of gastroscopy in pet ferrets have been reported.[6,17,29]

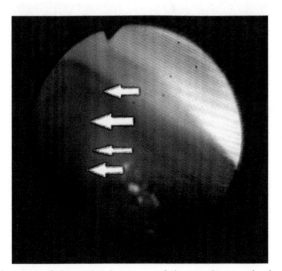

Fig. 22. Erosion (*arrows*) of the parietal mucosa of the esophagus of a ferret. (*Courtesy of* Charly Pignon, Maisons-Alfort, France.)

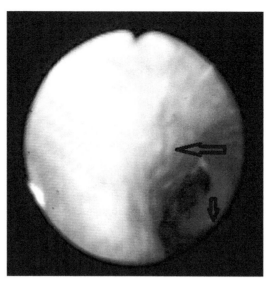

Fig. 23. Thickening and irregularity (*long arrow*) of the parietal mucosa of the esophagus with fibrin deposit (*small arrow*) in a ferret suffering esophagitis. (*Courtesy of* Charly Pignon, Maisons-Alfort, France.)

Chronic *H mustelae* infection may also result in the development of gastric adenocarcinoma or gastric mucosa-associated lymphoid tissue lymphoma.[37] Typically, the disease manifests as chronic gastritis with or without gastric or duodenal ulcers (**Fig. 24**). Recent stress (eg, surgery) may precipitate ulcer formation. The diagnosis is made by gastric biopsy, histologic examination, and culture of the organism from the stomach. *H mustelae* is identified with special silver stain on histologic examination. Contrast barium radiography can be used before endoscopy to depict ulcers.[37]

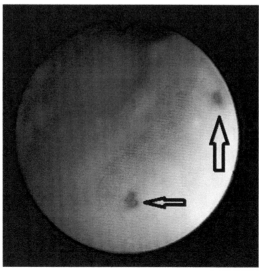

Fig. 24. Two punctiform gastric ulcers (*arrows*) in a ferret. (*Courtesy of* Charly Pignon, Maisons-Alfort, France.)

Other common causes of gastric disease are foreign bodies (including trichobezoars) and gastric tumors. Foreign bodies can be retrieved from the ferret esophagus or stomach. In ferrets, most of the foreign bodies have a soft consistency (eg, trichobezoar), facilitating endoscopic removal.[17,35] The foreign body can be firmly grasped with sharp rat-tooth grasping forceps, gasping snares, or wire basket retrieval devices. The entire stomach should be explored for additional foreign bodies. Ultrasonographic evaluation before the endoscopic procedure is valuable to count the number of foreign bodies and locate them in case one or more have progressed further into the duodenum or jejunum.

LOWER GASTROINTESTINAL TRACT ENDOSCOPY

Endoscopy procedures of the lower gastrointestinal tract include colonoscopy and jejunoileoscopy. Because the large intestine is anatomically simple, colonoscopy is relatively easy to perform. It is a safe, minimally invasive, and high-yield diagnostic procedure. A 3.7 mm × 54 cm broncho-fiberscope (or smaller) and 2.8 mm × 70 cm flexible video endoscope can be used, because the colon is 10 cm long with a diameter of 0.6 cm in ferrets.[3]

Indications

Indications for performing a colonoscopy include chronic diarrhea, tenesmus, excess fecal mucus, and hematochezia that accompanies formed feces. Less commonly, colonoscopy may be indicated for ferrets with severe constipation or severe acute hematochezia, with or without diarrhea.

Contraindications

Before insertion of the endoscope, the practitioner needs to rule out a rectal obstruction, mass, or ulceration, into which inadvertent placement of the endoscope could lead to rectal perforation.

Complications

Because lower gastrointestinal endoscopy is rarely described in ferrets, no complications have been described to date. In cats and dogs, colonoscopy is a relatively safe procedure when performed properly. Major complications in cats and dogs include fatal aspiration of a gastrointestinal lavage solution, colonic perforation, and excessive hemorrhage after biopsy of an adenocarcinoma with rigid forceps.[13]

Colonoscopy and Jejunoileoscopy Procedure

The well-lubricated endoscope should be advanced several centimeters into the rectum; air should be insufflated to distend the colon, and the endoscope should be advanced slowly as long as a patent lumen can be visualized (**Fig. 25**A). An assistant should grasp the perianal tissues tightly around the endoscope to prevent insufflated air escaping from the colon and to allow the rectal mucosal folds to distend. Advancement of the endoscope, with a clear view of the center of the colonic lumen, will reduce the possibility of colonic damage or perforation. The central portion of the lumen should be visualized by turning the angulation control knobs and rotating the fiberscope as needed. Air should be insufflated to distend the lumen and flatten the mucosa, and the insertion tube should be advanced as long as the lumen is clearly visible. If the central view of the lumen cannot be located, the endoscope should be slowly withdrawn until the lumen becomes visible. Inability to distend the colon may indicate severe fibrosis secondary to chronic inflammation or the presence of a stricture.

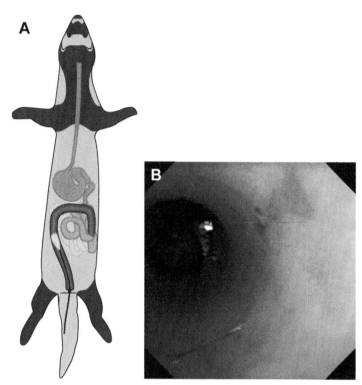

Fig. 25. (*A*) To perform colonoscopy in ferrets, a well-lubricated endoscope is advanced into the rectum and then the colon while insufflating with air. (*B*) Normal colonic mucosa of the descending colon in a ferret. Note the residual trace of brown feces. (*Courtesy of* Charly Pignon, Maisons-Alfort, France; and Eric Pignon, Maisons-Alfort, France.)

As the endoscope is advanced through the rectum, a partial fold, or flexure, located on the left side of the abdomen is encountered as the distal colon leaves the midline of the pelvic canal. In cats and dogs, passing this flexure requires sustained air insufflation and a slight directional change of the endoscope's tip. However, in ferrets, the slight directional change of the endoscope's tip is not necessary, and the endoscope can easily progress cranially.

As the endoscope is advanced into the proximal part of the descending colon (see **Fig. 25**B), the splenic flexure (the junction of the descending and transverse colons) is encountered. This flexure represents an approximate 90°change of direction as the transverse colon courses across the abdomen from the left to the right side (**Fig. 26**). Continued air insufflation will reduce the angle of this flexure and allow the passage of the fiberscope as it is deflected to the right side of the animal. Another fold, the hepatic flexure, will be reached at the junction of the transverse colon and the ascending colon. The tip of the endoscope must be deflected caudally (toward the anus), and the endoscope should be slowly advanced into the ascending colon. The jejunoileal-colic junction will often appear straight ahead (**Fig. 27**). The sphincter is likely to be open because of inflation, and the passage into the jejunoileum may be missed. Passage into the jejunoileum (**Fig. 28**) can be performed with a small-size endoscope (2.8 mm, 70 cm).

Complete evaluation of the colon is performed as the endoscope is slowly withdrawn. Often the visualization is of a better quality than during the insertion of the

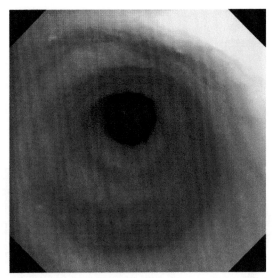

Fig. 26. Normal mucosa of the transverse colon in a ferret. Note the circular fold present when the lumen in not sufficiently insufflated. (*Courtesy of* Charly Pignon, Maisons-Alfort, France.)

endoscope, because the insufflation is ideal. The tip of the endoscope should be slowly rotated to ensure that the entire circumference of the colon is observed (**Fig. 29**). In dogs, a retroflexion of 180° is described as the endoscope is withdrawn into the rectum from the colon. However, to date, this has not been possible in ferrets. Instead, the endoscope should be slowly withdrawn toward the terminal rectum (**Fig. 30**) and then the anus.

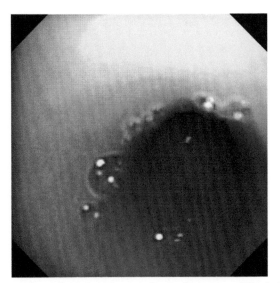

Fig. 27. Normal jejunoileo-colonic junction in a ferret. (*Courtesy of* Charly Pignon, Maisons-Alfort, France.)

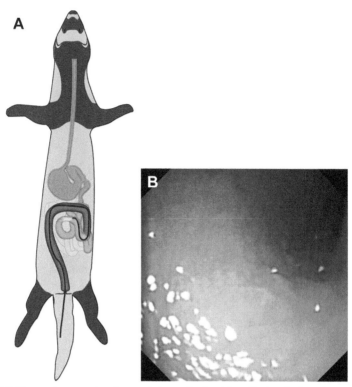

Fig. 28. (A) The endoscope is advanced through the jejunoileal-colic junction, which will allow the passage into the jejunoileum. (B) Visualization of the jejunoileum mucosa in a healthy ferret. (*Courtesy of* Charly Pignon, Maisons-Alfort, France; and Eric Pignon, Maisons-Alfort, France.)

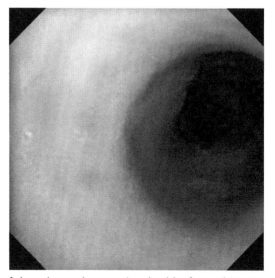

Fig. 29. Junction of the colon and rectum in a healthy ferret. (*Courtesy of* Charly Pignon, Maisons-Alfort, France.)

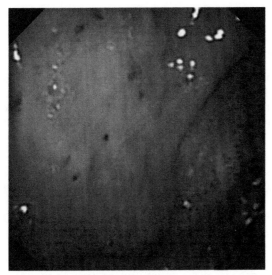

Fig. 30. Normal rectal mucosa in a ferret. (*Courtesy of* Charly Pignon, Maisons-Alfort, France.)

Biopsy

Multiple biopsy specimens from all abnormal-appearing areas and from normal areas of each segment of the colon (ascending colon, transverse colon, descending colon) should be collected. This procedure has been described in the ferret using 1.8-mm biopsy forceps and was found effective in diagnosing proliferative bowel disease.[43] Biopsy samples deeper than the submucosa are rarely obtained when a flexible endoscope is used in cats and dogs; the procedure has not been evaluated in ferrets. Excess pressure should not be applied as the flexible forceps approach the mucosa as perforation through an abnormal colonic wall can occur.

Brush cytology is a useful diagnostic technique if neoplasia is suspected. A guarded cytology brush can be advanced into the biopsy channel, extended from its protective sheath, and rubbed back and forth across the suspected neoplastic area, gently exfoliating cells. The brush is withdrawn into its protective sheath, and the entire accessory is withdrawn from the endoscope. The brush is extended from its protective sheath and gently rolled across a glass slide. Staining with a Romanowsky stain and microscopic evaluation can often provide a rapid diagnosis of colonic tumors.

Diseases of the Lower Intestinal Tract

Conditions of the lower intestinal tract described in the ferret include eosinophilic gastroenteritis,[44] proliferative bowel disease caused by *Lawsonia intracellularis*,[5,43] and neoplastic disease (lymphoma,[45] stromal tumor,[46] adenomatous polyp[47]). However, currently, flexible endoscopy has only been used to obtain colonic biopsies for diagnosing proliferative bowel disease in ferrets.[43]

SUMMARY

Endoscopy is widely used in cats and dogs. However, despite its frequent application in cats and dogs, it is surprisingly underused in ferrets. Practitioners should be aware of endoscopy as a useful procedure for diagnosing gastrointestinal disease in ferrets and for removing gastric foreign bodies.

ACKNOWLEDGMENTS

The authors would like to thank Eric Pignon for providing the illustrations of ferret anatomy, Valerie Freiche for helping to perform the endoscopies, Laurence Melony and Ludovic Valente of Karl Storz Endoscopie France SAS for the loan of the endoscopes used in preparing this article, and Thomas Donnelly for editing the article.

REFERENCES

1. Maurer KJ, Fox JG. Diseases of the gastrointestinal system. In: Fox JG, Marini RP, editors. Biology and diseases of the ferret. 3rd edition. Ames (IA): Wiley Blackwell; 2014. p. 363–75.
2. Hoefer HL, Fox JG, Bell JA. Gastrointestinal diseases. In: Quesenberry KE, Carpenter JW, editors. Ferrets, rabbits, and rodents: clinical medicine and surgery. 3rd edition. St Louis (MO): Elsevier; 2012. p. 27–45.
3. Evans H, Nguyen QA. Anatomy of the ferret. In: Fox JG, Marini RP, editors. Biology and diseases of the ferret. 3rd edition. Ames (IA): Wiley Blackwell; 2014. p. 23–67.
4. Sum S, Ward CR. Flexible endoscopy in small animals. Vet Clin North Am Small Anim Pract 2009;39(5):881–902.
5. Fox JG, Murphy JC, Ackerman JI, et al. Proliferative colitis in ferrets. Am J Vet Res 1982;43(5):858–64.
6. Divers SJ. Exotic mammal diagnostic endoscopy and endosurgery. Vet Clin North Am Exot Anim Pract 2010;13(2):255–72.
7. Fodor K, Prohaczik A, Andrasofszky E, et al. Determination of transit time in ferret and domestic cat. Magyar állatorvosok lapja 2006;128(11):674–9.
8. Poddar S, Murgatroyd L. Morphological and histological study of gastrointestinal-tract of ferret. Acta Anat 1976;96(3):321–34.
9. Brown SA, Powers LV. Basic anatomy, physiology, and husbandry. In: Quesenberry KE, Carpenter JW, editors. Ferrets, rabbits, and rodents: clinical medicine and surgery. 3rd edition. St Louis (MO): Elsevier; 2012. p. 1–12.
10. Bueno L, Fioramonti J, More J. Is there a functional large intestine in the ferret? Experientia 1981;37(3):275–7.
11. Scheidecker S. Anatomie clinique du furet: réalisation d'un atlas photographique [DVM thesis]. Maisons-Alfort (France): Ecole Nationale Vétérinaire d'Alfort; 2012.
12. Sherding RG, Johnson SE. Esophagoscopy. In: Tams TR, Rawlings CA, editors. Small animal endoscopy. 3rd edition. St Louis (MO): Elsevier/Mosby; 2011. p. 41–95.
13. Leib MS. Colonoscopy. In: Tams TR, Rawlings CA, editors. Small animal endoscopy. 3rd edition. St Louis (MO): Elsevier/Mosby; 2011. p. 217–44.
14. Smith AA, Posner LP, Goldstein RE, et al. Evaluation of the effects of premedication on gastroduodenoscopy in cats. J Am Vet Med Assoc 2004;225(4):540–4.
15. Weil AB. Anesthesia for endoscopy in small animals. Vet Clin North Am Small Anim Pract 2009;39(5):839–48.
16. Tams TR. Gastroscopy. In: Tams TR, Rawlings CA, editors. Small animal endoscopy. 3rd edition. St Louis (MO): Elsevier/Mosby; 2011. p. 97–172.
17. Wagner R, Finkler MR. Diagnosing gastric hairballs in ferrets. Exotic DVM 2008; 10(2):19–23.
18. Evans SE, Bonczynski JJ, Broussard JD, et al. Comparison of endoscopic and full-thickness biopsy specimens for diagnosis of inflammatory bowel disease

and alimentary tract lymphoma in cats. J Am Vet Med Assoc 2006;229(9): 1447–50.

19. Guilford WG. Upper gastrointestinal endoscopy. In: McCarthy TC, editor. Veterinary endoscopy for the small animal practitioner. St Louis (MO): W.B. Saunders; 2005. p. 279–321.

20. Tahara T, Shibata T, Nakamura M, et al. Gastric mucosal pattern by using magnifying narrow-band imaging endoscopy clearly distinguishes histological and serological severity of chronic gastritis. Gastrointest Endosc 2009;70(2):246–53.

21. Uedo N, Ishihara R, Iishi H, et al. A new method of diagnosing gastric intestinal metaplasia: narrow-band imaging with magnifying endoscopy. Endoscopy 2006; 38(8):819–24.

22. Jergens AE, Willard MD, Day MJ. Endoscopic biopsy specimen collection and histopathologic considerations. In: Tams TR, Rawlings CA, editors. Small animal endoscopy. 3rd edition. Saint Louis (MO): Elsevier Mosby; 2011. p. 293–309.

23. Day MJ, Bilzer T, Mansell J, et al. Histopathological standards for the diagnosis of gastrointestinal inflammation in endoscopic biopsy samples from the dog and cat: a report from the World Small Animal Veterinary Association Gastrointestinal Standardization Group. J Comp Pathol 2008;138(Suppl 1):S1–43.

24. Washabau RJ, Day MJ, Willard MD, et al. Endoscopic, biopsy, and histopathologic guidelines for the evaluation of gastrointestinal inflammation in companion animals. J Vet Intern Med 2010;24(1):10–26.

25. Willard MD, Moore GE, Denton BD, et al. Effect of tissue processing on assessment of endoscopic intestinal biopsies in dogs and cats. J Vet Intern Med 2010; 24(1):84–9.

26. Percie du Sert N, Andrews PLR. The ferret in nausea and vomiting research: lessons in translation of basic science to the clinic. In: Fox JG, Marini RP, editors. Biology and diseases of the ferret. Ames (IA): Wiley Blackwell; 2014. p. 735–78.

27. Blackshaw LA, Staunton E, Lehmann A, et al. Inhibition of transient LES relaxations and reflux in ferrets by GABA receptor agonists. Am J Phys 1999;277(4 Pt 1):G867–74.

28. Lennox AM. Gastrointestinal diseases of the ferret. Vet Clin North Am Exot Anim Pract 2005;8(2):213–25.

29. Huynh M, Pignon CP. Gastrointestinal disease in exotic small mammals. J Exotic Pet Med 2013;22(2):118–31.

30. Johnson-Delaney CA. Ferret nutrition. Vet Clin North Am Exot Anim Pract 2014; 17(3):449–70.

31. Smid SD, Page AJ, O'Donnell T, et al. Oesophagitis-induced changes in capsaicin-sensitive tachykininergic pathways in the ferret lower oesophageal sphincter. Neurogastroenterol Motil 1998;10(5):403–11.

32. Blanco MC, Fox JG, Rosenthal K, et al. Megaesophagus in nine ferrets. J Am Vet Med Assoc 1994;205(3):444–7.

33. Weisse C, Berent A, Kaae J, et al. Preliminary evaluation of esophageal stenting for recurrent benign esophageal strictures in 1 ferret and 2 dogs. 26th Annual Forum of the American College of Veterinary Internal Medicine. San Antonio, TX, June 4-7, 2008.

34. Graham JE, DeCubellis J, Hobbs J, et al. Diagnosis and management of esophageal strictures in a ferret (Mustela putorius furo). 12th Annual Conference of the Association of Exotic Mammal Veterinarians. Indianapolis, IN, September 14-19, 2013.

35. Mullen HS, Scavelli TD, Quesenberry KE, et al. Gastrointestinal foreign body in ferrets: 25 cases (1986 to 1990). J Am Anim Hosp Assoc 1992;28(1):13–9.

36. Garner MM, Ramsell K, Schoemaker NJ, et al. Myofasciitis in the domestic ferret. Vet Pathol 2007;44(1):25–38.
37. Fox JG, Marini RP. Helicobacter mustelae infection in ferrets: pathogenesis, epizootiology, diagnosis, and treatment. Semin Avian Exot Pet Med 2001;10(1): 36–44.
38. Fox JG, Correa P, Taylor NS, et al. Helicobacter mustelae-associated gastritis in ferrets. An animal model of Helicobacter pylori gastritis in humans. Gastroenterology 1990;99(2):352–61.
39. Perkins SE, Fox JG, Walsh JH. Helicobacter mustelae-associated hypergastrinemia in ferrets (Mustela putorius furo). Am J Vet Res 1996;57(2):147–50.
40. Cuenca R, Blanchard TG, Czinn SJ, et al. Therapeutic immunization against Helicobacter mustelae in naturally infected ferrets. Gastroenterology 1996;110(6): 1770–5.
41. Batchelder M, Fox JG, Hayward A, et al. Natural and experimental Helicobacter mustelae reinfection following successful antimicrobial eradication in ferrets. Helicobacter 1996;1(1):34–42.
42. Cabot EB, Fox JG. Bile reflux and the gastric mucosa: an experimental ferret model. J Invest Surg 1990;3(2):177–89.
43. Krueger KL, Murphy JC, Fox JG. Treatment of proliferative colitis in ferrets. J Am Vet Med Assoc 1989;194(10):1435–6.
44. Fazakas S. Eosinophilic gastroenteritis in a domestic ferret. Can Vet J 2000;41(9): 707–9.
45. Li X, Fox JG, Padrid PA. Neoplastic diseases in ferrets: 574 cases (1968–1997). J Am Vet Med Assoc 1998;212(9):1402–6.
46. Girard-Luc A, Prata D, Huet H, et al. A KIT-positive gastrointestinal stromal tumor in a ferret (Mustela putorius furo). J Vet Diagn Invest 2009;21(6):915–7.
47. Castillo-Alcala F, Mans C, Bos AS, et al. Clinical and pathologic features of an adenomatous polyp of the colon in a domestic ferret (Mustela putorius furo). Can Vet J 2010;51(11):1261–4.

Endoscopic Ovariectomy of Exotic Mammals Using a Three-Port Approach

Stephen J. Divers, BSc(Hons), BVetMed, DZooMed, DipECZM (Herpetology, Zoo Health Management), DACZM, FRCVS

KEYWORDS

- Mammal • Laparoscopy • Ovariectomy • Sterilization

KEY POINTS

- Laparoscopic ovariectomy should be considered the sterilization technique of choice for zoologic mammals.
- Knowledge of species-specific anatomy is essential because herbivores and omnivores have more extensive, obstructive gastrointestinal systems compared with dogs and other simple monogastrics.
- A three-port approach offers greatest application and flexibility, with fewer complications.

INTRODUCTION

With more than 10 million pet rabbits (*Oryctolagus cuniculus*), ferrets (*Mustela putorius furo*), and rodents (order Rodentia) in the United States, these exotic mammals represent the third largest group of companion mammals (behind dogs and cats).[1] In addition to these small common species, the zoologic practitioner may also be called on to sterilize exotic felids, canids, ursids, suids, and primates. The current (best practice) sterilization recommendation for dogs and cats is ovariectomy, without the need for hysterectomy.[2–4] Indeed, ovariohysterectomy is technically more complicated, time consuming, and is probably associated with greater morbidity (larger incision, more intraoperative trauma, increased discomfort) compared with ovariectomy.[2] Furthermore, despite the increased demands of equipment and personnel, laparoscopic ovariectomy is now the surgical technique of choice in the dog because of reduced postoperative pain.[5] For a detailed discussion of standard methodology the reader is referred to the laparoscopy literature, because only exotic mammal specifics are highlighted here.[6–8] Laparoscopic techniques including ovariectomy have been previously described for several zoologic species including rabbits, pigs, bears, lions, and

The author has nothing to disclose.
Department of Small Animal Medicine and Surgery, College of Veterinary Medicine, University of Georgia, 2200 College Station Road, Athens, GA 30602, USA
E-mail address: sdivers@uga.edu

tigers.[9–15] In general, the author has been particularly impressed with the faster recovery and return to normal behaviors following laparoscopic ovariectomy versus traditional laparotomy in these exotic species.

There are a variety of laparoscopic techniques available, specifically one-, two-, and three-port approaches to the abdomen. In the dog, the two-port technique has been preferred because of minor reductions in postoperative pain, and shorter surgery times compared with single-port technique (**Table 1**). However, this should be considered in light of the species. The dog is a simple monogastric, with the stomach the largest part of the alimentary canal. Therefore fasting and reducing the size of the gastrointestinal tract is practical in dogs, and the improved visualization permits the use of fewer ports and instruments. The same can be argued for zoologic carnivores including mustelids, felids, canids, and probably most ursids. However, it is virtually impossible to significantly reduce the gastrointestinal volume of herbivores, such as rabbits, and still difficult in many omnivores, such as pigs. Even with extensive fasting the intestinal tract remains a significant surgical obstruction. However, the use of a three-port approach to the abdomen of herbivores and omnivores permits the use of additional instruments to help retract visceral structures and aid localization of the ovaries. In at least two situations the author has witnessed (rabbit and pig), it proved impossible to identify at least one ovary using a two-port technique and conversion to a three-port or laparotomy approach was required.

Another disadvantage of the two-port system is the need to extend the ventral midline clip far laterally up the body wall (to secure the ovary). This may be considered a significant cosmetic issue for a display animal. Finally, the three-port technique offers wider application in practice. The two-port technique is really only useful for routine ovariectomy in simple monogastrics, and in situations that require greater tissue manipulation, a three-port approach is required. Therefore, performing routine ovariectomy in all species using a three-port approach creates a skill set that is transferable between species, and for many other nonroutine clinical situations. Given the variability in species anatomy that zoologic practitioners face, the development of a skill that has wider application is likely to result in more frequent use and improved surgical competency.

Uterine adenocarcinoma is related to reproductive hormones and is the leading neoplasia of female rabbits.[16] Therefore, concerns might exist regarding the development of neoplasia despite ovariectomy. The author is unaware of any evidence regarding the development of uterine cancer following ovariectomy; however, it is possible for microscopic neoplasms or precancerous cells to be present at the time of ovariectomy in mature animals, which further develop following ovariectomy. Such cases do not represent a failure of ovariectomy to prevent neoplasia, but rather a failure to identify pre-existing neoplasia at the time of ovariectomy. The author's own

Table 1 Comparison between one-, two-, and three-port laparoscopic ovariectomy techniques in the dog			
Parameter	Single-Port	Two-Port	Three-Port
Surgery time	24–36 min	14–22 min	16–22 min
Postoperative pain scores (low 0–high 18)	2 (0–6)	1 (0–5)	3 (0–8)
Owner comfort scores (1 worst pain–10 normal comfort)	8.5	10	8

Data from Case JB, Marvel SJ, Boscan P, et al. Surgical time and severity of postoperative pain in dogs undergoing laparoscopic ovariectomy with one, two, or three instrument cannulas. J Am Vet Med Assoc 2011;239(2):203–8.

experiences and those of numerous European colleagues have indicated that ovariectomy seems to be protective against uterine neoplasia. Nevertheless, given the risks of uterine adenocarcinoma detailed, evaluation of the uteri should precede ovariectomy in adult rabbits. The author's current recommendation is to perform ovariectomy before 9 months of age (and ovariohysterectomy after 9 months of age).

Endoscopic ovariectomy is likely to take longer than a traditional approach until the surgeon gains experience; however, with practice, endoscopic ovariectomy can be faster. More equipment and personnel are required, specifically to hold the telescope and endovideo camera while the surgeon manipulates the two instruments. In a large teaching institution, interns and residents are available, but in private practice a trained technician is effective as a surgical assistant. There is also the option of using a table-clamped mechanical arm to hold the telescope.

EQUIPMENT

A list of recommended equipment is provided in **Box 1**. In addition to the usual endovideo camera and monitor, a second slave monitor is positioned on the opposite side of the operating table to enable the surgeon to see the endoscopic image from either side of the table (**Fig. 1**). To permit the rapid insertion and removal of laparoscopic instruments, ports into the abdomen are created using cannulae (**Fig. 2**). Through these cannulae, instruments ranging from 2 to 10 mm in diameter can be used (**Fig. 3**). A large variety of instrument end-pieces are available in the 5-mm size, less so in 3 mm, but fortunately only a few are routinely required (**Fig. 4**). These end-pieces can also be used with a variety of interchangeable handles (**Fig. 5**). To maintain intracorporeal hemostasis, surgical devices including monopolar and bipolar radiosurgery or electrocautery are routinely used (**Fig. 6**).

For animals less than 10 kg (eg, many primates/felids, rabbits, rodents), the 2.7-mm telescope and 3-mm instrumentation are preferred. For animals 10 to 100 kg (eg, most suids and canids), the 5-mm telescope and instrumentation are more applicable. The major advantage of moving to 5-mm instrumentation is the time-saving use of a combined sealing and cutting device (eg, Ligasure Atlas, Covidien [Minneapolis, MN, USA]; **Fig. 7**), instead of separate bipolar forceps and scissors. **Box 1** details the preferred equipment for performing laparoscopic ovariectomy. Invariably there is a need to rotate the laparoscopic patient into left and right dorsolateral positions to facilitate access to the dorsal ovaries, and a tilting table greatly facilitates such intraoperative positioning (**Fig. 8**). Mechanical arms are also now available to hold the telescope and permit a single-surgeon three-port procedure.

ANESTHESIA AND PATIENT PREPARATION

Although some practitioners may still perform rabbit/rodent surgery under mask anesthesia, it is essential that the patient is intubated, ventilated, and more carefully monitored during abdominal insufflation and laparoscopy. In addition to normal precautions and monitoring, blood pressure, end-tidal capnography, and temperature are particularly important because of effects of CO_2 insufflation (**Fig. 9**). Following induction, intubation, and instrumentation, the animal is placed in dorsal recumbency on a tilting table. The ventral abdomen is shaved, aseptically prepared, and draped (**Fig. 10**).

ENDOSCOPIC OVARIECTOMY

A small 3- to 10-mm skin incision is made through in the ventral midline, at or just caudal to the umbilical scar. A minilaparotomy is undertaken to place the first cannula,

Box 1
Laparoscopy equipment for mammalian ovariectomy/ovariohysterectomy

Visualization and documentation

Endovideo camera and monitor

Xenon light source and light guide cable

Digital capture device (eg, AIDA-Vet)

Insufflation

Medical-grade CO_2

Insufflator with silicone tubing

Radiosurgery (or electrocautery)

3.8- or 4.0-MHz dual radiofrequency unit with foot pedal

Monopolar lead to connect to plastic instrument handles

Bipolar lead to connect to 3-mm Mahnes bipolar coagulation forceps

Instrument handles

Two clickline handles with rackets (Mahnes or hemostat dependent on surgeon preference) and radiosurgery connectors

Two clickline handles without racket, but with radiosurgery connectors

For animals less than 10 kg

2.7-mm × 18-cm telescope (30° or 0° view) housed within a 3.5-mm protection sheath

3.9-mm graphite and plastic cannula (accommodates telescope and sheath), with a CO_2-line connection

Two 3.5-mm graphite and plastic endotip cannula (accommodates 3-mm instruments); at least one should have a CO_2-line connection

3-mm fenestrated grasping forceps

3-mm short curved Kelly dissecting

3-mm Babcock forceps

3-mm scissors with serrated curved double-action jaws

3-mm Mahnes bipolar coagulation forceps

3-mm irrigation and suction cannula

For animals 10 to 100 kg

5-mm × 30-cm telescope (30° or 0° view)

Three 6-mm endotip cannulae and trocars (accommodates 5-mm instruments); at least one should have a CO_2-line connection

5-mm fenestrated grasping forceps

5-mm short curved Kelly dissecting

5-mm Babcock forceps

5-mm scissors with serrated curved double-action jaws

5-mm Mahnes bipolar coagulation forceps (or 5-mm Ligasure Atlas seal/cut device with ForceTriad unit)

5-mm irrigation and suction cannula

5-mm Ligasure device

For animals 100+ kg

10-mm × 45-cm telescope (30° or 0° view)

Three 12-mm endotip cannulae and trocars (accommodates 10-mm instruments); at least one should have a CO_2-line connection

10-mm Babcock forceps

10-mm scissors with serrated curved double-action jaws

10-mm irrigation and suction cannula

10-mm Ligasure device

which is secured in place using a mattress suture (Hasson technique, **Fig. 11**).[17] Alternatively, a Veress needle can be used to insufflate the abdomen before screwing in a threaded Ternamian endotip under telescopic guidance (**Fig. 12**). The telescope is advanced through the cannula and into the abdomen. Insufflation is maintained via the side port on a cannula at an appropriate flow rate (eg, 0.5 L/min for a 2-kg mammal; 5 L/min for a 35-kg mammal) to a pressure of 10 to 12 mm Hg. The surgeon examines the abdominal viscera for any abnormalities, and then proceeds to place the instrument cannulae on either side of the telescope, through the linea alba (**Fig. 13**). Following a 3- to 6-mm skin incision, the linea alba is penetrated using a trocar within the cannula. The telescope is used to visualize entry of each cannula. Once the telescope and both instrument cannulae are in position, the table is tilted 30° to 45° lateral, down on the side of the surgeon. This causes the viscera to displace toward the surgeon and away from the opposite body wall.

With the telescope held by an assistant mechanical arm, the right-handed surgeon inserts the grasping forceps through the left cannula and the scissors (with monopolar radiosurgery attached) or Ligasure Atlas through the right cannula. A left-handed

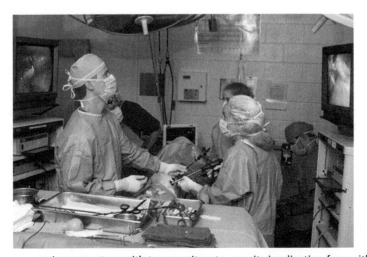

Fig. 1. Laparoscopic room set-up with two monitors to permit visualization from either side of the table. (*Courtesy of* Dr Stephen Divers, University of Georgia.)

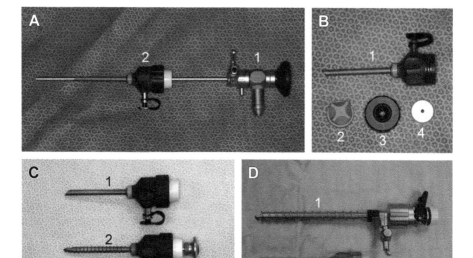

Fig. 2. Cannulae and trocars. (*A*) A 2.7-mm telescope within a 3.5-mm protection sheath (*1*) inserted through a 3.9-mm × 10-cm graphite/plastic cannula with insufflation side-port (*2*). (*B*) A 3.9-mm × 10-cm graphite/plastic cannula disassembled to illustrate the graphite cannula (*1*), leaflet valve (*2*), screw cap (*3*), and instrument seal (*4*). (*C*) A 3.9-mm × 10-cm graphite/plastic cannula with insufflation side-port (*1*), and 3.5-mm × 10-cm threaded cannula with insufflation side-port and trocar inserted (*2*). The 3.9-mm cannula can accommodate the 2.7-mm telescope housed in a 3.5-mm protection sheath, and the 3.5-mm cannula can accommodate 3-mm instruments, and thanks to the threaded design resists dislodgement in small exotic species. (*D*) Ternamian endotip cannulae; 6-mm × 15-cm with insufflation side-port and multifunctional valve (*1*), and 6-mm × 10.5-cm cannula with silicone leaflet valve (*2*). These metal cannulae are far heavier and best restricted to animals greater than 10 kg. (*Courtesy of* Dr Stephen Divers, University of Georgia.)

surgeon would typically reverse the position of the forceps and scissors, although a degree of ambidexterity often develops with experience. It may be necessary to gently move intestinal structures with the shaft of the instrument or a distendable (fan) retractor to reveal the ovary, which is then grasped using forceps with the racket engaged to ensure that the gonad is not dropped. As the ovary is elevated, the mesovarium is exposed so the vascular supply becomes obvious. In small, immature animals, the monopolar scissors are used to coagulate the vessels before dissecting the ovary from its ligamentous attachments. It must be appreciated that, unlike bipolar forceps, which only affect tissue between the jaws, anything a monopolar device touches is coagulated. For larger, more vascular pedicles, bipolar forceps or Ligasure Atlas are preferred to coagulate before transection.

Once the ovary is free, the left cannula is slid up the shaft of the grasping forceps, and the ovary is manipulated out of the hole in the body wall using hemostats to stretch the hole if necessary (**Fig. 14**). The ovary is not drawn through the cannula. The left cannula is replaced and the telescope used to check the ovarian pedicle

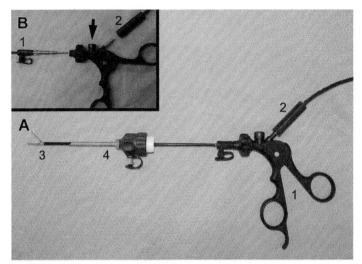

Fig. 3. (*A*) Typical laparoscopic instrument composed of an interchangeable handle (*1*) with radiosurgical connector (*2*) and terminal end-piece (*3*), being passed through a cannula (*4*). (*B*) Close-up of the handle demonstrating how the terminal end-piece (*1*) can be removed by pressing the button (*arrow*), and the radiosurgical connection that enables monopolar use (*2*). (*Courtesy of* Dr Stephen Divers, University of Georgia.)

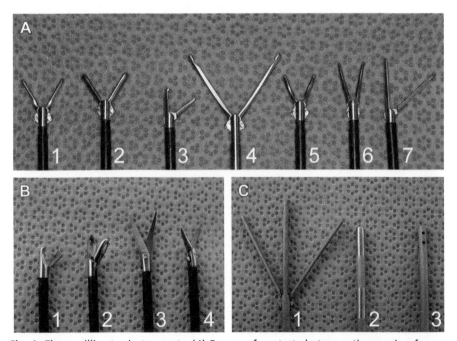

Fig. 4. Three-millimeter instruments. (*A*) Forceps: fenestrated atraumatic grasping forceps (*1*), Reddick-Olsen dissecting forceps (*2*), small Babcock forceps (*3*), large Babcock forceps (*4*), short curved Kelly dissecting and grasping forceps (*5*), long curved Kelly dissecting and grasping forceps (*6*), atraumatic dissecting and grasping forceps with single-action jaws (*7*). (*B*) Scissors and biopsy instruments: micro hook scissors with single action jaws (*1*), Blakesley dissecting and biopsy forceps (*2*), scissors with long sharp curved double-action jaws (*3*), scissors with serrated curved double-action jaws (*4*). (*C*) Probes: distendable palpation probe (*1*), palpation probe with centimeter markings (*2*), irrigation and suction cannula (*3*). (*Courtesy of* Dr Stephen Divers, University of Georgia.)

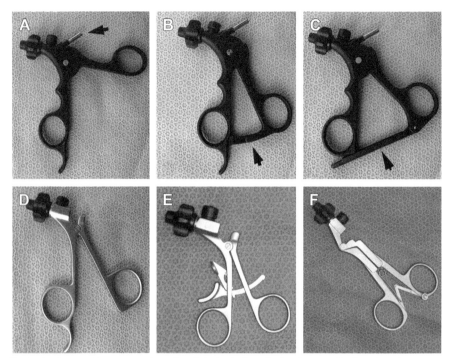

Fig. 5. Endoscopy instrument handles. (*A*) Plastic handle (without racket) with radiosurgery connector (*arrow*). (*B*) Plastic handle with hemostat-style racket (*arrow*). (*C*) Plastic handle with Mahnes-style racket (*arrow*). (*D*) Metal handle without racket or radiosurgery connection. (*E*) Metal handle with disengageable racket but no radiosurgical connection. (*F*) Metal Y-handle with spring action. (*Courtesy of* Dr Stephen Divers, University of Georgia.)

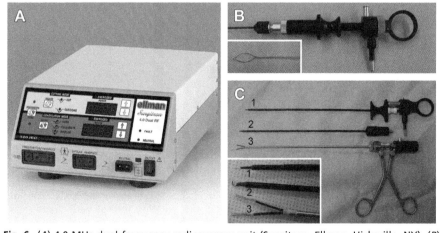

Fig. 6. (*A*) 4.0-MHz dual-frequency radiosurgery unit (Surgitron, Ellman, Hicksville, NY). (*B*) Polypectomy snare hand-piece with extended end shown (*insert*). (*C*) Various radiosurgical endoscopic devices: retractable needle (*1*), dissecting hook (*2*), and biplolar forceps (*3*). Close-up of instrument ends also shown (*insert*).

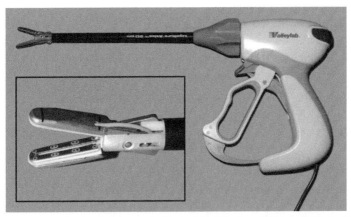

Fig. 7. The LigaSure Atlas (Covidien Surgical Solutions, Medtronic) is available in 20- and 37-cm lengths, and is a human disposable vessel sealing/cutting system that is frequently cleaned and resterilized for repeated veterinary use.

for hemorrhage. The animal is then rotated into the opposite dorsolateral, and the surgeon moves around the table to repeat the procedure. On completion, both cannulae and the telescope are removed and all insufflation gas is evacuated (by using manual external pressure and/or mild vacuum applied to the cannula side port). If the telescope cannula was placed using the Hasson technique, the linea alba is closed with a single suture (the other punctures through the linea alba do not need to be). The skin incisions are closed using single simple interrupted sutures (or tissue adhesive).

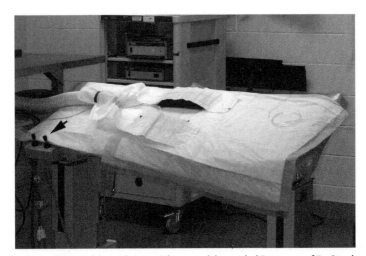

Fig. 8. Electronic tilting table with joy-stick control (*arrow*). (*Courtesy of* Dr Stephen Divers, University of Georgia.)

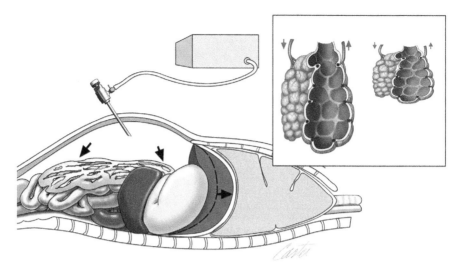

Fig. 9. Diagram illustrating the compressive effects of insufflation (*arrows*) on abdominal viscera and lung alveoli. (*Courtesy of* Educational Resources, University of Georgia.)

RECOVERY AND POSTOPERATIVE CARE

Laparoscopic procedures, including ovariectomy, have been credited with reduced pain and more rapid recovery compared with traditional laparotomy. Consequently, animals typically recover faster and commence normal behaviors including return to

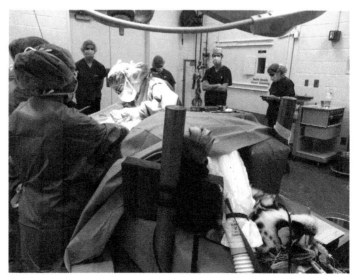

Fig. 10. Siberian tiger (*Panthera tigris*) positioned in dorsal recumbency on a large tilting table in preparation for laparoscopic ovariectomy. (*Courtesy of* Dr Stephen Divers, University of Georgia.)

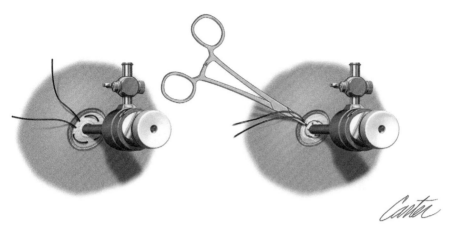

Fig. 11. Diagram illustrating the Hasson technique for the placement of the initial cannula. The mattress suture can either be secured using hemostats or tied. (*Courtesy of* Educational Resources, University of Georgia.)

eating more quickly. Postoperative analgesics (opiates and/or nonsteroidal anti-inflammatory drugs) are provided routinely.

COMPLICATIONS

Most endoscopy issues are caused by operator error until experience and ability have been gained. In the dog, complications have been rarely reported, but have

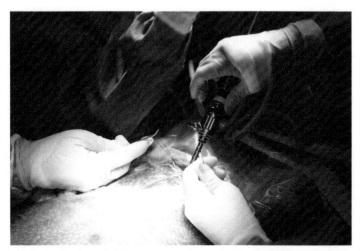

Fig. 12. Placement of a threaded 6-mm Ternamian endotip cannula in a pot-bellied pig (*Sus scrofa*) under intraluminal telescopic guidance. (*Courtesy of* Dr Stephen Divers, University of Georgia.)

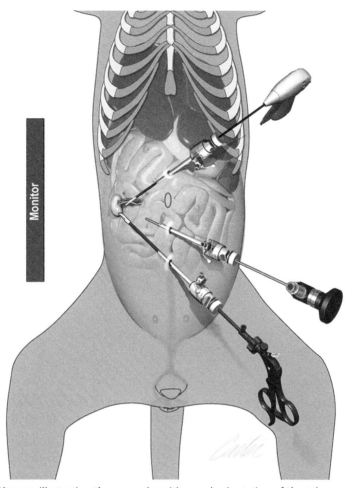

Fig. 13. Diagram illustrating the general position and orientation of the telescope and two instruments for access to the right dorsolateral ovary in a generic carnivore. (*Courtesy of Educational Resources, University of Georgia.*)

included hemorrhage, splenic trauma, and subcutaneous emphysema.[18] In those species prone to remove sutures (eg, primates, rabbits), complete removal of all skin sutures has not resulted in wound dehiscence and infection. To date the author has been involved with more than 30 laparoscopic ovariectomy procedures in exotic mammals, and has been impressed with the reduced morbidity associated with this approach.

To facilitate endoscopy caseload without compromising clients or patients, it is recommended that the surgeon retains the option to convert to a traditional surgical approach if required. Dedicated laparoscopy training is recommended and is available at various conferences and universities, including the University of Georgia (www.vet.uga.edu/CE/index.php).

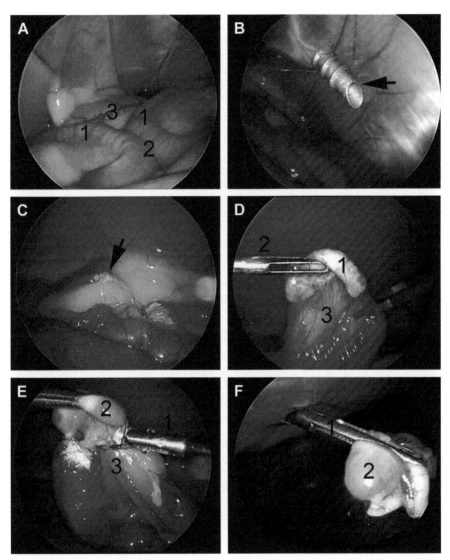

Fig. 14. Endoscopic ovariectomy in a rabbit (*Oryctolagus cuniculus*). (*A*) Initial view of the caudal abdomen revealing normal uteri (*1*), vagina (*2*), and bladder (*3*). (*B*) Placement of a 3.5-mm graphite/plastic threaded cannula (*arrow*) under endoscopic guidance. (*C*) View of the right ovary (*arrow*) at 30° lateral tilt. (*D*) View of the ovary (*1*) elevated using atraumatic (fenestrated) grasping forceps (*2*) to reveal the vasculature within the mesovarium (*3*). The bipolar forceps (*4*) are advanced to coagulate the vessels before transection in this large rabbit. (*E*) Monopolar scissors (*1*) being used to coagulate and cut to dissect the ovary (*2*) free from the mesovarium (*3*). (*F*) The cannula has been slid up the shaft of the grasping forceps (*1*) and is no longer visible. The forceps and ovary (*2*) are gently withdrawn through the hole in the body wall. (*Courtesy of* Dr Stephen Divers, University of Georgia.)

SUMMARY

Laparoscopic ovariectomy should be considered the sterilization technique of choice for many zoologic mammals. Knowledge of species-specific anatomy is essential, and a three-port approach offers greatest application and flexibility. Costs associated with additional equipment and surgical assistance result in higher fees, but many clients appreciate the improved benefits of minimally invasive surgery and are prepared to pay for higher standards of care.

ACKNOWLEDGMENTS

The author thanks Drs Clarence Rawlings and Mary-Ann Radlinsky for help and advice on modifying domestic animal laparoscopy for zoologic species. He also thanks Ashley Schuller and Carol McElhannon for their technical support. The author thanks the following UGA zoologic medicine house officers who were involved in a variety of laparoscopic procedures for their assistance: Drs David Perpinan, Foon Seng Choy, Johanna Meija-Fava, Rodney Schnellbacher, Laila Proenca, and Izidora Sladakovic.

REFERENCES

1. AVMA. U.S. pet ownership & demographics sourcebook. Schaumburg (IL): American Veterinary Medical Association; 2007.
2. Van Goethem B, Schaefers-Okkens A, Kirpensteijn J. Making a rational choice between ovariectomy and ovariohysterectomy in the dog: a discussion of the benefits of either technique. Vet Surg 2006;35(2):136–43.
3. Howe LM. Surgical methods of contraception and sterilization. Theriogenology 2006;66(3):500–9.
4. Okkens AC, Kooistra HS, Nickel RF. Comparison of long-term effects of ovariectomy versus ovariohysterectomy in bitches. J Reprod Fertil Suppl 1997;51: 227–31.
5. Culp WTN, Mayhew PD, Brown DC. The effect of laparoscopic versus open ovariectomy on postsurgical activity in small dogs. Vet Surg 2009;38(7):811–7.
6. Tams TR. Small animal endoscopy. 2nd edition. MO: Mosby; 1999.
7. McCarthy TC. Veterinary endoscopy for the small animal practitioner. St Louis (MO): Elsevier; 2005.
8. Monnet E, Twedt DC. Laparoscopy. Vet Clin North Am Small Anim Pract 2003; 33(5):1147–63.
9. Emerson JA, Case JB, Brock AP, et al. Single-incision, multicannulated, laparoscopic ovariectomy in two tigers (Panthera tigris). Vet Q 2013;33(2):108–11.
10. Steeil JC, Sura PA, Ramsay EC, et al. Laparoscopic-assisted ovariectomy of tigers (Panthera tigris) with the use of the LigaSure device. J Zoo Wildl Med 2012;43(3):566–72.
11. Hartman MJ, Monnet E, Kirberger RM, et al. Laparoscopic sterilization of the African lioness (Panthera leo). Vet Surg 2013;42(5):559–64.
12. Kolata RJ. Laparoscopic ovariohysterectomy and hysterectomy on African lions (Panthera leo) using the ultracision harmonic scalpel. J Zoo Wildl Med 2002; 33(3):280–2.
13. Bush M, Wildt DE, Kennedy S, et al. Laparoscopy in zoological medicine. J Am Vet Med Assoc 1978;173(9):1081–7.
14. Divers SJ. Exotic mammal diagnostic and surgical endoscopy. In: Quesenberry KE, Carpenter JW, editors. Rabbits, ferrets and rodents: clinical medicine and surgery. 3rd edition. Philadelphia: Elsevier; 2012. p. 485–501.

15. Divers SJ. Clinical technique: endoscopic oophorectomy in the rabbit (Oryctolagus cuniculus): the future of preventative sterilizations. J Exot Pet Med 2010; 19(3):231–9.
16. Asakawa MG, Goldschmidt MH, Une Y, et al. The immunohistochemical evaluation of estrogen receptor-alpha and progesterone receptors of normal, hyperplastic, and neoplastic endometrium in 88 pet rabbits. Vet Pathol 2008;45(2): 217–25.
17. Toro A, Mannino M, Cappello G, et al. Comparison of two entry methods for laparoscopic port entry: technical point of view. Diagn Ther Endosc 2012;2012: 305428.
18. Case JB, Marvel SJ, Boscan P, et al. Surgical time and severity of postoperative pain in dogs undergoing laparoscopic ovariectomy with one, two, or three instrument cannulas. J Am Vet Med Assoc 2011;239(2):203–8.

Oculoscopy in Rabbits and Rodents

Vladimir Jekl, DVM, PhD, Dip ECZM (Small Mammal)*, Karel Hauptman, DVM, PhD,
Zdenek Knotek, DVM, PhD, Dip ECZM (Herpetology)

KEYWORDS

- Oculoscopy • Ophthalmoscopy • Ocular pathology • Imaging • Rabbit • Rodent

KEY POINTS

- Ophthalmic diseases are common in rabbits and rodents.
- Pain and discomfort are common clinical signs of ocular disorders and have been associated with anorexia, a life-threatening condition in rabbits and rodents.
- Fast and definitive diagnosis is imperative for successful treatment of ocular diseases.
- Oculoscopy is an easy and simple technique that requires minimal training, and it allows detailed visualization and magnification of the ocular structures.
- Oculoscopy allows detailed examination of the periocular area and anterior eye segment, and an improved evaluation of the lens and retina.

INTRODUCTION

The European rabbit and rodent population has grown in the last years because of their increasing popularity as laboratory and pet animals. This popularity stimulates clinicians and researchers to study their anatomy, physiology, and diseases, including ophthalmology aspects.[1–6]

Ophthalmic disease in rabbits and rodents is diagnosed based on clinical history, physical and ophthalmic examinations, and ancillary diagnostic tests. The term oculoscopy refers to the examination of the ocular structures with a telescope, while still following the same basic principals of the traditional ophthalmic examination.

Ophthalmic examination in rabbits and rodents can be challenging due to the small size of the eye, restraint difficulties, and the use of large conventional diagnostic instruments.[6] Oculoscopy offers great magnification for the examination of the ocular

The authors have nothing to disclose.
This article was supported by specific research of the Faculty of Veterinary Medicine, University of Veterinary and Pharmaceutical Sciences Brno, Czech Republic (2014/2015).
Avian and Exotic Animal Clinic, Faculty of Veterinary Medicine, University of Veterinary and Pharmaceutical Sciences Brno, 1-3 Palackeho Street, Brno 61242, Czech Republic
* Corresponding author.
E-mail address: jeklv@vfu.cz

structures in such animals, including the evaluation of cornea, anterior eye chamber, limbus, iris, lens, and retina.

To date, oculoscopy has been described only sporadically and/or under experimental conditions.[7,8] However, the authors have used this endoscopic technique in exotic companion mammals for more than 10 years with great success. They feel it is an easy technique requiring minimal training.[9,10]

Oculoscopy can replace some of the traditional ophthalmic equipment (such as direct ophthalmoscope). If a practitioner is not sure about the diagnosis, consultation with veterinary ophthalmologists is recommended.

The purpose of this article is to describe the oculoscopy technique, normal and abnormal ocular findings, and the most common eye disorders diagnosed with the aid of endoscopy.

INDICATIONS/CONTRAINDICATIONS

Oculoscopy is indicated for the evaluation of animals with ocular clinical signs, including vision deficits, traumatic injury, ocular discharge, and exophthalmos. This noninvasive modality allows visual examination of the cornea, anterior eye chamber, iris, pupil, iridocorneal angle, ciliary bodies, vitreous, and retina.

To the authors' knowledge, there are no contraindications for oculoscopy. However, any ophthalmic disease causing loss of transparency of ocular structures (eg, corneal opacity or cataract) may prevent the ocular evaluation (**Fig. 1**).

Equipment includes

- Standard 2.7 -mm rigid endoscope with a 0° or 30° viewing angle; an endoscope with a 30° viewing angle is particularly useful for ciliary body examination or in case of problematic mydriasis.
- Endocamera
- Light source and cable; the best light sources for ocular examination are xenon or light emitting diode (LED) sources, as they do not produce excessive heat at the tip of the telescope
- Imaging recording device; images and/or video sequences should be recorded for further client education, clinical case follow-up, and comparison.

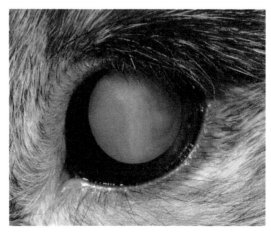

Fig. 1. Cataract in a 5-year-old rabbit prevents the examination of the retina with the endoscope.

- The endoscopic images presented in this study were performed with the use of a rigid endoscope, xenon lamp, and endocamera (Endovision Telekam SL 20212001; Karl Storz, Germany)
- Tropicamid, or atropine eye drops are recommended as mydriatic agents
- Nonantibiotic eye gel or saline should be used to keep the eyes lubricated during the evaluation

PATIENT PREPARATION AND POSITIONING

In rabbits and rodents, many ophthalmologic disorders are associated with dental disease or other systemic diseases, so thorough clinical examination, oral cavity inspection and skull radiography/computed tomography should precede oculoscopy, if indicated.

General anesthesia is required for oculoscopy. Because the procedure is relatively quick, a combination of opioid analgesics (butorphanol, buprenorphine), benzodiazepines (midazolam), ketamine and isoflurane/sevoflurane is recommended. Patient intubation is generally not necessary; the use of laryngeal mask (V-gel, Docsinnovent Limited, London, United Kingdom) or facemask is sufficient. If injectable anesthesia is used, oxygen supplementation should be provided. However, as anesthesia impacts the physical ocular properties (eg, intraocular pressure), intraocular pressure should be measured before anesthesia.

The anesthetized patient is placed on a heating pad in a right or left lateral recumbency, depending on the eye to be examined. Just prior to the examination, topical oxybuprocain (0.4%, Unimed Pharma s.r.o., Bratoslava, Slovak Republic) or other topical anesthetic, should be applied on the cornea. Transparent tear replacement drops or sterile saline should be used topically to provide the necessary fluid interface between the cornea and the terminal telescope lens.

If any corneal erosions are suspected, corneal fluorescent staining should be performed after the oculoscopic examination.

OCULOSCOPY TECHNIQUE

The tip of the telescope is slowly moved toward the eye and is supported by the operator's fingers (**Fig. 2**). The tip of the telescope should always be kept approximately 1 to 2 mm from the cornea and should never touch the corneal surface due to possible

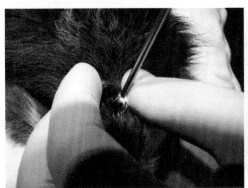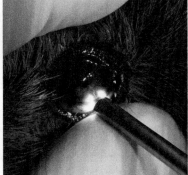

Fig. 2. Oculoscopy in a guinea pig using a 2.7 mm telescope 30° angle unsheathed telescope. Tip of the telescope is supported to allow proper telescope manipulation and to prevent potential corneal injury.

corneal damage. The eye should be examined in various angles, by gently moving the telescope in different directions. The conjunctiva, eyelids, lacrimal puncta, corneal surface, anterior eye chamber, and iris are evaluated by this technique (see **Fig. 2**).

The light necessary for the examination depends on the density of the pigmentation of the iris and retina. For most oculoscopies, the percentage of light set on the equipment (Xenon Nova 175, Karl Storz, Germany) is about 75% to 100%, which corresponds to 130 to 175 lumens. In albinotic animals, the percentage of light set on the equipment is lower, 50% to 75%, which corresponds to 87 to 130 lumens. Light reflectance, if present, can be controlled by slightly changing the endoscope tip position.

For detailed visualization of the lens, vitreous, and retina, a mydriatic agent (0.5%–1% tropicamide, Unitropic, Bratislava, Slovak Republic) is applied topically to the cornea of rabbits. In rats (*Rattus norvegicus*), atropine 1% (Atropin-PO, Ursapharm Arzneimittel GMBH & Co., Saarbrücken, Germany) is preferred over tropicanamid because of its better mydriatic effect.[11] In case of uveitis in rabbits and rodents, inflamed irides usually resist mydriasis and often require multiple doses of tropicanamid, atropine, or the addition of phenylephrine as described in other mammals.[11] However, because of the small size of the patient, care must be taken (especially in cases of conjunctival hyperemia or injury) to not induce systemic effects by the excessive application of local mydriatic agents.

At the end of the procedure, administration of topical ophthalmic gels containing retinol or dexpanthenol is recommended to ensure that the corneal surface will not get dry and that any minor corneal damage will heal. The complete examination of each eye takes approximately 5 minutes.

COMPLICATIONS

Numerous studies have described the negative influence of light on corneal and retinal morphology and function, especially in laboratory animals.[12–14] The light spectrum of a standard endoscope light source is limited to 400 to 750 nm; ultraviolet light is filtered. Short-term oculoscopies did not appear to pose a threat to the retina, even in fetal lamb eyes.[8] Xenon light, which is used for oculoscopy, has been used during vitrectomy and panretinal photography in rats and mice and has been found to be safe.[15,16]

Albinotic animals (especially rats) are more prone to light-induced degenerative retinal changes.[12] Therefore, in albinotic animals (**Fig. 3**), minimizing the light level (but still maintaining sufficient light to allow the clinician to optimally evaluate the retinal surface) is recommended. Continuous telescope-fluid-cornea interface should be maintained to prevent possible thermal injury.

The authors of this article (VJ, KH) did not observe any changes in vision, behavior, and/or ocular function change associated with oculoscopy in any of the examined animals.

RABBIT OCULAR ANATOMY

The orbits of the rabbit (*Oryctolagus cuniculus*) are situated in either side of the skull, and their openings are directed at an 85° angle to the transverse plane of the head. Rabbit eyes appear compressed in the anteroposterior dimension and possess, in contrast to people, and active retractor bulbi muscles and acinotubular glands of the third eyelid (Harder gland) are present. The conjunctiva is divided in palpebral and bulbar conjunctiva and is relatively thin (10–40 μm). The cornea of an adult rabbit has a power of 40 to 43 diopters. The rabbit lens accommodation is limited (0–1.5 diopters). The external ophthalmic artery is the chief arterial supply to the orbital structures, including the bulbus. The venous sinus completely surrounds the muscle cone and covers Harder gland.[3]

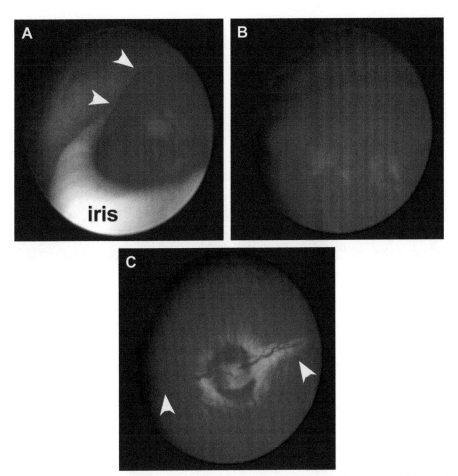

Fig. 3. Oculoscopy of a normal iris, lens. and retina in a 2-year-old albino rabbit. (*A*) Iris and lens bulging out (*arrowheads*) of the pupil (caudorostral view). (*B*) View of a lens and lateral part of the retina (caudorostral view). (*C*) merangiotic retina; note the presence of large vessels forming wing-ling structure (*arrowheads*). (*Courtesy of* Vladimir Jekl, DVM, PhD, Dip ECZM (Small Mammal), Brno, Czech Republic.)

The cornea is large, occupying 30% of the globe. Rabbits are able to resist blinking for long intervals, because they have a very stable tear film. Tears of a rabbit are a clear and slightly alkaline solution, with an average pH of 7.5 with electrolyte concentration similar to that of plasma.

The rabbit has only 1 lacrimal punctum, which is located in the inferior eyelid, 3 to 5 mm from the medial eye canthus and 3 to 5 mm from the inner eyelid margin.[3] Rabbitspossess a well-developed third eyelid (nictitating membrane) that moves across the cornea. The pupil is circular. Lagomorphs are the only species with a merangiotic fundus (see **Fig. 3**; **Fig. 4**), in which the retinal blood vessels radiate horizontally from the optic disc, which is situated in the superior fundus (temporal quadrant).

RODENT OCULAR ANATOMY

The eyes are located on the lateral sides of the head allowing the animal to have a large visual field with limited binocular vision. The eyes of rats, mice (*Mus musculus*), and

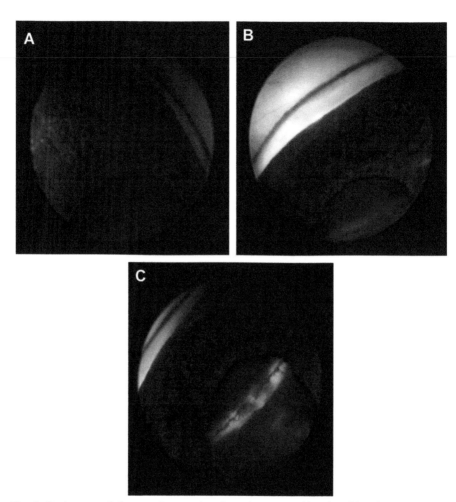

Fig. 4. Oculoscopy of the anterior eye chamber of a 4-year old male rabbit showing normal anterior eye chamber, iris, and pupil (*A, B*) and merangiotic retina (*C*). Mydriatics were not used. (*Courtesy of* Vladimir Jekl, DVM, PhD, Dip ECZM (Small Mammal), Brno, Czech Republic.)

hamsters protrude more from the skull than those of degus (*Octodon degus*) and guinea pigs (*Cavia porcellus*).[3]

The globes of rodents have a large corneal surface (approximately 40%–50%) with the largest in chinchillas (*Chinchilla lanigera*). The orbital shape is almost circular in guinea pigs, chinchillas, and degus, in contrast to the ovoid shape of small pocket rodents (eg, rats, mice, and gerbils). Small rodents and chinchillas have an orbit that is shallower, which may predispose these animals to traumatic eye injury. *Tapetum lucidum* has only been described in the lowland paca (*Cuniculus paca*).

The Harderian gland is located within the bony orbit. In contrast to rabbits, secretions from this gland include the reddish-to-brownish pigment, porphyrin. In case of stress or any disease, excessive porphyrin secretion is called chromodacryorrhoea.

Mice have extensive periorbital venous sinuses behind the globe of the eye, while rats have a more discrete plexus of vessels. The third eyelid is vestigial, and the pupil is circular in guinea pigs, rats, mice and gerbils, and vertical in chinchillas and degus. In the guinea pigs (**Fig. 5**), chinchillas, and degus the retinal blood vessels are minute and restricted to the direct neighborhood of the optic disc (paurangiotic pattern). Rats (**Fig. 6**), mice, and gerbils have holangiotic retinal vascular pattern (the retina contains a compact plexus of blood vessels located in the major part of the light-sensitive portion of the retina).[17]

CLINICAL IMPLICATIONS

Oculoscopy has been shown to effectively evaluate corneal ulceration, foreign body and laceration, the iris, and the structures of the limbus in dogs.[7] Fundoscopy was recently described under experimental conditions in conscious mice and in anesthetized selected exotic companion mammals.[9,10,18]

Oculoscopy allows safe, detailed, magnified visualization of the ocular structures in rabbits and rodents, including the periocular area and anterior eye segment (**Fig. 7**). Moreover, it allows an improved evaluation of the lens (**Figs. 8 and 9**) and retina.[7,9,10]

Fundoscopic and evaluation of retinal periphery is possible in rabbits and all rodents. Several anatomic factors may contribute to the evaluation of the peripheral retina in rodents and lagomorphs. Among these factors are the large angle between the peripheral retina and the iris due to the presence of the lens and the posterior position of the ciliary process compared with people.[3,18]

Congenital and acquired disorders of the posterior segment have been described in rabbits and rodents, such as persistence of the hyaloid vasculature, coloboma, preretinal loops, saccular aneurysm, tortuous retinal vessels, retinal dystrophy, retinal detachment (**Fig. 10**) and optic nerve hypoplasia/aplasia. In rats, retinal dystrophy is a common problem.[19,20]

Oculoscopy could be used also as a method for video-ophthalmography[21] for the measuring and recording of eye movements. This could be helpful, especially in case of nystagmus associated with vestibular disease or with other neurologic disorders.

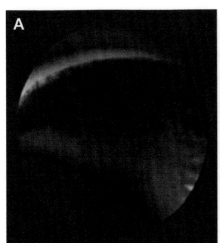
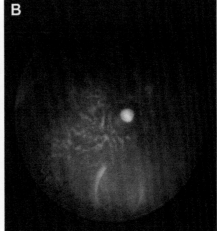

Fig. 5. Endoscopic view of the normal iris and retina of a 2-year-old male guinea pig showing detailed surface of the iris (*A*) and paurangiotic pattern of retinal vessels (*B*). (*Courtesy of* Vladimir Jekl, DVM, PhD, Dip ECZM (Small Mammal), Brno, Czech Republic.)

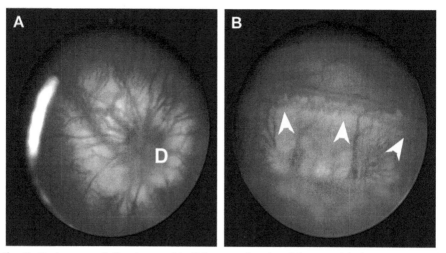

Fig. 6. Oculoscopy of the 1-year-old albino rat showing (*A*) normal holangiotic retinal vascular pattern with optic disc (*D*) and (*B*) ciliary bodies (*arrowheads*). (*Courtesy of* Vladimir Jekl, DVM, PhD, Dip ECZM (Small Mammal), Brno, Czech Republic.)

The magnification provided by the endocamera allows the clinician to view even the smallest structure, such as the retina of a rat. Therefore, even minor pathologies can be seen. The use of an imaging capture device permits recording and re-evaluation by different clinicians.[9,10]

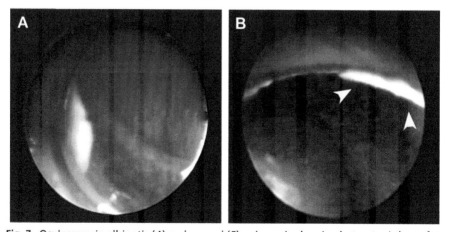

Fig. 7. Oculoscopy in albinotic (*A*) and normal (*B*) guinea pig showing heterotopic bone formation in the ciliary body (*arrowheads*). Incidental finding. It has been suggested that guinea pigs over supplemented with vitamin C have a higher probability of developing such lesions,[2] but this theory has not been proved yet. (*Courtesy of* Vladimir Jekl, DVM, PhD, Dip ECZM (Small Mammal), Brno, Czech Republic.)

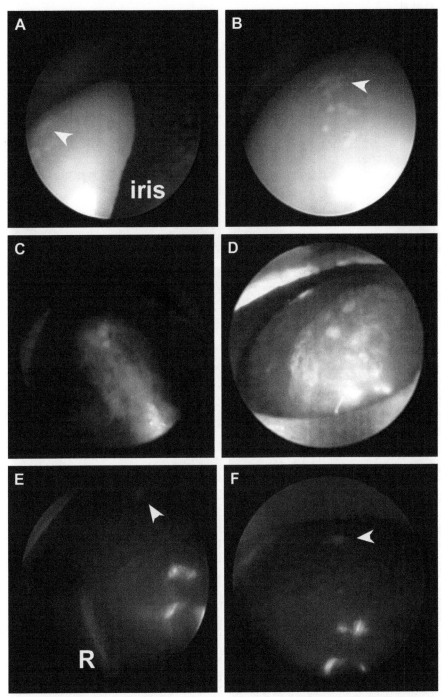

Fig. 8. Oculoscopy in 3 different rabbits showing different stages and types of cataracts. (*A, B*) Hypermature cataract with the presence of crystalline particles (*arrowheads*) from degraded lens fibers and proteins in cortical region in a 5-year-old rabbit. (*C, D*) Immature cataract in a 3-month-old rabbit, and (*E, F*) presence of lacalized corneal opacity (*arrowheads*) in a 4-year-old animal. Cataract etiology in rabbits could be congenital, postinflammatory, parasitic (*Encephalitozoon cuniculi*), metabolic, or idiopathic in origin. R, retina. (*Courtesy of* Vladimir Jekl, DVM, PhD, Dip ECZM (Small Mammal), Brno, Czech Republic.)

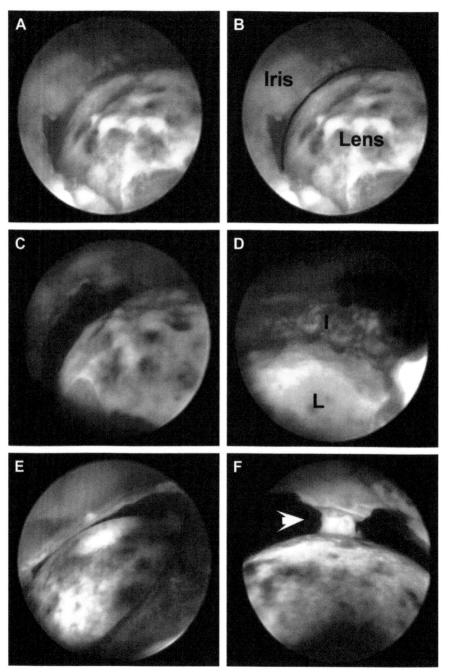

Fig. 9. Oculoscopy in a 4-year-old guinea pig suffering from uveitis (*A–C*) associated with superficial lens (*L*) opacity, iris inflammation with fibrin accumulation (*I*), and hyphema. Images (*D–G*) show evolution of the clinical case after 7 days of treatment with obvious less inflammatory changes. Superficial lens opacity is still present. *Arrowheads* indicate synechias between iris and lens (*F, G*). Ciliary bodies (*C*) could be also visible using oculoscopy. (*Courtesy of* Vladimir Jekl, DVM, PhD, Dip ECZM (Small Mammal), Brno, Czech Republic.)

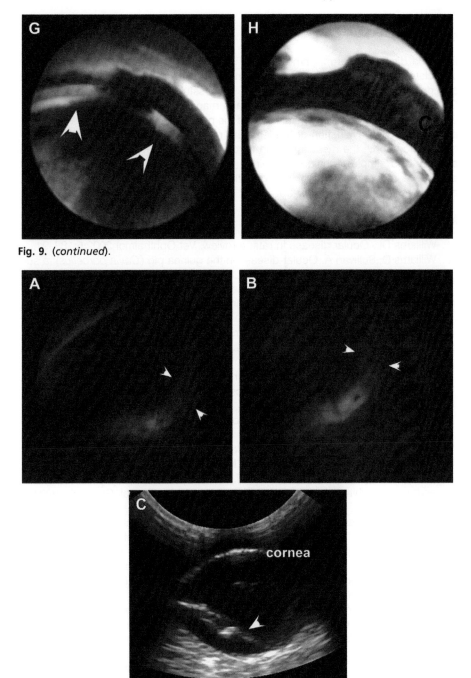

Fig. 9. (*continued*).

Fig. 10. Fundoscopy of a 3-year-old rabbit that was presented for acute onset of incoordination. *Arrowheads* (*A*, *B*) indicate asymmetry of the merangiotic membrane and unilateral major retinal vessel loss associated with retinal detachment (*C*). Retinal detachment confirmed on ultrasonography (*arrowhead*). Retinal detachment is relatively rare in exotic companion mammals and is mostly associated with traumatic injury. (*Courtesy of* Vladimir Jekl, DVM, PhD, Dip ECZM (Small Mammal), Brno, Czech Republic.)

SUMMARY

Pain and discomfort are common clinical signs of ocular disorders and have been associated with anorexia, a life-threatening condition in rabbits and rodents. Fast and definitive diagnosis is imperative for successful treatment of ocular diseases. Oculoscopy allows detailed visualization and magnification of the ocular structures. Oculoscopy allows detailed examination of the periocular area, anterior eye segment, and an improved evaluation of the lens and retina. The telescope allows for video-ophthalmography, the measuring and recording of eye movements. Oculoscopy is an easy and simple technique, requiring only minimal training. Video oculoscopy and image recording improve the educational experience of students and clients, and allow accurate case follow-up.

REFERENCES

1. Williams DL. Ocular disease in rats: a review. Vet Ophthalmol 2002;5:183–91.
2. Williams D, Sullivan A. Ocular disease in the guinea pig (*Cavia porcellus*): a survey of 1000 animals. Vet Ophthalmol 2010;13(Suppl):54–62.
3. Williams DL. Laboratory animal ophthalmology. In: Gellat KN, editor. Veterinary ophthalmology. Oxford (United Kingdom): Blackwell Publishing; 2007. p. 1336–69.
4. Montiani-Ferreira F. Rodents: ophthalmology. In: Keeble E, Meredith A, editors. BSAVA manual of rodents and ferrets. Gloucester (United Kingdom): BSAVA; 2009. p. 169–80.
5. Müller K, Mauler DA, Eule JC. Reference values for selected ophthalmic diagnostic tests and clinical characteristics of chinchilla eyes (Chinchilla lanigera). Vet Ophthalmol 2010;13(Suppl):29–34.
6. Kern TJ. Rabbit and rodent ophthalmology. Semin Avian Exot Pet Med 1997;6: 138–45.
7. McCarthy TC. Otheroscopies. In: McCarthy TC, editor. Veterinary endoscopy for the small animal practitioner. St Louis (MO): Elsevier Saunders; 2005. p. 423–46.
8. Deprest JA, Luks FI, Peers KH, et al. Natural protective mechanisms against endoscopic white-light injury in the fetal lamb eye. Obstet Gynecol 1999;94: 124–7.
9. Jekl V, Hauptman K, Rauser P, et al. 2012 rabbit ophthalmology. In: BRAVO Meeting Proceedings, British Association of Veterinary Ophthalmologists, Spring Meeting. Birmingham (United Kingdom): Bravo; 2012. 6(1). p. 11–13.
10. Jekl V. Rodent ophthalmology. In: BRAVO Meeting Proceedings, British Association of Veterinary Ophthalmologists, Spring Meeting. Birmingham (United Kingdom): Bravo; 2012. 6. p. 7–9.
11. Ollivier FJ, Plummer CE, Barrie KP. Ophthalmic examination and diagnostics. Part 1-The eye examination and diagnostic procedures. In: Gellat KN, editor. Veterinary ophthalmology. Oxford (United Kingdom): Blackwell Publishing; 2007. p. 438–83.
12. Katz ML, Eldred GE. Retinal light damage reduces autofluorescent pigment deposition in the retinal pigment epithelium. Invest Ophthalmol Vis Sci 1989;30:37–43.
13. Haritoglou C, Priglinger S, Gandorfer A, et al. Histology of the vitroretinal interface after indocyanine green staining of the ILM, with illumination using a halogen and xenon light. Invest Ophthalmol Vis Sci 2005;46:1468–72.
14. Framme C, Flucke B, Birngruber R. Comparison of reduced and standard light application in photodynamic therapy of the eye in two rabbit models. Graefes Arch Clin Exp Ophthalmol 2006;244:773–81.

15. Yanagi Y, Iriyama A, Woo-Dong J, et al. Evaluation of the safety of xenon/band-pass light in vitrectomy using A2E-laden RPE model. Graefes Arch Clin Exp Ophthalmol 2007;245:677–81.
16. van Biesen PR, Berenschot T, Verdaasdonk RM, et al. Endoillumination during vitrectomy and phototoxicity thresholds. Br J Ophthalmol 2000;84:1372–5.
17. De Schaepdrijver L, Simoens P, Lauwers H, et al. Retinal vascular patterns in domestic animals. Res Vet Sci 1989;47:34–42.
18. Paques M, Guyomard JL, Simonutti M, et al. Panretinal, high-resolution color photography of the mouse fundus. Invest Ophthalmol Vis Sci 2007;48:2769–74.
19. Wagner F, Fehr M. Common ophthalmic problems in pet rabbits. J Exot Pet Med 2007;16:158–67.
20. Williams D. Rabbit and rodent ophthalmology. Eur J Companion Anim Pract 2007;17:242–52.
21. Jacobs JB, Dell'Osso LF, Wang ZI, et al. Using the NAFX to measure the effectiveness over time of gene therapy in canine LCA. Invest Ophthalmol Vis Sci 2009;50:4685–92.

Video Otoscopy in Exotic Companion Mammals

Vladimir Jekl, DVM, PhD, Dip ECZM (Small Mammal)*, Karel Hauptman, DVM, PhD,
Zdenek Knotek, DVM, PhD, Dip ECZM (Herpetology)

KEYWORDS

- Otoscopy • Endoscopy • Otitis • Ear disorders • Rabbit • Rodent

KEY POINTS

- Ear disease is a common reason for presentation of exotic companion mammals to the practitioner.
- Video otoscopy is a valuable diagnostic and therapeutic tool for the complete evaluation of the external ear and tympanic membrane of exotic companion mammals.
- Video otoscopy enables foreign object retrieval, external ear canal flushing, intralesional drug administration, myringotomy, and middle ear cavity flushing.
- Video otoscopy is an easy and simple technique requiring minimal training.
- Video otoscopy and photo documentation improve the educational experience of students and clients, and allow accurate case follow-up.

INTRODUCTION

Ear disease is often associated with systemic conditions in exotic companion mammals, such as infections, trauma, neoplasia, and abnormal behavior (**Fig. 1**).[1] Otoscopy is essential for the evaluation of the external ear and tympanic membrane, but other diagnostic modalities are also used for the complete evaluation of ear disease, including radiography, computed tomography, and magnetic resonance imaging.[2]

Specific otoscopes were design for the examination of the dog and cat ear; however, because of to the variety and anatomic differences of exotic mammals, the use of the 2.7-mm rigid endoscope is often preferred.

Otoscopic applications in exotic companion mammals are wide,[3] as these species commonly suffer from peripheral vestibular disease (rabbits, rats, gerbils), ear mites

The authors have nothing to disclose.
This article was supported by specific research of the Faculty of Veterinary Medicine, University of Veterinary and Pharmaceutical Sciences Brno, Czech Republic (2015).
Avian and Exotic Animal Clinic, Faculty of Veterinary Medicine, University of Veterinary and Pharmaceutical Sciences Brno, 1-3 Palackeho Street, Brno 61242, Czech Republic
* Corresponding author.
E-mail address: jeklv@vfu.cz

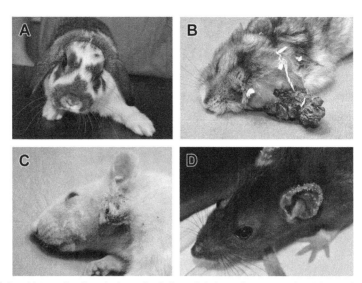

Fig. 1. (*A*) Rabbit with a head tilt to the left with bilateral otitis media. (*B*) Aural neoplasia (squamous cell adenocarcinoma) in a hamster. (*C*) Otic abscess with fistulation in a rat. (*D*) Severe otitis caused by ear mites (*Notoedres muris*) in a rat.

(ferrets, rabbits), and ear neoplasia (hamsters). Early evaluation and diagnosis not only help in the treatment of ear disease but can also be valuable for excluding ear disease in cases of head tilt or other vestibular disorders.[4]

When compared with conventional otoscopy, video otoscopy allows a more thorough and detailed external ear and tympanic membrane evaluation because of the magnification provided by the endocamera. Moreover, the ergonomics of examination using a monitor are preferred over bending over the animal. Photo documentation improves the educational experience of students and clients and facilitates accurate case reevaluation over time.

The purpose of this article is to describe the video otoscopy technique and main findings in common exotic companion mammals, such as ferrets, rabbits, chinchillas, guinea pigs, degus, rats, hamsters, and mice.

INDICATIONS AND CONTRAINDICATIONS

Indications for otoscopy are any suspected ear disease or the exclusion of ear disease in cases of central vestibular/neurologic problems. Clinical signs may include hemorrhagic or purulent discharge, presence of pruritus, nervousness, head shaking, rictus, unilateral chewing, vestibular syndrome (head tilt, circling, nystagmus), or unilateral dry eye syndrome (see **Fig. 1**).

There are no known contraindications for this technique. Standard anesthetic risks exist, and any animal should be stabilized beforehand. Treatment of ear disease should not be started until after otoscopy. Any bleeding, discharge, or the presence of a large mass in the external ear canal that cannot be flushed might hinder otoscopic examination.

INSTRUMENTATION AND EQUIPMENT

- A video otoscope or rigid endoscope can be used for external ear examination.
  - A standard veterinary video otoscope is seen in **Fig. 2** (5 mm × 8–10 cm, 0° telescope with 3-way stopcock, irrigation adaptor, and an integrated

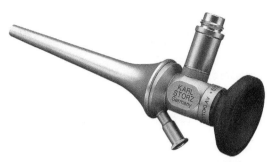

Fig. 2. A 5-mm otoscope (with 0° forward-oblique telescope and a 3-way stopcock with integrated working channel and adaptor to irrigation) attached to an endovideo camera. This device would only be useful for animals greater than 500 g. (*Courtesy of* KARL STORZ GmbH & Co. KG, Tuttlingen, Germany.)

2F–5F working channel for instrument use). The shape of the telescope is similar to that of conventional otoscopes. The working channel and small endoscope size allows optimal external ear and tympanic membrane examination, irrigation and suction, and sample collection using various types of biopsy forceps. Xenon or light-emitting diode light sources are preferred over the halogen light because of their more natural white light.[5]
  - A rigid endoscope can also be used (1.9–2.7 mm operating or forward-oblique telescope of working length of 10–18 cm and viewing angle 0° or 30°, with operating/integrated sheath, irrigation ports, and 3F–5F working channel for instrument use).
- Suction and irrigation system is recommended for larger exotic companion mammals (eg, rabbits and guinea pigs). Irrigation and suction pressures should be regulated separately (**Fig. 3**). For smaller animals or when specific pumps are not available, the use of syringes and catheters (eg, tomcat catheters, red rubber catheters) is possible.

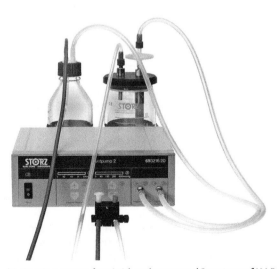

Fig. 3. Suction and irrigation pump for rigid endoscopes. (*Courtesy of* KARL STORZ GmbH & Co. KG, Tuttlingen, Germany.)

- Miscellaneous instruments
  - Various endoscopic forceps are available for sampling for cytology, bacteriology/mycology, and histopathology (eg, biopsy forceps or grasping forceps, 3F or 5F, length of 28 or 34 cm).
  - Endoscopic scissors (3F to 5F, length 34 cm), myringotomy needle (1.5 mm, length 31 cm), brushes (5F, length 19 cm) or intravenous catheters are used for myringotomy, if indicated. For irrigation, 1- or 1.3-mm, tomcat catheters can be used. For tumor removal, the polypectomy snare (5F, length 32 cm) is valuable.
- Image and video documentation requires an endocamera, monitor, and digital capture device. Several commercial systems are available (including high-definition resolution). Images or video sequences should be recorded for further client education, clinical case follow-up, and comparison

PATIENT PREPARATION, ANESTHESIA, AND POSITIONING
Clinical Examination

A complete medical history and physical examination are required. Facial symmetry is recorded, and the jaws, temporomandibular joints, areas around the eyes and ear pinna, and whole skeleton are thoroughly palpated. Ear pinna should be palpated and any signs of discharge, discoloration, or masses recorded. The oral cavity is examined using pediatric laryngoscope or otoscope.

Patient Preparation and Anesthesia

General anesthesia is recommended to minimize head movement and the risks of injury or telescope damage. Detailed evaluation of the narrow external ear, especially in small rodents, is also improved with anesthesia. The authors commonly use the combination of benzodiazepines, opioids, and inhalant or injectable anesthesia. Tracheal intubation and intravenous access are strongly recommended if patient size permits. Tracheal intubation is especially important in cases of tympanic membrane perforation to prevent aspiration of the tympanic bulla content via the Eustachian tube. In small rodents, in which intubation is difficult, the head should be positioned in a head down position with nostrils close to the examination table. The volume of fluid administered for tympanic membrane flushing should not exceed 1 to 3 mL/kg.

Positioning

The patient is positioned in lateral or sternal recumbency. The authors prefer the patient in lateral recumbency with the dorsum toward the clinician (**Fig. 4**). Consequently, ventral ear structures will appear dorsal in the endoscopy image and vice versa.

VIDEO OTOSCOPY

It is important not to attempt sample collection just before otoscopy, as such procedures may have a negative effect on visualization and sample collection.

- The pinna is elevated to minimize external ear canal folding (especially the border between vertical and horizontal parts).
- The tip of the telescope is gently placed on the incisura intertragica. From this point, the telescope is carefully advanced proximally into the vertical and horizontal canal toward the tympanic membrane. When using a 30° telescope, greater appreciation of the external ear and tympanic membrane can be accomplished by rotating the telescope around its longitudinal axis (**Fig. 5**).

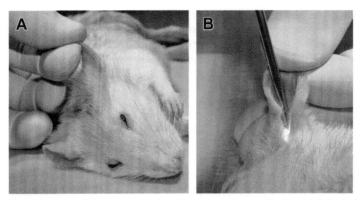

Fig. 4. Optimal fixation of the rat ear during the otoscopic examination. (*A*) Rostral view. (*B*) Endoscope is inserted into the external ear can. Mask with oxygen supply was removed from the patient for illustrative reasons.

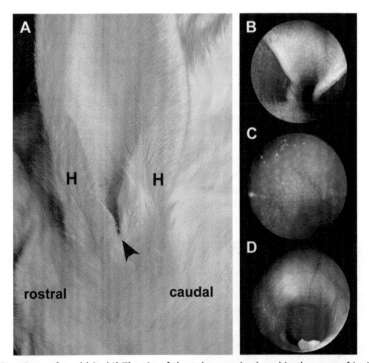

Fig. 5. Ear pinna of a rabbit. (*A*) The tip of the telescope is placed in the area of incisura intertragica (*arrowhead*). The auricular cartilage provides the ear's typical appearance with helix (*H*) formation. (*B–D*) Endoscopic images of a normal rabbit external ear canal. (*B*) Tragus is seen immediately when the telescope is inserted in the incisura intertragica. (*C*) Hair follicles are magnified and in case of infection are more reddish in color and are bulging form the mucosal surface. (*D*) Endoscopic view of the external ear canal.

- The tip of the telescope should be advanced within the center of the lumen, as any mucosal bruising could cause bleeding and hinder evaluation (see **Fig. 5**; **Figs. 6–9**).
- Complete assessment of the external ear includes evaluation of
  - Excessive debris and cerumen accumulation (see **Fig. 8**)
  - Discharge (color, consistency)
  - Hemorrhage
  - Discoloration of mucosa or skin
  - Patency or stenotic changes
  - Erosive or ulcerative changes
  - Foreign bodies
  - Ectoparasites
  - Nodules or masses (**Fig. 10**)
- Complete assessment of the tympanic membrane includes evaluation of
  - Integrity
  - Opacity and color changes
  - Vascularization (quantity and quality)
  - Hemorrhage (see **Fig. 9**)
  - The malleus
  - Foreign bodies
  - Middle ear cavity content (if any)

If necessary, samples for cytology, histology, or bacterial and fungal cultures should be obtained. If a particular amount of debris or cerumen is obstructing the external ear canal, flushing with warm sterile saline is recommended. Lavage of the external ear canal is especially helpful in ferrets and rodents. In rabbits, the cerumen is very thick and requires manual removal, as cerumenolytics are not always effective. Removal of foreign body can be performed with the use of endoscopy. In some cases, removal of parasites is also possible (see **Fig. 7**).

During irrigation with saline, gravity usually provides sufficient pressure[5]; however, it can be difficult to control the volume of fluid administered, especially when flushing the middle ear. Therefore, the use of a syringe system may be preferable.

Irrigation and suction could be performed via the sheath ports. Alternatively, because of the small external ear canal diameter of most exotic companion mammals, tomcat catheters (1.3 mm in diameter), red rubber catheters (up to 2 mm/6F) or intravenous cannulas (21–24 gauge) are used (see **Fig. 8**).

If the tympanic membrane is perforated, the content of the middle ear can be aspirated for further laboratory examination. The middle ear cavity should be flushed;

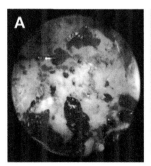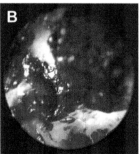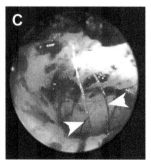

Fig. 6. (*A, B*) Endoscopic images of a ferret external ear canal with overproduction of brownish cerumen. (*C*) The ferret was presented for mild ear pruritus, which resolved after hair removal (*arrowheads*) from the proximal part of the external ear canal.

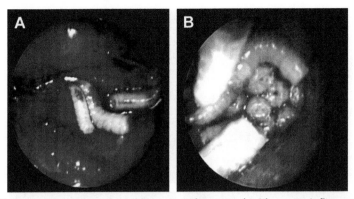

Fig. 7. (A) Endoscopic image of a rabbit external ear canal with severe inflammation and myasis. (B) Fly larvae completely obstructed the proximal part of the external ear canal.

however, care must be taken to prevent tracheal aspiration of excessive fluid and debris coming down the Eustachian tube (see **Fig. 10**). Intralesional drug administration is possible in cases of neoplastic or other proliferative lesions.

Myringotomy

In exotic companion mammals, middle ear infections can be caused by ascending bacterial infections via Eustachian tube without perforation of the tympanum.[6–8] When evaluating the middle ear through the intact tympanic membrane, the surgeon

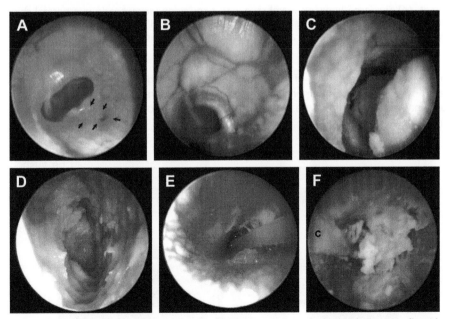

Fig. 8. (A) Endoscopic image of a normal rabbit tympanic membrane with the pars flaccida depicted by arrows. (B) Endoscopic image of a normal rabbit external ear canal. (C, D) Presence of large amount of yellowish to whitish cerumen can be a normal finding in rabbits. (E) Hyperemia of the external ear canal in a rabbit. (F) Ear canal is irrigated with warm saline using tomcat catheter (C) and debris is removed using fluid flow and ear curettage.

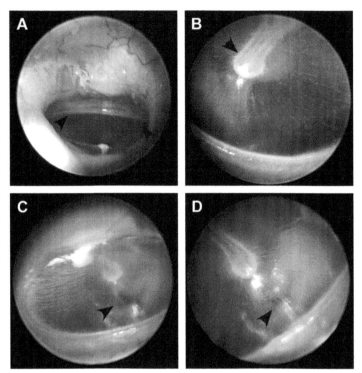

Fig. 9. (A) The large tympanic membrane with bony ridge (*arrowheads*) in a normal chinchilla. (B) Manubrium of the malleus (*arrowhead*) in a chinchilla. (C, D) Tympanic membrane with hemorrhage (*arrowhead*) associated with traumatic head injury in a chinchilla.

may visualize the presence of yellowish exudate behind the pars tensa. Particularly in rats, otitis media is commonly presented with the pars flaccida bulging into the external ear canal, therefore, hindering the evaluation of the pars tensa (**Figs. 11** and **12**).

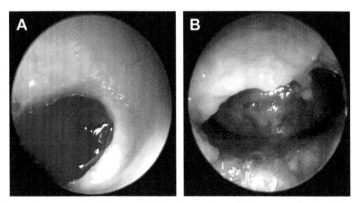

Fig. 10. External ear canal of 2 rats. (A) Bleeding after middle ear cavity flushing. (B) Presence of neoplastic mass within the lumen. Biopsy found Zymbal gland carcinoma.

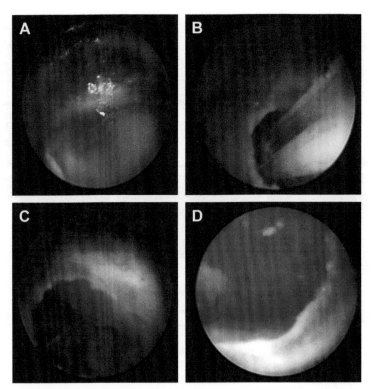

Fig. 11. (*A*) Accumulation of inflammatory debris (pus) in the external ear canal of a degu associated with otitis media and tympanic membrane rupture. (*B, C*) All the material was gently removed by irrigation using intravenous catheter and syringe. (*D*) Middle ear cavity was then evaluated for the presence of any foreign bodies or pathologic masses, but only granulation of the soft tissue was found.

The tympanic membrane can be perforated with a myringotomy needle, biopsy forceps, or an intravenous catheter/spinal needle (with stylet). The external ear canal should be thoroughly cleaned and flushed with sterile saline before the pars tensa or pars flaccida is incised. After aspiration (see **Fig. 12**) of the contents, the middle ear cavity is flushed with sterile saline.

Based on the author's experience, a larger incision is often necessary, as a small hole will not allow adequate lavage of debris and exudate from the middle ear. Instead, the contents might be directed into the Eustachian tube. In cases of otitis media, antibiotics (guided by Gram stain) or anti-inflammatory drugs (indomethacin, 0.1% eye drops) could be administered directly to the middle ear cavity. Subsequent antibiotic choice is based on culture and sensitivity test results.

Complications

- Debris or cerumen can hinder visualization, necessitating frequent cleaning of the endoscope with the use of moist and dry gauze.
- Iatrogenic mucosal bruising and hemorrhage hinder evaluation of the external ear canal and tympanic membrane. In these cases, lavage of the external ear canal with sterile saline can be helpful.
- Hemostasis can be achieved by applying topical pressure with a cotton-tipped applicator or with the use of collagen hemostatic materials.

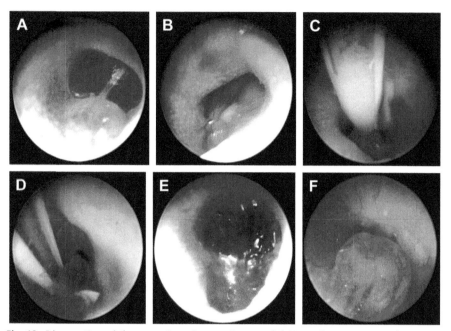

Fig. 12. Diagnostic and therapeutic endoscopy in a rat. (*A*) Normal tympanic membrane. (*B*) Tympanic membrane is slightly bulging into the external ear cavity and lost its concavity; accumulation of greenish debris/pus in the middle ear cavity is apparent. (*C*) Intravenous catheter is introduced into the external canal, and tympanic membrane is incised with a stylet. Content of the middle ear cavity is aspirated for cytology and bacteriology. (*D*) Then, middle ear cavity is gently flushed with warmed saline. (*E*) Follow-up of the affected tympanic membrane after 7 days; a formation of a crust is seen. (*F*) Otitis media could be also presented with bulging of the pars flaccida into the external ear canal and completely obscure view of pars tensa.

- In the author's experience, perforation is mostly done by unexperienced operators or by head movement of sedated but unanesthetized patients. This is a particular risk in small rodents with short external ear canals. Although the tympanic membrane heals by second intention, deeper structures may be affected, and hearing could be reduced.
- With high output xenon light sources, the tip of the telescope can heat up quickly causing thermal damage. The use of saline irrigation prevents thermal injury.
- Fogging of the telescope is best prevented by soaking the scope in warm sterile saline 39°C to 40°C (102°F –104°F) or by the application of antifog to the terminal lens of the telescope.

NORMAL ANATOMY OF THE EXTERNAL EAR AND TYMPANIC MEMBRANE OF THE RABBIT
External Ear

- The external ear consists of the pinna and the external ear canal. The pinna functions to collect and direct sound waves via the external ear canal to the tympanic membrane, visual interactions, and, especially in rabbits, important thermoregulatory functions. The external part of the ear pinna is covered by mobile skin and fine hair, whereas the skin on the inner side of the pinna is adhered to cartilage with less hair.

- Three cartilages support the pinna and distal part of external ear canal, the auricular, scutiform, and annular cartilages. These cartilages are connected by fibrous tissue that permits some degree of movement. The auricular cartilage is broad dorsally and funnels to the narrow external ear canal. In lop-eared rabbits, there is a 3- to 5-mm soft tissue gap between the cartilaginous external ear canal and the tragus, giving the floppy ear appearance and promoting cerumen accumulation.[8] The proximal part of the external ear canal is supported by osseous part of the temporal bone.
- The external ear canal consists of a proximal vertical portion, which bends to a shorter horizontal region. Because the external ear is elastic, the ear canal can be straightened enough to permit otoscopic examination. In the non–lop-eared rabbits, the ear canal appears wide and conical shaped and allows clear visualization of the tympanic membrane, whereas in the lop-eared breeds, the ear canal is smaller and visualization more difficult.[9]
- The general anatomy of the external ear of other exotic companion mammals is similar to that of rabbits. However, size and shape of the pinna and its cartilages and size of the external ear canal differ among species.

Normal Ear Cerumen

The external ear canal is lined by skin containing sebaceous and ceruminous glands and hair follicles. Cerumen in rabbits and some rodents appears white to yellow, brown in ferrets, and almost black in guinea pigs (see **Figs. 6** and **8**). Therefore, cytologic examination of the external ear canal content is recommended.

Tympanic Membrane

- The middle ear is separated from the external ear by the tympanic membrane (ear drum), which is circumscribed by a fibrocartilaginous annulus (**Figs. 13–15**). This ring is attached to the osseous part of the external ear canal and is complete in ferrets, rabbits, chinchillas, guinea pigs, and degus but U shaped in rats and mice. The tympanic membrane is thin, oval to circular in shape, and 2 to 9 mm in diameter, depending on species (eg, tympanic diameter in the chinchilla is 8.32–8.53 mm and in the rat 2.2–2.4 mm).[10]
- The external aspect of the tympanic membrane is concave because of traction on the medial surface by the manubrium of the malleus. The outline of the manubrium of the malleus is usually visible through the tympanic membrane as the

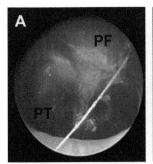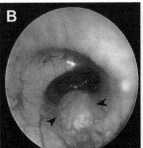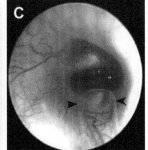

Fig. 13. (*A*) Tympanic membrane in rabbits is elliptical and is divided in 2 indistinctive portions—pars tensa (PT) and pars flaccida (PF). (*B*) Pars flaccida can significantly distend (*arrowheads*) and then (*C*) collapse (*arrowheads*) with breathing forming a large bubble.

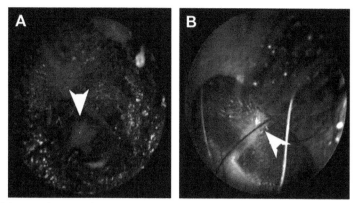

Fig. 14. (*A*) Normal external ear canal (*arrowhead*) and (*B*) tympanic membrane in a guinea pig (*arrowhead* indicates insertion of malleus). Tympanic membrane in guinea pigs lacks the pars flaccida.

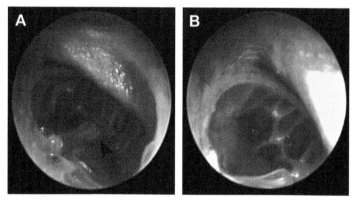

Fig. 15. (*A, B*) Tympanic membrane in the degus is transparent (*arrowhead* indicates insertion of malleus). Middle ear cavity in the degus has unique structure and is compartmentalized in several saclike structures. Care must be taken to not perforate transparent tympanic membrane.

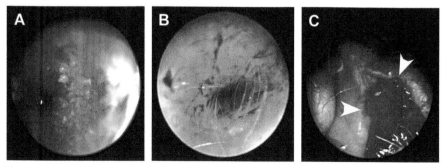

Fig. 16. Yeast otitis externa in a ferret (*A*) before and (*B*) after treatment. (*C*) Proliferative mass (*arrowheads*) is present in the external ear canal of a ferret. Biopsy found squamous carcinoma.

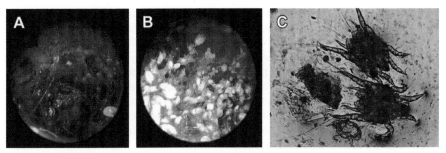

Fig. 17. (A) Parasitic otitis externa in a ferret with (B) detailed view. (C) Ear cytology showed the presence of the ear mites (*Otodectes cynotis*).

stria mallearis. Opposite to the distal end of the manubrium, the depressed point on the external surface of the tympanic membrane is called the *umbo membrane tympani*.[2]

- The tympanic membrane is divided into 2 distinguishable portions, the pars flaccida and pars tensa. The pars flaccida, if present, is located dorsally and pars tensa ventrally. The pars flaccida is more opaque and has richer vascular supply than the pars tensa and, therefore, heals more rapidly when injured.[10]

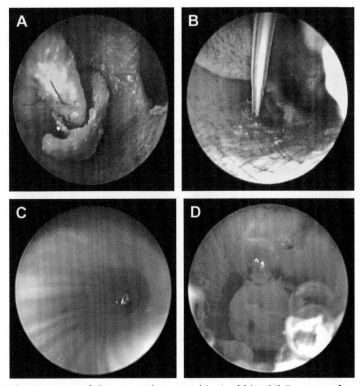

Fig. 18. Video otoscopy of the external ear canal in 4 rabbits. (A) Presence of a ceruminal plug close to the tragus. (B) Insertion of the irrigation cannula into the blind ear sac—cannula reinsertion is necessary. (C) Stenosis of the ear canal is the indication for radiography or computed tomography examination. (D) Bruising of the mucosal surface should be avoided, as it is painful, and part of the mucosa could interfere with the visual field of the endoscope.

- The pars tensa in ferrets, rabbits, and guinea pigs is slightly opaque and transparent in chinchillas, degus, rats, gerbils and mice (see **Figs. 9** and **15**). The pars tensa is composed of 4 main layers. The 2 middle layers, unique to mammals, consist of circumferentially oriented and radially oriented collagen fibers, both contributing to the mechanical stiffness of the tympanum. The other layers consist largely of relatively flexible epidermal and mucosal.[11]
- Ferrets have small pars flaccida and larger pars tensa.
- Rabbits (see **Fig. 13**), rats, mice, and gerbils have a large pars flaccida, which can significantly distend with breathing, forming a large bubble, which may occupy almost all the pars tensa.[10,12]
- Guinea pigs only have a pars tensa and a dorsal bony segment called the *supratympanic crest* (see **Fig. 14**).

EAR DISEASES

Ear disease is a common reason for presentation to the veterinarian. Examples of other pathologic changes are depicted in **Figs. 16–18**.

Chronic sneezing in rats, guinea pigs, and rabbits could also be one of the presenting signs of otitis media. Otitis media is often subclinical, especially in chinchillas and guinea pigs.[6,7]

FUTURE CONSIDERATIONS

Future considerations comprise the use of high-definition equipment, which will increase the detail and improve photo and video documentation.

SUMMARY

Ear disease is a frequent complaint of exotic companion mammals presented to the veterinarian. Video otoscopy facilitates accurate diagnosis of diseases affecting the external ear canal or middle ear. It is relatively easy to learn and apply in clinical practice. The tip of the telescope should always be advanced within the center of the canal, as any mucosal bruising or bleeding can hinder evaluation. Therapeutic video endoscopy facilitates foreign body removal, external ear canal flushing, intralesional drug administration, myringotomy, and middle ear cavity flushing. Resulting images and video are useful for clients and student education and for clinical case consultation and posttreatment evaluations.

REFERENCES

1. Paterson S. Skin diseases of exotic pets. Hoboken (NJ): Blackwell Science; 2007.
2. Gotthelf LN, editor. Small animal ear diseases: an illustrated guide. 2nd edition. St Louis (MO): Elsevier Saunders; 2005. p. 434.
3. Divers SJ. Exotic mammal diagnostic and surgical endoscopy. In: Quesenberry KE, Carpenter JW, editors. Ferrets, rabbits and rodents. Clinical medicine and surgery. 3rd edition. St Louis (MO): Elsevier Saunders; 2012. p. 485–501.
4. Jeklova E, Jekl V, Kovarcik K, et al. Usefulness of detection of specific IgM and IgG antibodies for diagnosis of clinical encephalitozoonosis in pet rabbits. Vet Parasitol 2010;28:143–8.
5. Rosychuk RA. Video-otoscopy. In: McCarthy TC, editor. Veterinary endoscopy for the small animal practitioner. St Louis (MO): Elsevier Saunders; 2005. p. 387–411.

6. Mans C, Donnelly TM. Update on diseases of chinchillas. Vet Clin North Am Exot Anim Pract 2013;16(2):383–406.

7. Wagner JE, Owens DR, Kusewitt DF, et al. Otitis media of guinea pigs. Lab Anim Sci 1976;26(6 Pt 1):902–7.

8. Chitty J, Raftery A. Ear and sinus surgery. In: Harcourt-Brown FM, Chitty J, editors. BSAVA manual of rabbit imaging, surgery and dentistry. Gloucester (United Kingdom): BSAVA; 2013. p. 212–32.

9. Capello V. Lateral ear canal resection and ablation in pet rabbits. Proceedings of the North American Veterinary Conference. 2006. Available at: http://www.ivis.org. Accessed October 3, 2015.

10. Puria S, Fay RR, Popper AN, editors. The middle ear: science, otosurgery, and technology. Springer handbook of auditory research, vol. 46. Heidelberg (Germany): Springer-Verlag GmbH; 2013.

11. Wang AY, Shen Y, Wang JT, et al. Animal models of chronic tympanic membrane perforation: "A 'time-out' to review evidence and standardize design". Int J Pediatr Otorhinolaryngol 2014;78:2048–55.

12. Castagno LA, Lavinsky L. Tympanic membrane healing in myringostomies performed with argon laser or microknife: an experimental study in rats. Rev Bras Otorrinolaringol 2006;72(6):794–9.

Endoscopy and Endosurgery in Nonhuman Primates

Norin Chai, DVM, MSc, PhD

KEYWORDS

- Nonhuman primate • Endoscopy • Diagnosis • Minimally invasive surgery
- Salpingectomy

KEY POINTS

- Endoscopy in nonhuman primates is of great value for the diagnostic process, minimally invasive surgery, and research applications.
- Knowledge of the specific anatomy, physiology, anesthesiology, and management are mandatory before performing endoscopy in nonhuman primates.
- Valuable information may be gained from the human endoscopy literature.
- Endoscopy is a tool that often provides a definitive diagnosis.
- Endosurgery is the obvious choice for nonhuman primates because self-mutilation of surgical wounds is common.

INTRODUCTION

The most recent compilation by the International Union for Conservation of Nature/Species Survival Commission Primates Specialist Group recognizes 16 families, 77 genera, 479 species, and 681 taxa of nonhuman primates (NHPs).[1] NHPs can be divided in prosimians, monkeys, and apes, with most being monkeys (70%). Great apes account for only 2% of all taxa, even though they are the most commonly known by the general public.[1] Laparoscopy in NHPs was first described in the 1970s.[2] Minimally invasive surgery has resulted in improvements in research and clinical care. As in human surgery, endoscopy will have an expanding role in the future.[2–4] The endoscopic indications and procedures performed in nonhuman primates are similar to those in humans.

The author has nothing to disclose.
Ménagerie du Jardin des Plantes, Muséum national d'Histoire naturelle, 57 Rue Cuvier, Paris 75005, France
E-mail address: chai@mnhn.fr

Vet Clin Exot Anim 18 (2015) 447–461
http://dx.doi.org/10.1016/j.cvex.2015.04.004
1094-9194/15/$ – see front matter © 2015 Elsevier Inc. All rights reserved.

The approach is also similar to that used for dogs and cats, and much can be learned and applied from the domestic animal and the human literature. Limitations are related to equipment availability and surgeon training. This article presents selected endoscopic procedures that are frequently performed in NHPs, including rhinoscopy, tracheobronchoscopy, gastrointestinal endoscopy, laparoscopy, and endoscopic salpingectomy.

Indication/Contraindication

The most common indications and contraindications for the selected endoscopy procedures performed in NHP are listed in **Table 1**.

EQUIPMENT

Given the diversity in patient size and the variety of endoscopy procedures, different scopes and instruments may be required. Basic endoscopy equipment necessary for the performance of the selected procedures discussed here in NHP between 500 g and 250 kg consist of:

- A 2.7-mm diameter, 18-cm length, 30° angle oblique rigid telescope with a 4.8-mm operating sheath
- Endovideo camera and monitor

Table 1
Most common indications and contraindications for the selected endoscopy procedures performed in nonhuman primates

Procedure	Principal Indications	Contraindications
Rhinoscopy	Sneezing; nasal discharge; epistaxis; and sampling tissues for cytology, histology, and culture Minimally invasive surgery (see **Fig. 2**)	Clotting disorders
Tracheobronchoscopy	Acute or chronic cough that is unanticipated or unresponsive to standard medical therapy, unexplained radiographic infiltrates, tissue sampling, bronchoalveolar lavage	The procedure should not be performed in patients that are not candidates for general anesthesia and unless oxygenation can be maintained
Gastrointestinal endoscopy (esophagus, stomach, duodenum, and large intestine)	Weight loss, vomiting, diarrhea, intestinal bleeding, unexplained anemia, anorexia, sialorrhea, melena, foreign body removal	Complete intestinal obstruction; in that case, traditional laparotomy is preferred
Laparoscopy	Abnormal results from laboratory work or abnormalities diagnosed on imaging (abdominal radiographs and ultrasonography)	The main contraindications are obesity and pregnancy
Endoscopic salpingectomy	Elective sterilization	Pregnancy, large reproductive mass

- Xenon light source and light cable
- Flexible biopsy and alligator grasping forceps, 1.7-mm diameter
- Flexible bronchofiberscope, 5.2-mm or 3.7-mm diameter, 85-cm length, or 54-cm length, respectively (for respiratory endoscopy)
- Flexible 9.8-mm diameter endoscope, 140-cm length, with a 2.2-mm instrument channel and 4-way tip deflection capability (for gastroscopy)

For laparoscopy and reproductive endosurgery, additional equipment items are:

- Veress needle
- Carbon dioxide (CO_2) insufflator, silicone tubing, and medical grade CO_2
- Electrical surgical unit (eg, electrocautery, radiosurgery)
- Set of 3 trocars: threaded (or sharp) cannulas (3.5-mm diameter, 5-cm length)
- Kelly grasping forceps (3-mm diameter, 20-cm length, curved)
- Endoscopic Metzenbaum scissors, 3 mm, with serrated, curved blades, blunted tips, double-action jaws
- Endoscopic bipolar coagulating forceps, 3-mm

The 2.7-mm diameter and 18-mm long telescope with a 30° offset viewing angle allows exploration of body cavities by simply rotating the scope around its longitudinal axis. Although a 30° offset viewing angle scope can be used, for reproductive minimally invasive surgery, a 0° offset viewing angle scope may be preferred by some clinicians.

Flexible endoscopes are available in diameters ranging from 1 mm to 14 mm. Most flexible scopes greater than 2 mm in diameter have an accessory channel and a deflectable tip. Endoscopic instruments (eg, biopsy forceps) can be used through the working channel. The practitioner must ensure before use that the instruments have a sufficient length to reach the end of the flexible scope. The insufflator delivers medical CO_2 into the abdomen of the patient, to create a working space and maintain a steady intra-abdominal pressure (eg, about 12 mm Hg for an adult female *Macaca fascicularis* of 6–8 kg body weight).

PATIENT PREPARATION

The usual preoperative examination of the patient is mandatory to evaluate the anesthetic risks, although this is often restricted to a visual appraisal for many species. Starving should be in accordance with body size and feeding habits. The amount of time necessary to withhold food before anesthesia varies by species and ranges from 3 to 4 hours in the ruffed lemur (*Varecia variegata*), a frugivorous species, to up to 24 hours in eastern lesser bamboo lemurs (*Hapalemur griseus*) and Coquerel's sifaka (*Propithecus verreauxi coquereli*), species that are highly folivorous. Great apes should be starved (including water) for 12 hours before anesthesia.

Anesthesia

Most anesthetic induction agents are given via intramuscular injection (hand or remote dart). In general, ketamine in combination with (dex)medetomidine is typically used, with dose rates varying between species. Small species like marmosets or juvenile Old World monkeys can be masked down or put directly in an induction chamber with the inhalation agent. After induction, all animals should be intubated with cuffed (if possible) endotracheal tubes. General anesthesia maintenance may be provided either by gas anesthesia or injectable anesthesia (by repeated injections or continuous infusion). For bronchoscopy, the animal is extubated for a brief period; long enough to allow the respiratory track examination and then reintubation of the animal.

Human safety precautions should be kept in mind to avoid disease transmission between the endoscopist and NHP, especially when investigating respiratory diseases (eg, use of surgical mask and biofilters for inhalant anesthesia).

Analgesia

Analgesia should be considered in all painful procedures, and meloxicam and buprenorphine are recommended, especially following major surgical procedures. Buprenorphine may provide prolonged relief for up to 8 hours in some NHPs. Both oxymorphone and hydromorphone have also been used postoperatively with good results. Butorphanol is not used in combination with other anesthetics because of commonly seen respiratory depression. However, it can be used alone for short periods.[5]

Monitoring and Positioning

General physical examination is performed after induction of the anesthesia. An intravenous catheter is placed and intravenous fluids are given. The patient's reflexes, temperature, heart rate and rhythm (electrocardiogram), respiratory rate, end-tidal CO_2, oxygen saturation levels, and blood pressure are closely monitored. Positioning of the animal depends on the procedure.

PROCEDURES

Specific anatomic and physiologic features should be reviewed carefully. Anatomic pictures and illustrations can also be helpful during the examination.

Rhinoscopy

Patients are best placed in a seated position, if possible, with adequate restraint equipment (foldable surgery table, ophthalmic mattress). If this is not possible, they can be either in dorsal, lateral, or sternal recumbency (**Fig. 1**). The use of a cuffed endotracheal tube is paramount and the cuff should be rechecked before any flushing. The oropharynx is packed with moistened gauze. Care must be taken not to impede the movement of fluid from the nasopharynx into the mouth, in order to prevent aspiration. This prevents any potential contamination of the gastrointestinal tract from the upper respiratory tract and adds another precaution against false swallowing.

Before passing the scope, the patient's nose is anesthetized with a topical anesthetic (the author uses oxymetazoline-soaked gauze, followed by lidocaine spray). The nasal cavities are then flushed using warm sterile saline to remove any debris and excess mucus. A rigid telescope is used for the procedure. If possible, an operating sheath should be used to enable intraoperative flushing to maintain visualization.

The scope is passed gently along the floor of the nasal cavity and into the nasopharynx to examine the inferior meatus and the inferior turbinates (**Fig. 2**). As the endoscope is advanced caudally, surfaces are closely examined for abnormalities, including inflammation, ulcers, plaques, foreign bodies, and masses. Nasal secretions and blood may be removed by flushing the nose with sterile saline to improve visualization. Medication can also be injected directly into nasal cavity or sinus for treatment of fungal infections.

Bronchoscopy

Patients are seated or placed in dorsal recumbency. The tongue is gently extended. The endoscope is inserted into the larynx, past the vocalis muscle, and into the

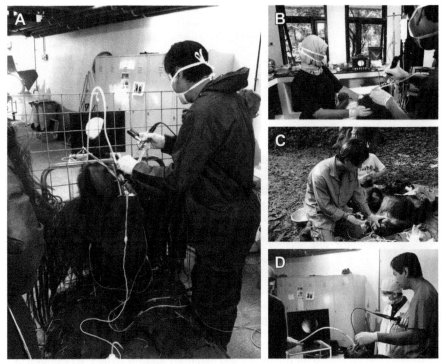

Fig. 1. Rhinoscopy in apes. (*A*) Position of an orangutan (*Pongo pygmaeus*) in a seated position for rhinoscopy. (*B*) Performing rhinoscopy in an orangutan in dorsal recumbency. (*C*, *D*) Performing rhinoscopy in chimpanzees (*Pan troglodytes*) in field conditions and in a zoo. (*Courtesy of* Norin Chai, DVM, MSc, PhD, Paris, France.)

trachea (**Fig. 3**). The scope is then advanced past the primary tracheal bifurcation into the primary bronchus, and further into the upper lobar bronchus (see **Fig. 3**). Patients should always be given 100% oxygen for 10 to 15 minutes before tracheobronchoscopy and again for 10 to 15 minutes after the procedure. Because the animal is not supplied with oxygen while processing the bronchoscopy, the procedure should not exceed 2 to 3 minutes.

For bronchoalveolar lavage, warm saline is pushed through the operating channel by use of a syringe. The volume depends on the size of the animal (and the length of the bronchoscope), but 10 mL have been showed to be sufficient to perform total and differential cell analysis in normal rhesus (*Macaca mulatta*).[6] The lavage fluid is visualized through the camera, and immediately suctioned and placed into a sterile collection cup for cytologic examination and bacterial/fungal cultures. After examination and sampling, the bronchoscope is carefully removed. Lung auscultation is performed to check for crackles or any indication of liquid.

Endoscopy of the Upper Digestive System

Animals are placed into dorsal or left lateral recumbency. A bite guard (dog or cat mouth gag, hard plastic tube) is placed to prevent damage to the endoscope (**Fig. 4**). Lubrication facilitates are introduction into the esophagus. For a better visualization, air insufflation is preferred. Once past the lower esophageal sphincter, the stomach is slightly inflated. The tip of the endoscope is slid along the greater curvature

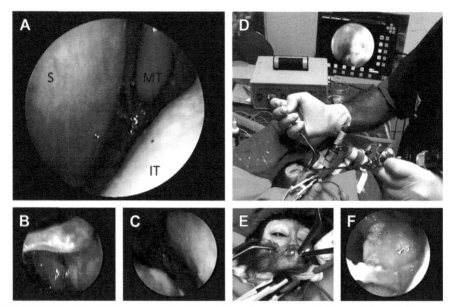

Fig. 2. Performing rhinoscopy and minimally invasive surgery. (*A*) Normal view of the anterior third of the left nasal cavity in a gorilla (*Gorilla gorilla*). Nasal septum (S), inferior turbinate (IT), and middle turbinate (MT). (*B*) Advanced allergic sinusitis with secondary infection in an orangutan. (*C*) The same orangutan after treatment. (*D*) Position of a sooty mangabey (*Cercocebus atys lunulatus*) for rhinoscopy and minimally invasive surgery. (*E*) Removal of a hamartoma in a sooty mangabey. (*F*) A hamartoma on rhinoscopy in a sooty mangabey. (*Courtesy of* Norin Chai, DVM, MSc, PhD, Paris, France.)

wall. At this point, the endoscope tip can be deflected fully in the upward direction to observe the gastric fundus (**Fig. 5**). Still along the greater curvature, the endoscope is eventually advanced into the antrum until the pylorus is seen.[7] If the gastric wall is too stretched, finding the pylorus may prove difficult.

The stomach can stretch to accommodate and respond to the presence and the movement of the endoscope and air insufflation. The greater curvature may then be displaced caudally in the abdomen.[8] In such cases, it is advisable to retract the endoscope, decrease the stomach volume by aspirating the air, and rotate the patient to alter the approach angle to the antrum.[8]

Colonoscopy

Colonoscopy is the endoscopic examination of the large intestine and the distal part of the small intestine. Before the colonoscopy, enema is gently performed with warm saline in order to trigger the evacuation of stool. The animal is placed in dorsal, sternal, or left lateral recumbency (see **Fig. 4**B). The scope is lubricated and inserted 8 to 25 cm (depending on the animal's size) proximally through the rectum and into the colon. In apes, a 13.3-mm diameter, 168-cm length fiberscope may be inserted approximately 100 cm to reach the cecocolic junction. For callithricids, the author uses a flexible bronchofiberscope of 3.7-mm diameter, 54-cm length, with a working channel of 1.2 mm. The use of a pediatric bronchoscope with a 4.8-mm diameter has been described.[9] Spontaneous colitis is a major cause of poor welfare and premature death of callitrichids.[9] Regular examination of the colon is advised. However, endoscopic

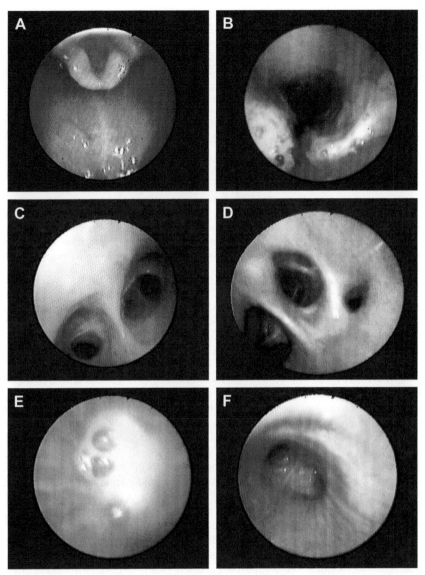

Fig. 3. Tracheobronchoscopy in nonhuman primates. (A) Entry of the glottis in a gray-cheeked mangabey (*Lophocebus albigena*). (B) Tracheitis in an orangutan (*P pygmaeus*). (C) Normal view of the bronchi in an orangutan. (D) Normal view of the secondary lobar bifurcation of the bronchi in an orangutan. (E) Presence of pus in the bronchi in an orangutan. (F) Same bronchi after aspiration of the pus for culture. (*Courtesy of* Norin Chai, DVM, MSc, PhD, Paris, France.)

evaluation has to be gentle, because iatrogenic complications such as perforation of the colon may occur.

Laparoscopy

Patients are surgically prepared and placed in dorsal recumbency for laparoscopy (**Fig. 6**). Following aseptic preparation, a 3-mm skin incision is made on the midline,

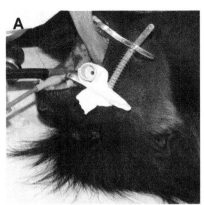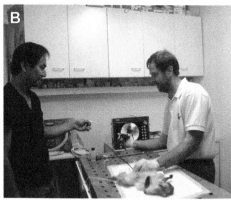

Fig. 4. Positioning of primates for endoscopy of the digestive system. (*A*) A gray-cheeked mangabey (*L albigena*) intubated and placed on dorsal recumbency with a mouth gag ready for upper gastrointestinal endoscopy. (*B*) Colonoscopy in a golden-headed lion tamarin (*Leontopithecus chrysomelas*). The animal is placed in dorsal recumbency. (*Courtesy of* Norin Chai, DVM, MSc, PhD, Paris, France.)

just caudal to the umbilicus. A Veress needle is then inserted through the linea alba. Care is taken to avoid puncturing underlying organs or blood vessels by lifting the body wall before insertion of the needle. Once the Veress needle is in place, CO_2 is insufflated into the peritoneal cavity at a rate of 4 L/min to a pressure of 10 to 12 mm Hg. The pneumoperitoneum is maintained by a constant gas flow of 200 mL/min (see **Fig. 6**). The Veress needle is removed, and a trocar for the telescope is inserted through the same opening. A characteristic sound is heard, indicating that the abdominal cavity has been reached. Another option for initial insufflation, also preferred by the author, is the Hansson technique. Instead of the Veress needle, the surgeon can place the first cannula through a minilaparotomy. A 1-cm to 2-cm skin incision is made on the midline just caudal to the umbilicus. The subcutaneous tissues are smoothly dissected and the linea alba and the body wall incised before placing the cannula. A mattress suture secures the cannula and maintains the necessary seal.[10]

The 2.7-mm telescope, housed within its protection sheath, is then inserted through the cannula until the abdominal cavity and organs are visible on the video monitor. The laparoscopic examination can then be performed. Laparoscopy allows direct examination of the peritoneal cavity and organs (including sample collection) as well as endosurgical techniques. In the author experience, nearly all parenchymatous organs can be biopsied, similarly to traditional laparotomy (**Fig. 7**).

Endoscopic Salpingectomy

Endoscopic salpingectomy of female crab-eating macaques (*M fascicularis*) is described here. Before endosurgery, abdominal ultrasonography to evaluate the reproductive tract should be undertaken. In several cases, endoscopic salpingectomy is contraindicated because of pregnancy, endometrial disorder (hyperplasia, endometritis, neoplasia), or gross obesity. In those cases a traditional surgical approach is typically preferred. The decision to operate or not depends on the experience of the surgeon.

With the animal in dorsal recumbency, the pelvis is slightly elevated so that the abdominal organs are positioned cranially (reverse Trendelenburg position). This

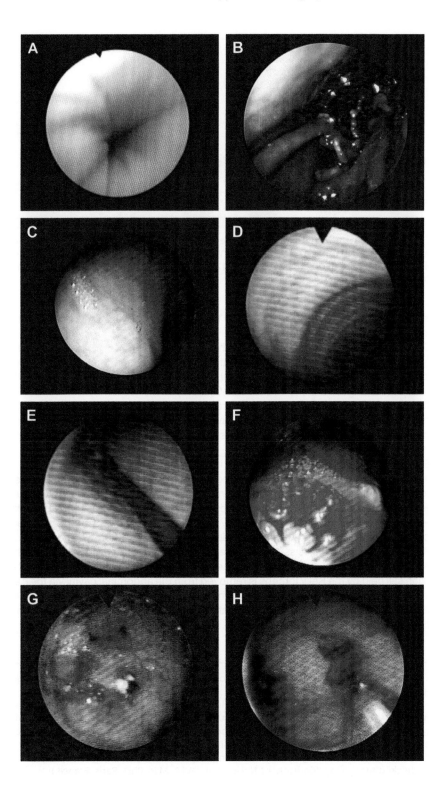

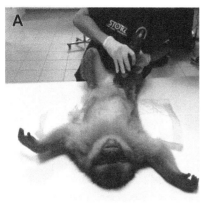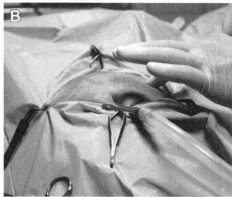

Fig. 6. Laparoscopy in a crab-eating macaque (*M fascicularis*). (*A*) Patients are extensively shaved, and placed in dorsal recumbency. (*B*) With the Veress needle in place, the abdominal cavity is insufflated with CO_2 to a pressure of 12 mm Hg. (*Courtesy of* Norin Chai, DVM, MSc, PhD, Paris, France.)

position helps to expose the reproductive tract. The screen is located caudal to the animal (**Fig. 8**).

Once pneumoperitoneum has been achieved, typically at 10 to 12 mm Hg, the 2.7-mm telescope with a protection sheath is inserted through the 3.5-mm cannula placed just caudal to the umbilicus. The abdominal cavity is then evaluated and the uterus, the salpinges, and the ovaries identified.

The second cannula is placed under direct telescope visualization and guided by transillumination of the body wall, thereby avoiding large vessels. The 3.5-mm cannula and trocar are inserted through a 2-mm skin incision (see **Fig. 8**). A third trocar is placed in the same manner (see **Fig. 8**).

Short, curved Kelly forceps (3-mm) are inserted through the cannula and used to locate and isolate the salpinx by gently lifting the uterus. The salpinx appears as a delicate thin pink structure. Bipolar forceps (3-mm) are inserted through the third cannula. The fallopian tube held with the Kelly forceps is then cauterized at both ends using the bipolar forceps until the tissue turns white, indicating that the blood supply has been occluded (**Fig. 9**). After cauterization, the bipolar forceps are withdrawn and the 3-mm Metzenbaum endoscopic scissors is inserted to dissect the cauterized tissue. Only the tips of the scissors are used so that the resection is carefully monitored. The resected section still held by the Kelly forceps is removed from the abdominal cavity via the cannula. The contralateral fallopian tube is removed using the same technique. The surgical sites are observed to ensure adequate hemostasis. The pneumoperitoneum is deflated before removing the cannulas.[10]

Fig. 5. Esophagostomy and gastroscopy in nonhuman primates. (*A*) Normal air-distended esophagus of a gray-cheeked mangabey (*L albigena*). (*B*) Severe, acute esophagitis in an orangutan (*P pygmaeus*) with gastric reflux caused by the insufficiency of the lower esophageal sphincter. (*C*) Normal stomach mucosa at the proximal greater curvature of a gray-cheeked mangabey. (*D, E*) The endoscope tip has been deflected fully in the upward direction, cranially to observe the gastric fundus. (*F, G*) Chronic, bacterial, hemorrhagic, and ulcerative gastritis in a gray-cheeked mangabey. (*H*) Biopsy of the gastric mucosa of a gray-cheeked mangabey. (*Courtesy of* Norin Chai, DVM, MSc, PhD, Paris, France.)

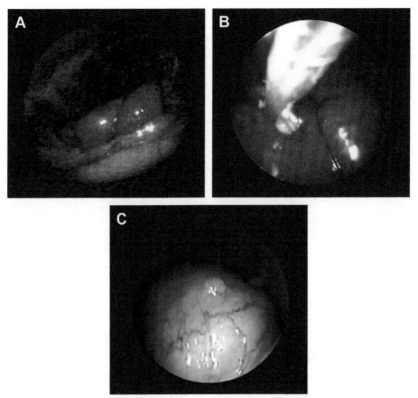

Fig. 7. Laparoscopy in nonhuman primates. (*A, B*) Hepatomegaly and biopsy of the liver in a macaque (*Macaca sylvanus*). (*C*) Hypertrophy of the cervix in a Diana monkey (*Cercopithecus diana*) that presented with chronic hypermenorrhea, acute lower abdominal pain, and episodes of diarrhea. Chronic endometritis was diagnosed on histology. (*Courtesy of* Norin Chai, DVM, MSc, PhD, Paris, France.)

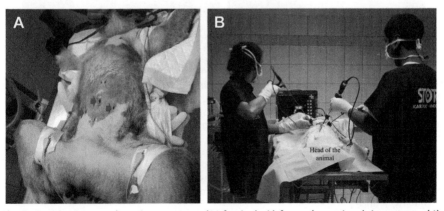

Fig. 8. Positioning a crab-eating macaque (*M fascicularis*) for endoscopic salpingectomy. (*A*) Animal in dorsal recumbency, with the pelvis slightly elevated to displace the abdominal organs cranially (reverse Trendelenburg). Red arrows show the entry sites of 3 cannulas. (*B*) The head of the animal is toward the camera. (*Courtesy of* Norin Chai, DVM, MSc, PhD, Paris, France.)

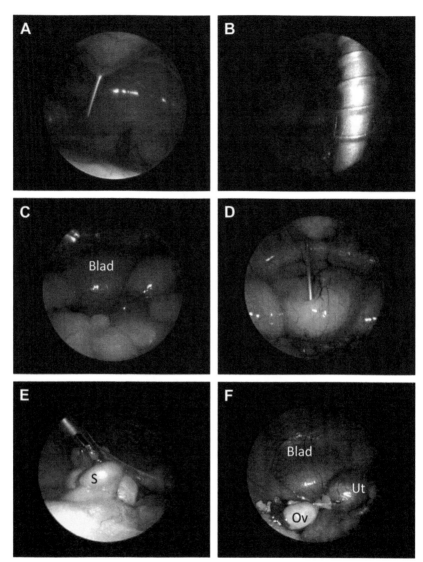

Fig. 9. Endoscopic salpingectomy in a crab-eating macaque (*M fascicularis*). (*A* and *B*) Placement of the secondary cannulas via direct visualization. (*C*) Examination of the abdominal cavity. (*D*) Cystocentesis via direct visualization. (*E, F*) The short curved Kelly forceps are used to locate the salpinx (S) and to gently lift the uterus (Ut) for a more close and complete examination of the ovary (Ov). (*G*) The salpinx is grasped with the Kelly forceps. (*H*) The salpinx is cauterized with bipolar forceps. (*I*) Only the tips of the scissors are used to gently dissect the salpinx. (*J*) The peritoneum at the portal site after removing the trocar. The clinician must ensure that the mesentery is not pulled into the subcutaneous space while the trocar is taken out. Blad, bladder. (*Courtesy of* Norin Chai, DVM, MSc, PhD, Paris, France.)

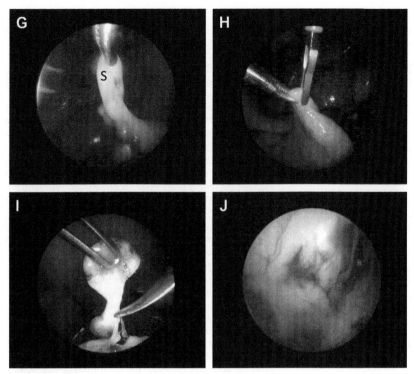

Fig. 9. (*continued*)

Care is taken to ensure that the mesentery is not pulled into the subcutaneous space as the cannula is removed from the portal site (see **Fig. 9**). Only the skin layer is closed, using a single absorbable suture.

BENEFITS OF ENDOSCOPY

The benefits of endoscopic investigations are similar to those described for domestic species and humans, and include the minimally invasive approach reducing trauma, postoperative pain, and recovery time. Thus, endosurgery is an obvious choice for primates because self-mutilation of a standard laparotomy wound is common.

Concerning the described salpingectomy procedure, a study concluded that endoscopic salpingectomy was a more suitable surgical choice for macaque sterilization, compared with endoscopic ovariectomy, because of the lower incidences of hemorrhage and inflammation of the severed ends of the fallopian tubes and the associated reproductive organs, and shorter surgical times associated with salpingectomy.[11] Furthermore, although reversal of sterilization with ovariectomy is impossible, laparoscopic tubal sterilization reversal/recanalization is theoretically possible in NHP, as it is in humans.[12]

COMPLICATIONS AND POTENTIAL ADVERSE OUTCOMES

It is essential to remain mindful that the endoscope itself may cause trauma to the mucosa of the organs, potentially resulting in misdiagnosis. The most common complications and potential adverse outcomes for selected endoscopy procedures performed in NHPs are discussed in **Table 2**.

Table 2
Most common complications for the selected endoscopy procedures performed in nonhuman primates

Procedure	Complications and Potential Adverse Outcome
Rhinoscopy	Rhinoscopy is generally considered a safe procedure. In addition to risks or limitations of endoscopy in general, the most common finding is that bleeding may persist for a short period after the procedure, but it is generally inconsequential. In the rare event of severe, persistent bleeding, dilute epinephrine instilled into the nose can help arrest bleeding
Tracheobronchoscopy	Hypoxemia may develop if the procedure is too long (probably more than 2–3 min); 100% oxygen can be delivered at 1–2 L/m through the biopsy channel of the endoscope. Alternatively, oxygen flow may be delivered through a separate tube (cat or dog urinary catheters) passed alongside the endoscope
Gastrointestinal endoscopy	The main risks are perforation, or a tear of the gastrointestinal mucosa. Care must be taken not to overdistend the stomach with insufflation, which may result in significant cardiopulmonary compromise
Laparoscopy	Insufflation creates a positive pressure within the abdominal cavity, which can result in cardiac arrhythmias, including tachycardia with decreased cardiac output caused by lower body venous return. Bradycardia with direct sympathetic stimulation from peritoneal stretching may also occur. Abdominal insufflation displaces the diaphragm and reduces lung volume, leading to a reduction in oxygenation and potential acid-base balance.[2] The absorption of insufflation CO_2 can result in hypercarbia and acidemia. However, CO_2 is rapidly absorbed and excreted by the body and therefore is much less likely to cause gas embolism
Endoscopic salpingectomy	Postoperative complications of endoscopic salpingectomy in Formosan macaques (*Macaca cyclopis*) have been documented.[13] Major complications included difficult entry into the abdominal cavity using the Veress needle, intraoperative hemorrhage, and inadvertent cauterization of uterus. Bleeding from the omentum as a result of Veress needle or trocar trauma has also been reported[13]

Postoperative Care

In most diagnostic procedures postoperative care and treatment depend on results of the diagnostic tests. The need for analgesia and antiinflammatory treatments should be evaluated individually, but these are often required. The aim is to return the animal to its enclosure as soon as possible. In case of laparoscopy and minimally invasive surgery, postoperative analgesia is paramount. Antimicrobial therapy should be used only when sterility is compromised or based on culture and sensitivity.

CONTROVERSIES/FUTURE CONSIDERATIONS

Because noninvasive techniques are particularly suitable in NHPs, endoscopy should be encouraged for most veterinarians working with NHPs. This goal can only be accomplished with the collaboration of small animal practitioners, zoo and wildlife veterinarians, and human surgeons.

SUMMARY

Endoscopy in NHPs is of great value for disease diagnosis, minimally invasive surgery, and research studies. Primate-specific anesthesiology, case management, and surgical anatomy are important prerequisites before performing any endoscopic procedure. Knowledge may be gained from the human literature. Endoscopy is generally used in conjunction with other investigations, but often facilitates definitive diagnosis through biopsy. For NHPs, endosurgery is an obvious choice because self-mutilation of laparotomy wounds is common.

ACKNOWLEDGMENTS

We thank our friends and colleagues Aude Bourgeois and Muriel Kohl DVM from the Ménagerie du Jardin des Plantes, Leonor Camacho Sillero DVM in Spain, Thierry Petit DVM from the Palmyre Zoo, Rui Bernadino DVM from Lisbon Zoo, and Sarah Ouard DVM from the Refuge de l'Arche for their time in sharing experience and unforgettable endoscopic time. Many thanks also to Karl Storz France for their assistance.

REFERENCES

1. Mittermeier RA, Rylands AB, Wilson DE. Handbook of the mammals of the world. Vol. 3. Primates. Barcelona (Spain): Lynx Edicions; 2013.
2. Fanton JW. Rigid endoscopy. In: Wolfe-Coote S, editor. The laboratory primate. London: Elsevier; 2005. p. 316–47.
3. Dukelow WR. The morphology of follicular development and ovulation in nonhuman primates. J Reprod Fertil Suppl 1975;22:23–51.
4. Nigi H. Laparoscopic observations of ovaries before and after ovulation in the Japanese monkey (*Macaca fuscata*). Primates 1977;18:243–59.
5. Unwin S. Anaesthesia. In: Wolfe-Coote S, editor. The laboratory primate. London: Elsevier; 2005. p. 275–315.
6. Tate MK, Rico PJ, Roy CJ. Comparative study of lung cytologic features in normal rhesus (*Macaca mulatta*), cynomolgus (*Macaca fascicularis*), and African green (*Chlorocebus aethiops*) non-human primates by use of bronchoscopy. Comp Med 2004;54:393–6.
7. Authier S, Chaurand F, Legaspi M, et al. Comparison of three anesthetic protocols for intraduodenal drug administration using endoscopy in rhesus monkeys (*Macaca mulatta*). J Am Assoc Lab Anim Sci 2006;45(6):73–9.
8. Tams TR. Gastroscopy. In: Tams TR, Rawlings CA, editors. Small animal endoscopy. 3rd edition. St Louis (MO): Elsevier; 2011. p. 97–171.
9. Clapp NK, Mc Arthur AH, Carson RL. Visualisation and biopsy of the colon in tamarins and marmosets by endoscopy. Lab Anim Sci 1987;37:217–9.
10. Chai N, Wedlarski R, Rigoulet J. Endométrite chez un cercopithèque Roloway (*Cercopithecus diana roloway*). Prat Ani Sauv Exotiques 2007;7(1):17–9.
11. Kumar V, Kumar V. Clinical evaluation of laparoscopic sterilization techniques in female rhesus macaques (*Macaca mulatta*). Arch Vet Sci 2012;17:20–6.
12. Yashoda RA. A study on tubal recanalization. J Obstet Gynaecol India 2012;62: 179–83.
13. Yu PH, Weng CC, Kuo HC, et al. Evaluation of endoscopic salpingectomy for sterilization of female Formosan macaques (*Macaca cyclopis*). Am J Primatol 2015; 77(4):359–67.

The Value of Endoscopy in a Wildlife Raptor Service

Marion R. Desmarchelier, DVM, IPSAV, DES, MSc, DACZM[a],*,
Shannon T. Ferrell, DVM, DABVP (Avian), DACZM[b]

KEYWORDS

- Birds of prey • Endoscopy • Raptors • Rehabilitation • Wildlife

KEY POINTS

- Endoscopic equipment can be purchased at lower cost on the used market or donated by human hospitals to nonprofit wildlife centers.
- For many respiratory conditions, endoscopy is the diagnostic and therapeutic modality of choice (eg, debridement of aspergillomas).
- Endoscopy is also useful to diagnose conditions such as esophageal trauma, mycobacteriosis, viral hepatitis, and neoplasia.
- Endoscopy allows for the noninvasive removal of foreign bodies, such as pieces of metal and porcupine quills, as well as cloacoliths.
- Endoscopy equipment is now available for the use in field research and conservation projects.

INTRODUCTION

Endoscopy has been used in raptor medicine for decades.[1,2] It was first developed for the purposes of gender identification and rapidly became a popular diagnostic and therapeutic tool. Endoscopy is now routinely used in most veterinary hospitals that treat falconry birds and other privately owned raptors and it is often recommended as a component of prepurchase examinations.[3,4] Yet, many wildlife rehabilitation centers that handle raptors are not using endoscopy to its maximum potential for a host of reasons.

Primarily, some centers do not have access to the equipment because of financial or space reasons. In addition, endoscopic examinations are sometimes thought to be time consuming and, therefore, inappropriate in the typical busy, hectic schedule of a rehabilitation center. Conversely, radiography is often mistakenly considered to be

The authors have nothing to disclose.
[a] Zoological Medicine Service, Faculté de médecine vétérinaire, Université de Montréal, C.P. 5000, Saint-Hyacinthe, Quebec J2S 7C6, Canada; [b] Granby Zoo, 525, rue Saint-Hubert, Granby, Quebec J2G 5P3, Canada
* Corresponding author.
E-mail address: marion.desmarchelier@umontreal.ca

a sufficient diagnostic test in wild birds, although it rarely provides a definitive diagnosis other than orthopedic injuries. Endoscopy, however, has multiple indications for the diagnosis and treatment of wild raptor conditions. In many cases, the prognosis can be considerably improved when endoscopy is available.

Before detailing the value of the use of endoscopy in a wildlife raptor service, the authors demonstrate how to overcome the most common difficulties encountered by rehabilitation centers in regards to the access to the appropriate equipment. Techniques for patient preparation and positioning are presented, as well as the different approaches used for diagnosis and treatment of various diseases, removal of foreign bodies, and gender identification. In this article, the term raptor or bird of prey refers to any bird belonging to the orders Accipitriformes (including the Cathartidae family [New World Vultures]), Falconiformes, and Strigiformes.[5]

EQUIPMENT ACQUISITION
General Suggestions

The type of equipment required for avian endoscopy has been previously reviewed in detail.[4,6] The following discussion focuses mostly on rigid endoscopy equipment but could also apply to flexible endoscopy. The main limitation in any wildlife rehabilitation setting is the actual procurement and maintenance of endoscopy equipment. Funds are limited, and the actual purchase price of a new standard rigid endoscopy set can be quite substantial. After determining the equipment needs, there are various avenues available to obtain the required items at a reduced cost.

First, the veterinarian should contact local hospitals and ask to speak with the biomedical engineers responsible for the medical equipment maintenance and storage at the facility. These individuals are a great resource for medical equipment advice and possible donations. Many hospitals routinely disperse older, but functional, equipment to charities or to the used medical equipment market with little to no reimbursement to the hospital. A strategic discussion with the chief of the biomedical department, detailing the existing needs, might result in the donation of used endoscopy equipment or other useful medical equipment (eg, anesthetic monitors, portable blood gas analyzers, surgical tables, supplies). An additional avenue is to contact a local endoscopy equipment sale representative. Many times, the representatives have access to used equipment that might be donated to nonprofit facilities or available at a considerably reduced cost.

A clinician with time and interest in researching equipment can also use various Internet sources such as eBay, Craigslist, and federal/state government auction sites (eg, GovSales, GSA Auctions). Used and new medical equipment are available on the referred Web sites through reputable dealers and sources who may offer warranties, inspections, and full refunds. Other times, no such guarantees exist, and detailed, knowledgeable questions are needed to avoid the purchase of an incorrect or broken item. However, these channels have become popular among physicians and veterinarians because of the discounts offered.

Before any acquisition, it is imperative to garner an understanding of the equipment offered, the current prices on new equipment, quality, compatibility, and product support from the various manufacturers. Catalogs that contain such information and are useful to have are available on-line, especially when checking into compatibility issues between the products from different companies. It is uncommon to find a complete endoscopic package on the used market.

Many times, there is reasonable compatibility between the major manufacturers or, at least, the availability of any needed adapter. A potential means to avoid some of these issues is to purchase equipment that is described as universal or comes with adapters. For example, some light sources accommodate a light cable only from the same manufacturer, whereas others have either a rotating turret of adapters for the light cables from the major manufacturers or at least an adjustable diaphragm that accepts any common light cable size, hence becoming a universal light source.

Specific Comments on the Purchase of Used Endoscopic Components

Rigid endoscope
A used endoscope should be immediately functional with no defects in the optics, the frame, or seals. The cost of repairs and inspection by a repair company can equal the cost of a new endoscope. Ideally, the scope should be autoclavable, as seen in the newer models. Some of the older scopes are not autoclavable and require soaking in disinfection solutions such as glutaraldehyde. The scope should have fittings to attach to the brand of light cable being used in the hospital. Some scopes on the used market come with the appropriate adapters already attached over the original fittings. If none are present, the adapters should be ordered through the relevant manufacturer to ensure correct fitment. The approximate cost of a used 2.7-mm rigid endoscope, 30° angle, 18 cm length was $800 to $1500 as of January 2015.

Light cable
The light cable should be free of breaks in the optical fibers. Each fractured filament diminishes the light available for visualization. Attach the cable up to a light source and focus the beam about 4 to 6 in from a piece of white paper on a table. The field should appear bright and homogenous. Dark spots are filament breaks. Consider bypassing any cable with multiple filament breaks. Make sure the cable attaches correctly to the scope and the light source. The approximate cost of a used light cable with no obvious defects was $100 to $300 as of January 2015.

Light source
Many types of older light sources are available now. Incandescent and halogen light sources are the cheapest units, but only halogen should be considered. Ideally, one would purchase a used xenon unit, as the quality of illumination is superior. Used xenon units on the market now are capable of varying the light intensity automatically or manually based on user preference. Again, it is imperative to test the equipment fully, making sure all buttons and electronics respond correctly. It is also important to consider the costs of bulb replacement. Sometimes, one can acquire a junk unit for a small sum and then harvest the bulb for immediate use or as a spare in a current functional light source. New xenon bulbs can cost from $500 to $1000. The approximate cost of a used xenon light source can vary from $500 to $1500 (January 2015).

Endoscopy camera
The current state of camera technology is high definition (HD). However, the system is costly, and all the components must be capable of HD transmission to reap the benefits. The 3-chip camera was the immediate predecessor to HD, and it offers, in many respects, image quality (but not size) similar to that of HD at a fraction of the cost. As human hospitals shift their inventory to HD, completely functional 3-chip cameras are available on the used market.

The camera should come with both the camera console (also called the controller or processor) and an actual camera head with coupler to attach to the rigid endo-scope.[7] For veterinary use, a universal C mount coupler should attach to the scope heads of the 1.9-, 2.7-, and 4-mm rigid scopes being used in most veterinary facilities. It is important to hook the camera up to a rigid scope to check for the C mount functioning and to a video monitor to ensure that the camera processor is operating correctly.

Finally, one should make sure the output video format for the processor is compatible with the monitor. In the United States and Canada, the output video format is analog NTSC (National Television System Committee), whereas in Europe, most of Asia, and Australia, the video format is analog PAL (Phase Alternating Line). The camera processor and video monitor must have the same video format, or the user cannot view the processor's video output. The digital HD format will eventually become the standard as the older equipment is replaced. The approximate cost of a used 3-chip camera with its respective camera controller varies from $600 to 2000 (January 2015).

Monitor

One can use a computer monitor, a television, an HD monitor, or a laptop as long as there is the correct connection from the camera processor to the output viewing device. This is an area of confusion, as there are different types of output signals and associated connectors. Output signals are commonly carried in 1 cable (composite), 3 cables (red-green-blue), or S-video (1 cable with multiple prongs, also known as Separate video or Y/C).[7] Many camera processors offer multiple types of outputs as some of the signal is sent to the light source and to the monitor simultaneously. Adapters can be purchased for the various cables and connectors to aid in the correct attachment of the output signal from the camera processor to the input connector on the monitor.

An alternative, for both visualization and image storage, is to use a laptop with image capture software. The video signal from the camera controller connects to the computer via a video/Universal Serial Bus (USB) cable that comes with the image capture software package. The software allows for real-time visualization of endoscopy, video capture as Audio Video Interleaved (AVI) or Moving Picture Experts Group (MPEG) files, and still images (Joint Photographic Experts Group [JPEG] format). Examples of such software packages are EZCap video and Elgato video capture.

Independent documentation systems are also available from the major manufacturers (eg, Karl Storz AIDA mini system [Karl Storz Veterinary Endoscopy America Inc, Goleta, CA, USA], Richard Wolf Medicap USB 200 [Richard Wolf Medical Instruments, Vernon Hills, IL, USA]), which can record both videos and still images onto an internal hard drive, USB drive, or server. The advantages of these systems are their ease of use, their storage capacity, and the Ethernet and USB connections that allow for easy transfer of patient materials to an individual computer or server. The main disadvantages compared with the aforementioned image capture software on a laptop are the necessity for a monitor and the cost of the systems.

Carts

Many endoscopy carts are available on the used market with or without specific platforms for the monitors. A stand or attachment for the monitor is recommended for safety when moving the cart. In addition, a built-in power strip is a useful item to organize cords and to centralize the power supply. The main drawback of buying any cart, used or new, is paying the freight for shipment. Finding a local medical equipment dealer on the aforementioned Internet sites who accepts local pickups can greatly decrease costs if one can pick up the item with a clinic vehicle. Finally, in the advent that no medical carts are available, a metal automotive tool chest on wheels, a microwave stand, or even a tiered Rubbermaid cart can be made to function as a viable endoscopy cart.

Storage

After the acquisition of the endoscopy equipment, all the components should be protected from damage. The major components listed earlier are best secured on a cart for transport around the clinic. Rigid endoscopes, sheaths, and endoscopy instruments should be stored in rigid plastic cases designed for endoscope storage and/or autoclaving. Rigid plastic composite cases such those made by Pelican are ideal for both storage and transport, as the interior foam can be cut to fit the needs of the equipment. Both types of storage cases can be found used.

Cleaning

Each manufacturer can provide specific information regarding their recommended means of endoscopy equipment cleaning and disinfection.[7] This material should be reviewed to promote the longevity of the equipment. Numerous other sources have reviewed this topic in detail.[8] As a general rule, the equipment should be rinsed or soaked in distilled or deionized water immediately after use to prevent any biological material from becoming adherent. Furthermore, an additional soaking in an enzymatic cleaner is recommended.[8] After rinsing again, any debris can be gently removed with isopropyl alcohol on a cotton gauze or alcohol on a cotton tip applicator for the optics.[7] The equipment can then either be soaked in appropriate concentrations of glutaraldehyde or autoclaved based on the manufacturer's recommendations for disinfection. Endoscopy equipment should not be soaked for longer than 45 minutes in glutaraldehyde solutions to avoid potential damage.[7] For both rigid and flexible endoscopy systems, courses are available from repair companies, the manufacturer, or local veterinary associations that teach hospital staff how to maintain endoscopy equipment. These courses are highly recommended to protect the monetary and time investment in the equipment, to enhance the skills of the employees, and to have functional equipment when needed.

PATIENT SELECTION: INDICATIONS AND CONTRAINDICATIONS

Injured and starving wild birds of prey often need intensive supportive care on arrival.[9] Depending on their presenting condition, they may require days to weeks before being stable enough to undergo anesthesia for endoscopic examination. Exceptions may include the endoscopic removal of a life-threatening foreign body (a rare occurrence in wild raptors) and some cases of aspergillosis that may require urgent debridement or topical treatment via endoscopy.

As many wild raptors are anemic or emaciated, a hematocrit and total solids determination are recommended before the procedure. A manual white blood cell count estimate can be performed in a few minutes with 1 drop of blood and can bring useful information. In case of a profound leukocytosis, a thorough celioscopic examination of both the right and the left sides is indicated to investigate the presence of an aspergilloma.[3] In the authors' center, radiography is also routinely performed on all birds shortly after arrival to evaluate for fractures, gunshots, and masses.

Contraindications to endoscopic examinations in wild raptors are similar to what has been reported in other avian species.[10–12] The most common and concerning contraindication for endoscopy is hemodynamic instability, which would make anesthesia a risky venture.

A second contraindication to endoscopy is the occasional presence of large fat deposits in the coelom of wild birds. Studies have shown that many raptors migrate with fat stores in the range of 4% to 18% to their body weight and that adult females have higher fat stores in the spring (up to more than 15% of their body weight).[13] Obesity is more common in birds that have been kept in captivity for several weeks or months. Even in birds with adequate body condition scores of 3 to 4 of 5 (1 being emaciated, and 5 being obese), internal fat accumulation can be significant in raptors and can impair good visualization during the endoscopic examination. High-fat diet, ad libitum feeding and restricted exercise (eg, after an orthopedic trauma) can contribute to fat accumulation; however, the authors have experienced this problem in birds that were kept on appropriate diets and allowed to exercise in large flight aviaries.

Thirdly, as celioscopy can lead to a fluid leak from the hepatic peritoneal cavity to the air sacs, ascites is another contraindication. Although this condition is rare in birds of prey, it should be ruled out in cases in which coelomic distension is noted.[10]

Finally, endoscopy should be avoided in females during the breeding season because of the risk of causing iatrogenic egg-yolk coelomitis.

Procedure Preparation

The key to a successful procedure is good organization. In rehabilitation centers, volunteers with variable levels of training and medical knowledge might be in charge of the room and equipment preparation. Developing a checklist decreases the amount of time allotted to procedure preparation and ensures that all the appropriate equipment and material are available once the bird is anesthetized.

Patient Preparation

Fasting
Assuming the bird's condition allows for it, a starvation period of 12 to 24 hours is recommended but varies with the size of the bird.[1] In the authors' experience, large birds such as turkey vultures might require a longer starvation period with a thorough aviary cleaning, as they have a tendency to hide food.

Anesthesia
General anesthesia is required and can be performed as previously described.[14,15] Inhalation anesthesia is generally preferred for many reasons, including faster recoveries.[14] Anesthesia protocols routinely used by the authors include mask induction with isoflurane, followed by intubation and manually assisted ventilation (target End-tidalco$_2$ of 35–45 mm Hg).[15] Butorphanol is used for analgesia.

When performing tracheoscopy in small species, inserting the endoscope in the endotracheal tube might not be possible. In these cases, propofol anesthesia can be used or a temporary air sac intubation can be performed (preferred for longer procedures, technique previously described).[9]

Anesthesia monitoring is accomplished using available equipment. The authors routinely use a Doppler ultrasonic blood flow detector placed on the palatine artery, a cloacal thermometer, and a capnograph for anesthetic monitoring. In the authors' experience, electrocardiography and pulse oximetry seem less practical and less reliable than the other previously cited monitoring tools.[16] However, capnography readings are unreliable if there is a leak in the air sacs to the outside environment, which is common during celioscopy and always present when using an air sac cannula.[17]

Appropriate tube diameter and careful manipulation of the head are critical to avoid a postintubation tracheal stenosis.[18] However, this condition seems to be rarely reported in raptors.[18] At the Bird of Prey Clinic, 1 case of tracheal stenosis has occurred in a short-eared owl (*Asio flammeus*) of more than 550 birds anesthetized and intubated for surgery and/or endoscopy (data from the Bird of Prey Clinic database, Dr Guy Fitzgerald, personal communication, 2014).

To prevent hypothermia, the use of a heating blanket, a heat lamp, heating pads, or fluid warmers have been recommended. Heating pads, covered with blue wraps (**Fig. 1**), can be used to maintain the wings in dorsal extension while keeping the bird and the fluid line warm. Sterile transparent plastic drapes placed over the bird during the procedure also help maintain an appropriate body temperature. As medical grade, disposable transparent drapes can be expensive, a cheaper alternative is to purchase plastic oven bags for roasting meat, cut the bags to the desired sizes, and then autoclave them with the rest of the surgical equipment. Fluid therapy is recommended even for short anesthesia procedures. Warm subcutaneous fluids can be administered preoperatively and postoperatively. Alternatively, for longer procedures, intravenous or intraosseous fluids can be given during the procedure. For catheter placement, the authors use the ulnar vein in most species (**Fig. 2**), as well as the medial metatarsal vein in larger species (eagles, vultures). In very small patients or severely dehydrated/hypotensive birds, an intraosseous catheter can be placed in the ulna or in the tibiotarsus.

Although some authors recommend the routine use of antibiotics for celioscopic examinations, preventive antibiotic administration is not recommended.[1,3] There have been no reported cases of bacterial infections related to an endoscopy procedure performed at the Bird of Prey Clinic of the University of Montréal in the past 10 years. Antibiotics should be used rationally in all species, especially in birds that will be released into the wild or are predisposed to fungal infections.

Positioning

Positioning for the different endoscopic approaches has been described in detail elsewhere.[3,10,12,19] Choosing to approach the coelomic cavity cranially to the leg (between the last 2 ribs) (see **Fig. 1**) or caudally to the leg (caudal to the last rib) (see **Fig. 2**) depends on the species, the individual animal, and the veterinarian's preference.[3,10,12,19] Manually ventilating the bird and observing the air sac insufflation can help make the decision as to which approach would be best in a particular case.

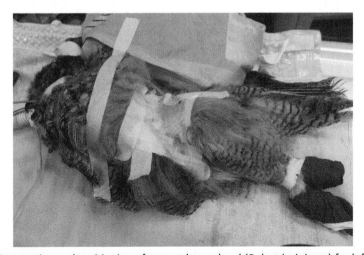

Fig. 1. Preparation and positioning of a great-horned owl (*Bubo virginianus*) for left lateral prefemoral celioscopy. Talons are wrapped to protect the heating pad. Heating bags (covered with blue wrap for protection) are used to keep the bird warm while placing the wings in an extended dorsal position. Masking tape is used to tape the feathers around the surgical site. Doppler ultrasonography, capnography, and an esophageal thermometer are used for anesthesia monitoring.

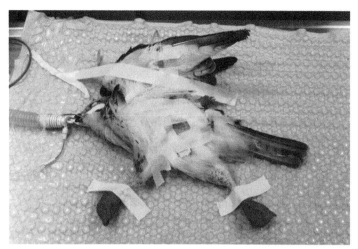

Fig. 2. Positioning of a broad-winged hawk (*Buteo platypterus*) for left lateral postfemoral celioscopy. An intravenous catheter is placed in the left ulnar vein.

In general, the authors find that Falconidae and Accipitrinae celioscopies are best examined through a prefemoral approach, whereas the Buteoninae and Haliaetinae are generally easier to examine through a postfemoral approach. As in other avian species, a midline approach is preferred for hepatic biopsies when ascites is present to prevent fluid leaking into the air sacs and lungs.[20]

The clavicular air sac can be approached between the clavicles (**Fig. 3**) with the bird positioned in dorsal recumbency. Tracheoscopy, otoscopy, upper gastrointestinal endoscopy, and cloacoscopy are performed through the same approaches described in other avian species.[3,10] Proper positioning of the bird can be achieved using masking tape and heating bags (see **Figs. 1** and **2**).

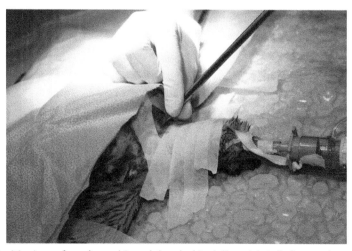

Fig. 3. Positioning of a sharp-shinned hawk (*Accipiter striatus*) for an interclavicular endoscopy.

PROCEDURES AND BENEFITS

Most endoscopic procedures in raptors are similar to what has been previously reported for other avian species.[10–12] Therefore, the authors focus only on a few procedures that are commonly seen in and specific to wild birds of prey.

Diagnosis and Treatment of Respiratory Conditions

Diseases of the respiratory system are common in raptors in rehabilitation settings and can rapidly become life-threatening.[9] An accurate diagnosis often requires endoscopy, as radiographs and even tomodensitometry do not allow for direct visualization of the lesions, precise biopsy procurement, or focal treatment (eg, granuloma debridement and topical antifungal therapy).[21] Endoscopy can be the diagnostic tool of choice in cases in which one suspects a respiratory foreign body, a tracheal stenosis, or aspergillosis.[21]

Tracheoscopy

In most medium to large raptorial species, tracheoscopy can be safely accomplished by inserting a 2.7-mm unsheathed rigid telescope directly through the preplaced endotracheal tube. In species with a smaller tracheal diameter, such as American kestrels (*Falco sparverius*), sharp-shinned hawks (*Accipiter striatus*), merlins (*Falco columbarius*), Northern saw-whet owls (*Aegolius acadicus*), and Eastern screech owls (*Megascops asio*), direct insertion of the unsheathed 2.7-mm endoscope into the trachea can be attempted, but the use of a 1.9-mm telescope might be necessary. As in all avian species, gentle insertion of the telescope is warranted.[3]

Tracheoscopy is mostly performed in wild birds of prey to investigate the presence of syringeal aspergillomas, tracheal foreign bodies, postintubation tracheal stenosis, tracheal trauma (snare), severe *Syngamus* infections, trichomoniasis, and bacterial tracheitis. All these conditions can cause moderate to severe nonspecific respiratory signs and require a rapid and accurate diagnosis.[21–24]

Instruments such as biopsy or grasping forceps can be used to retrieve foreign bodies or debride *Aspergillus* granulomas, following a single or multiple attempts, depending on the size and consistency of the material/tissue. An operating sheath is not commonly used in these situations because of the small tracheal diameter; therefore, the forceps must run along the side of the endoscope in a parallel fashion to reach the material of interest. The presence of complete tracheal rings in birds makes the trachea function as a rigid sheath. Some mucosal damage does occur from the endoscope and forceps, but this is usually negligible compared with the inciting problem. If the complete removal of a fungal granuloma is not possible in 1 procedure, topical antifungals can be applied and the procedure repeated a few days later.[3]

Celioscopy

Respiratory signs can be caused by a primary respiratory disease or by a space-occupying mass compressing the air sacs. If coelomic distension is present, radiography and/or ultrasonography should be performed before the endoscopic examination. Special precautions are needed if a highly vascularized mass is present in the caudal air sacs or if there is ascites.

Celioscopic entry via the caudal thoracic air sacs allows for visualization of most of the middle and caudal coelomic cavity up to the caudal part of the lungs.[10] Internal hemorrhage can often be visualized after a traumatic event. An increase in the thickness and opacity of the normally transparent air sacs can be a sign of air sacculitis, but can also be observed in fat animals. When opaque air sac membranes prevent visualization of the tissues in the adjacent cavity, biopsy forceps or endoscopic scissors can be used to gently incise the air sac membrane to allow inspection without the need for excessive force and the risks of causing damage to the tissues on the other side.

Biopsy of any abnormal air sac walls should be taken and has been used as an adjunct diagnostic tool for *Mycoplasma* detection.[25] In the presence of severe leukocytosis (>30 × 10^9 cells/L), endoscopy should be performed as soon as possible to look for the typical mycelial and caseous lesions of aspergillosis (**Fig. 4**) and potentially administer topical antifungals.[4] When typical aspergillosis lesions are not visible, submitting biopsies for histopathology and culture can be required.

Birds of prey can die of aspergillosis without showing severe respiratory signs, and prognosis is poor once caseous granulomas have formed. Early diagnosis and endoscopically assisted debridement and topical treatment may improve the prognosis, compared with systemic antifungal administration alone.[4,26] When aspergillosis is suspected, it is critical to examine both sides of the bird with a scope, as *Aspergillus* lesions can be widespread throughout the respiratory system.[3] In case of a coelomic

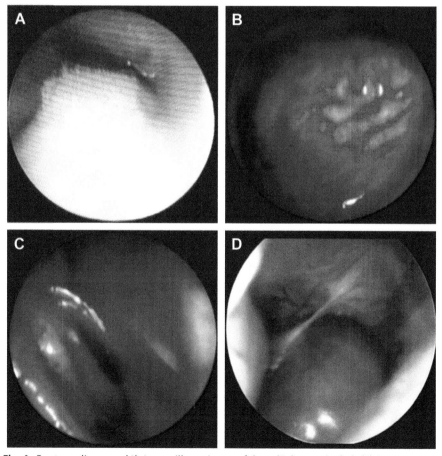

Fig. 4. Raptor celioscopy. (*A*) Aspergilloma in a gyrfalcon (*Falco rusticolus*). (*B*) Lung congestion in a sharp-shinned hawk (*Accipiter striatus*). (*C*) Normal syrinx in a sharp-shinned hawk. (*D*) Splenomegaly in a great-horned owl (*Bubo virginianus*) caused by *Leukocytozoon* infestation.

mass or organomegaly, biopsies should be taken. Nonfungal pneumonia and lung congestion (see **Fig. 4**) are occasionally observed in wild raptors. Caudal lung biopsies can be performed if needed.

Foreign Body Removal

Endoscopic removal of foreign bodies is often preferred over a surgical procedure for several reasons. This procedure is less invasive, and the postoperative prognosis is often better after endoscopic removal, especially compared with tracheostomy, proventriculotomy, or ventriculotomy.[10] The most common gastrointestinal foreign bodies found in wild raptors include plastic or metallic items. Soft plastic containers such as yogurt lids should not be used to offer food to raptors as they can ingest them. Although these items may be expelled with the pellet, large pieces can remain in the ventriculus and cause chronic irritation, requiring removal.

Feeding raptors with chicken necks is a common practice due its availability and low cost. However, the neck vertebrae need to be manually broken with a hammer before being fed to the birds. Failure to do so can cause crop impaction with secondary ingluvitis (**Fig. 5**). Removal of the vertebrae using an endoscope and grasping forceps is the treatment of choice. Foreign bodies can also be found in other systems, including the air sacs and the coelomic cavity. Bullets and porcupine quills can penetrate deeply into tissues and body cavities. Secondary inflammation and infection in some cases may warrant endoscopic removal. Great-horned owls, especially young, can attack porcupines and often get quills embedded in their face and neck. Careful inspection might reveal their presence in the coelomic inlet. In this case, endoscopy of the clavicular air sac (see **Fig. 4**) may be warranted, as quill migration into the clavicular air sac, just cranial to the heart, has been seen.

Diagnosis of Miscellaneous Conditions

Wild raptors are most commonly presented for trauma. Endoscopy is a minimally invasive technique, which can evaluate the extent of internal trauma, allowing for an

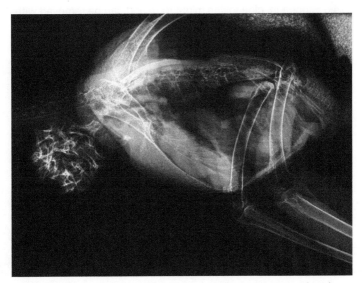

Fig. 5. Whole-body radiography of a red-tailed hawk (*Buteo jamaicensis*) with a crop impaction caused by chicken necks. Endoscopic removal was performed successfully in this case.

improved determination of prognosis. For example, when birds of prey are incidentally trapped in snares, which can be common in red-tailed hawks (*Buteo jamaicensis*) and bald eagles, upper gastrointestinal and tracheal endoscopy is recommended to assess potential extension of neck trauma to the esophagus (**Fig. 6**) and to the trachea. Tracheal and esophageal necrosis can have fatal consequences, and their early detection is required to an appropriate case management.

Noninfectious masses and neoplasia are rare in wild raptors. Upper gastrointestinal and cloacal masses are more commonly infectious in origin (eg, *Trichomonas, Capillaria, Salmonella*).[26] Organomegaly is rare in birds of prey. However, splenomegaly (caused by *Leukocytozoon* and *Chlamydophila psittaci*) (see **Fig. 4**) and hepatomegaly have been reported.[27,28]

Liver biopsies are important to differentiate between the multiple hepatic conditions that can affect wild raptors (eg, chlamydiosis, mycobacteriosis, amyloidosis, viral hepatitis, neoplasia).[4,27,29] Renal biopsies are best performed by a lateral approach through the thoracic caudal or abdominal air sacs.[30] The approach caudal to the ischium and dorsal to the pubis is not recommended in raptors, as they have large tail muscles that could bleed if penetrated.[30] Unless there is an obvious mass or abnormality on visual examination, kidney biopsies should be performed in the middle and caudal renal divisions, because the cranial renal artery lies more superficially than the middle and caudal ones.[30] However, biopsy of the cranial division of the kidney is also routinely performed by the authors. Biopsies of any abnormal mass or organ likely yields an etiologic diagnosis that will guide both therapy and prognosis.

Treatment of Miscellaneous Conditions

The value of the endoscopic removal of air sac nematodes (*Cyathostoma, Serratospiculum*) remains controversial.[4,23,26,30] Treatment with anthelmintics is currently recommended.[26,30] In case of a severe infestation, endoscopic removal of the worms might be considered to avoid profound air sacculitis secondary to parasite death.[4,19,22,30]

Neurologic signs are common sequelae of trauma and shock in wild raptors.[9] Leg paresis and paralysis are frequently seen with a concomitant cloacal dysfunction. Secondary to this dysfunction, cloacoliths might form and can be removed with the aid of the endoscope.[31]

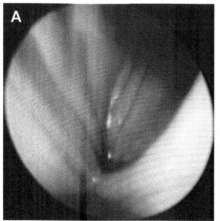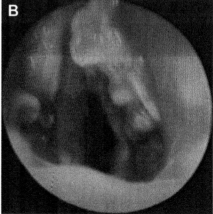

Fig. 6. (*A*) Normal esophagus in a red-tailed hawk (*Buteo jamaicensis*). (*B*) Severe esophageal necrosis following neck trauma in a red-tailed hawk.

Gender Identification

Although gender identification via DNA might be less invasive than endoscopy, it has not been validated for all wild raptorial species and, until recently, was not always reliable.[20] If amenable to captivity, nonreleasable birds can be relocated to breeding facilities and need to have their gender identified for breeding or foster pairs. When endoscopy equipment is available in a wildlife center, endoscopic gender identification could be preferred over DNA. However, gonad visualization can be challenging in obese or juvenile animals. As prices are progressively lower for DNA sexing and as newer techniques are providing more reliable results, endoscopy will likely be used less commonly for identifying the gender of wild raptors. Details on the methodology for gender identification in avian species by endoscopy have been previously reported.[4,12,20]

Research and Conservation

The use of endoscopy in research and conservation allows the rapid, antemortem acquisition of tissue samples from endangered species, including free-ranging animals. These animals can be caught and released within an hour because of the minimally invasive nature of endoscopy. Equipment has become more portable and can now be adapted for fieldwork. Portable light sources (such as the MLS1 mini light [Endoscopy Support Services, Brewster, NY, USA] and the Storz battery-operated light-emitting diode) and USB cameras (such as the iCap [Endoscopy Support Services, Brewster, NY, USA] and the eN-CAM [Laborie USA, Williston, VT, USA]) are now available and significantly reduce the weight and volume of the regular endoscopic equipment. Examples of endoscopic field procedures include liver biopsies for subclinical exposure to heavy metals and gonadal biopsy to study the impact of environmental toxins on reproductive activity. Early gender identification in captive-breeding programs is another example of how endoscopy can be used to promote conservation efforts.

POSTOPERATIVE CARE AND POTENTIAL COMPLICATIONS

Postoperative care is minimal after most endoscopic procedures. Birds usually recover quickly and eat the same day. Suture monitoring can be done daily for a few days if the bird has to be caught for other reasons or is not too stressed. Infection or dehiscence of the sutures has never been observed by the authors. Minor subcutaneous emphysema can occur but does not seem to be associated with pain or inflammation. Although some investigators recommend deflating subcutaneous emphysema, in the authors' experience, it resorbs within a few days without any further intervention.[12]

If the bird was hypotensive, anemic, or hypoproteinemic before the anesthesia, attention should be paid to providing adequate supportive care during and after the procedure.[9] Severe hemorrhage is rare when proper endoscopic technique is used. However, the biopsy of highly vascularized organs (spleen, lungs) should be avoided in critical cases. In case of an acute, severe hemorrhage during a procedure, transfusion might be considered.[32] Interspecies blood transfusion has been performed repeatedly by the authors in various species of birds without any adverse reaction.[32] In most cases, birds return to normal function within hours after the end of the procedure.

SUMMARY

Endoscopy is an underestimated and yet valuable diagnostic and therapeutic tool for wildlife raptor centers. Acquiring low-cost or free high-quality used equipment is easy and helps overcome financial restraints encountered by most wildlife rehabilitation programs. Endoscopy allows for the earlier diagnosis and treatment of potentially fatal conditions, improving the prognosis and general welfare of the animals in many cases. Although minimally invasive surgical equipment is unlikely to be part of the basic medical equipment for wild birds in the near future, the routine diagnostic and therapeutic use of endoscopy will become commonplace, as the standards of care are continuously improved.

ACKNOWLEDGMENTS

The authors thank Dr Guy Fitzgerald for sharing his broad experience in bird of prey medicine, endoscopy, and anesthesia; Dr Stéphane Lair for his extensive expertise in wild animal medicine and surgery; Dr Émilie Couture for her insightful reports; and the Union québécoise de réhabilitation des oiseaux de proie (www.uqrop.qc.ca) for supporting the Birds of Prey Clinic programs at the University of Montréal for now more than 27 years.

REFERENCES

1. Bush M. Diagnostic avian laparoscopy. In: Cooper JE, Greenwood AG, editors. Recent advances in the study of raptor diseases: international symposium proceedings. Asheville (NC): Chiron Publications Ltd; 1981. p. 97–100.
2. Böttcher M. Endoscopy of birds of prey in clinical veterinary practice. In: Cooper JE, Greenwood AG, editors. Recent advances in the study of raptor diseases: international symposium proceedings. Asheville (NC): Chiron Publications Ltd; 1981. p. 101–4.
3. Muller MG. Practical handbook of falcon husbandry and medicine. New York: Nova Science publishers; 2009.
4. Samour J. Endoscopy. In: Amour J, editor. Avian medicine. 2nd edition. Philadelphia: Elsevier; 2008. p. 122–35.
5. Gill F, Donsker D. IOC world bird list (v. 4.2). 2014. Available at: www.worldbirdnames.org. Accessed December 15, 2014.
6. Divers SJ. Endoscopy equipment and instrumentation for use in exotic animal medicine. Vet Clin North Am Exot Anim Pract 2010;13:171–85.
7. Chamness CJ. Instrumentation. In: Lhermette P, Sobel D, editors. BSAVA manual of canine and feline endoscopy and endosurgery. Gloucester (United Kingdom): British Small Animal Veterinary Association; 2008. p. 11–30.
8. Chamness CJ. Endoscopic instrumentation and documentation for flexible and rigid endoscopy. In: Tams TR, Rawlings CA, editors. Small animal endoscopy. 3rd edition. Saint Louis (MO): Mosby; 2011. p. 3–26.
9. Graham JE, Heatley JJ. Emergency care of raptors. Vet Clin North Am Exot Anim Pract 2007;10:395–418.
10. Divers SJ. Avian diagnostic endoscopy. Vet Clin North Am Exot Anim Pract 2010; 13:187–202.
11. Taylor M. Endoscopic examination and biopsy techniques. In: Ritchie BW, Harrison GJ, Harrison LR, editors. Avian medicine: principles and application. Fort Worth (FL): Harrison Bird Diets International; 1994. p. 327–54.
12. Lierz M. Diagnostic value of endoscopy and biopsy. In: Harrison GJ, Lightfoot TL, editors. Clinical avian medicine. Palm Beach (FL): Zoological Education Network; 2006. p. 631–52.
13. DeLong JP, Hoffman SW. Fat stores of migrant sharp-shinned and Cooper's hawks in New Mexico. J Raptor Res 2004;38:163–8.

14. Edling TM. Updates in anesthesia and monitoring. In: Harrison GJ, Lightfoot TL, editors. Clinical avian medicine. Palm Beach (FL): Zoological Education Network; 2006. p. 747–60.

15. Desmarchelier M, Rondenay Y, Fitzgerald G, et al. Monitoring of the ventilator status of anesthetized birds of prey by using end-tidal carbon dioxide measured with a microstream capnometer. J Zoo Wildl Med 2007;38:1–6.

16. Schmitt PM, Göbel T, Trautvetter E. Evaluation of pulse oximetry as a monitoring method in avian anesthesia. J Avian Med Surg 1998;12:91–9.

17. Touzot-Jourde G, Hernandez-Divers SJ, Trim CM. Cardiopulmonary effects of controlled versus spontaneous ventilation in pigeons anesthetized for coelioscopy. J Am Vet Med Assoc 2005;227:1424–8.

18. Sykes JM, Neiffer D, Terrell S, et al. Review of 23 cases of postintubation tracheal obstruction in birds. J Zoo Wildl Med 2013;44:700–13.

19. Heidenreich M. Birds of prey: medicine and management. Hoboken (NJ): Wiley-Blackwell; 1997.

20. Lierz M. Endoscopy, biopsy and endosurgery. In: Chitty J, Lierz M, editors. BSAVA manual of raptors, pigeons and passerine birds. Gloucester (United Kingdom): British Small Animal Veterinary Association; 2008. p. 139–42.

21. Bailey T. Raptors: respiratory problems. In: Chitty J, Lierz M, editors. BSAVA manual of raptors, pigeons and passerine birds. Gloucester (United Kingdom): British Small Animal Veterinary Association; 2008. p. 223–34.

22. Lacina D, Bird D. Endoparasites of raptors: a review and an update. In: Lumeij JT, Poffers J, editors. Raptor biomedicine III: including bibliography of birds of prey. Lake Worth (FL): Zoological Education Network; 2000. p. 65–99.

23. Lavoie M, Mikaelian I, Sterner M, et al. Respiratory nematodiases in raptors in Quebec. J Wildl Dis 1999;35:375–80.

24. Willette M, Ponder J, Cruz-Martinez L, et al. Management of select bacterial and parasitic conditions of raptors. Vet Clin North Am Exot Anim Pract 2009;12: 491–517.

25. Lierz M, Schmidt R, Goebel T, et al. Detection of mycoplasma spp. In: Lumeij JT, Poffers J, editors. Raptor biomedicine III: including bibliography of birds of prey. Lake Worth (FL): Zoological Education Network; 2000. p. 25–33.

26. Samour J. Management of raptors. In: Harrison GJ, Lightfoot TL, editors. Clinical avian medicine. Palm Beach (FL): Zoological Education Network; 2006. p. 915–56.

27. Johns JL, Luff JA, Shooshtari MP, et al. What is your diagnosis? Blood smear from an injured red-tailed hawk. Vet Clin Pathol 2009;38:247–52.

28. Forrester DJ, Greiner EC. Leucocytozoonosis. In: Atkinson CT, Thomas NJ, Hunter DB, editors. Parasitic diseases of wild birds. Oxford (United Kingdom): Wiley-Blackwell; 2008. p. 54–107.

29. Satterfield WC. Early diagnosis of avian tuberculosis by laparoscopic and liver biopsy. In: Cooper JE, Greenwood AG, editors. Recent advances in the study of raptor diseases: international symposium proceedings. Asheville (NC): Chiron Publications Ltd; 1981. p. 105–6.

30. Lumeij JT. Pathophysiology, diagnosis and treatment of renal disorders in birds of prey. In: Lumeij JT, Poffers J, editors. Raptor biomedicine III: including bibliography of birds of prey. Lake Worth (FL): Zoological Education Network; 2000. p. 169–78.

31. Beaufrère H, Nevarez J, Tully TN Jr. Cloacolith in a blue-fronted amazon parrot (Amazona aestiva). J Avian Med Surg 2010;24:142–5.

32. Shaw S, Tully T, Nevarez J. Avian transfusion medicine. Compend Contin Educ Vet 2009;31(12):E1–7.

Endoscopy in Amphibians

Norin Chai, DVM, MSc, PhD

KEYWORDS

- Amphibians • Endoscopy • Diagnosis • Biopsy

KEY POINTS

- The majority of endoscopy procedures described in reptiles (especially lizards) can be undertaken in most amphibians.
- Coelioscopy is a safe and effective technique to directly visualize visceral organs and collect tissue samples.
- Coelioscopy is a valuable complement to radiography and ultrasonography.
- Like other imaging methods, the large number of amphibian species requires special knowledge of anatomic differences.

INTRODUCTION

More than 7360 species of amphibians exist, of which 6488 belong to the Anura (frogs and toads), 673 to the Caudata (newts and salamanders), and 200 to the Gymnophiona (caecilians).[1] Only the commonly maintained companion animal species are discussed here; therefore, caecilians have been excluded.

There have been sporadic reports of amphibian endoscopy since the 1980s. Most previous reports describe the use of endoscopy to examine gender or retrieve foreign bodies.[2–5] In contrast with reptile medicine, where endoscopy has been well-developed, the literature is scarce in amphibians. The greatest limiting factor is probably equipment compatibility owing to the small size of most amphibians. In addition, anesthesia can also be challenging; however, valuable information may be gained by passing a small, rigid endoscope through the oropharynx into the stomach or into the coelomic cavity.

With appropriate equipment, many species of newts, salamanders, frogs, and toads can be examined internally with minimal trauma and discomfort. Endoscopy is a useful complementary tool to radiography and ultrasonography.[6] However, it is often difficult to interpret images in such small animals. Misdiagnosis is not uncommon. Endoscopy produces a 2-dimensional representation including size, color,

The author has nothing to disclose.

Ménagerie du Jardin des Plantes, Muséum national d'Histoire naturelle, 57 Rue Cuvier, Paris 75005, France

E-mail address: chai@mnhn.fr

Vet Clin Exot Anim 18 (2015) 479–491

http://dx.doi.org/10.1016/j.cvex.2015.04.006

contours, and spatial awareness of other structures. In this author's experience, endoscopy in amphibians permits visualization of almost all the coelomic organs from a single point of entry.

INDICATIONS

In the author experience, the main indications of endoscopy in amphibians are as follows.

- Gender identification.
- Retrieval of foreign bodies from the upper gastrointestinal tract.
- Rapid, magnified, ante mortem or post mortem assessment of intracoelomic lesions in cases of high mortality in a colony.
- Valuable diagnostic tool when confronted by nonpathognomonic clinical signs, such as anorexia, weight loss, or loss of pigmentation.
- Biopsies of tissues and coelomic organs.

CONTRAINDICATIONS

Given the application of the 2.7-mm or the 1.9-mm system, the small size of the animal is the most common limitation/contraindication. Sick animals with high anesthetic risks should not undergo endoscopy.

EQUIPMENT

Despite the variation in size and the nature of the procedures that may be performed, the basic endoscope system consist of the following.

- A 1.9-mm integrated telescope.
- A 2.7-mm diameter, 18-cm length, 30° oblique rigid telescope with a 4.8-mm operating sheath.
- An Endovideo camera and monitor.
- A xenon light source and light cable.
- A 1- or 1.7-mm endoscopic biopsy forceps and grasping forceps (an endoscopic needle is optional).
- Carbon dioxide (CO_2) insufflator with silicone tubing. Care must be taken when using CO_2 insufflation, because it can quickly dry out the organs and the mucosa. Therefore, in the author experience, the endoscopic procedure should not last more than 10 minutes. A simple syringe for air or saline infusion is also practical.

PATIENT PREPARATION

Because most amphibians are presented in a state of advanced disease, they need to be stabilized before undergoing anesthesia and endoscopy. The amphibian patient should be handled with care, and wrapping with a wet paper towel is a good technique to restrain an animal for a quick examination or for medication administration. Wearing moistened, powder-free gloves prevents the transfer of microorganisms or chemicals from the handler as well as protection against secreted toxins. Manual restraint is used for short and nonpainful procedures. As long as the animal is outside his natural environment, his integument should be moistened regularly with dechlorinated water. For a better visualization, it is advisable to fast large frogs and toads for 24 to 48 hours before anesthesia. Preoperative preparations include hydration of the animal in a shallow, dechlorinated water bath.

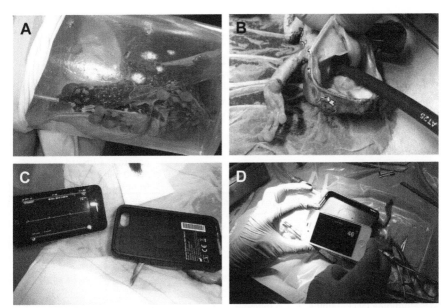

Fig. 1. Amphibian anesthesia and monitoring. (*A*) Anesthesia by bath with M-S222 of a milk frog (*Trachycephalus resinifictrix*). (*B*) Intubation of a 2-colored leaf frog (*Phyllomedusa bicolor*) with an uncuffed 4-mm diameter tube. (*C, D*) Monitoring of 2 amphibians with a portable electrocardiogram (AliveCor Veterinary Heart Monitor devices, Vetoquinol, PARIS, France). (*Courtesy of* Norin Chai, DVM, MSc, PhD, Paris, France.)

ANESTHESIA AND ANALGESIA

Because the procedures are very stressful and may be painful for the animal, general anesthesia with analgesia is required for endoscopy. In this author's experience, the drug of choice for sedation or anesthesia is tricaine methanesulfonate (MS-222; **Fig. 1**A). **Table 1** presents only protocols that have been used and evaluated by the author; additional options may be found elsewhere.[6,7] The righting reflex is used as a primary indicator to determine the stage of anesthesia. Loss of this reflex suggests a light stage of anesthesia. A surgical plane is indicated by the loss of withdrawal reflexes. Recovery from water-bath–based anesthesia (MS-222) can be accomplished by thoroughly rinsing the animal with anesthetic-free water. Aquatic animals should have their head out of water during recovery. The amphibian should be considered recovered when all of the reflexes have returned and heart and respiration rates have returned to preanesthetic levels.

If possible, animals are intubated (uncuffed tubes, red rubber catheters; see **Fig. 1**B). A low flow of oxygen (this author uses 0.5–0.75 L/min) may then be provided (with or without 0.5%–1% isoflurane saturation). Heart rate should be monitored and the use of portable electrocardiogram (AliveCor Veterinary Heart Monitor devices, Vetoquinol, Paris, France) is less traumatic and preferred over a standard electrocardiogram (see **Fig. 1** C, D). Doppler ultrasonography is also a good way to assess the heart rate.

ENDOSCOPY PROCEDURES

Most endoscopy procedures described in reptiles (mainly lizards) can be undertaken in the majority of amphibians if equipment can be matched to patient size. However, like other imaging methods, anatomic knowledge of a particular species is paramount.

Table 1
Protocols for anesthesia and analgesia in anurans

Drug	Dosage and Route	Comments
Tricaine methanesulfonate (MS-222)	Tadpoles and aquatic frogs 0.25–0.5 g/L (Bath) Adult frogs and toads 1 g/L (Bath)	Buffer MS-222 solutions before use. Induction times are variable. After induction, place the frog into a shallow amount of nonanesthetic water or on a wet towel. Recovery is generally achieved 30–90 min after removal from the anesthetic.
Isoflurane	5% in oxygen (inhalation or bubbling in bath; see **Fig. 1**) 2–3 mL/L (Bath) 0.01–0.06 mL/g (topical)	Gentle stimulation encourages continued respiration. Effective but slow induction. Isoflurane is sprayed directly into the water. Dilute in gel form or apply directly
Medetomidine (M)/ketamine (K)/meloxicam (Mel)/ butorphanol (But)	M 0.5 mg/kg + K 50 mg/kg + Mel 0.2 mg/kg + But 25 mg/kg (IM)	Effective protocol in *Xenopus laevis* for heart surgery Reversed with atipamezole hydrochloride at equal volume to medetomidine IM.
Meloxicam	0.1– 0.2 mg/kg (IM)	—

Abbreviation: IM, intramuscular.

Selected procedures to be discussed here include stomatoscopy, gastroscopy, coelioscopy, and biopsy of coelomic organs and lesions.

Stomatoscopy and Gastroscopy

The animal is placed in dorsal recumbency or, alternatively, held by an assistant during the procedure (**Fig. 2**A). The oral cavity is gently opened with radiographic film or a silicone or wooden spatula to avoid trauma. The telescope-sheath system can be used to examine the oral cavity, esophagus, and stomach. Once in the oral cavity, the choana can be observed and evaluated (see **Fig. 2**B). The oral cavity is separated from the esophagus by a strong upper sphincter (see **Fig. 2**C).[8] The oral cavity of adult amphibians is generally wide and large, but visualization of the sphincter can be difficult. Mucus, secreted by buccal epithelial glands, might also be normally present in the oral cavity.[8] Once past the upper esophageal sphincter, one may observe the esophageal mucosa (see **Fig. 2**D), followed by the lower esophageal sphincter (see **Fig. 2**E), and stomach.[9] Slight insufflation using air is often needed to allow passage of the telescope. The stomach can be evaluated for the presence of masses, ulcers, nodules, parasites, and foreign objects (**Fig. 3**). If needed, object removal can be accomplished using 1- or 1.7-mm endoscopic grasping forceps through the working channel. If not possible, traditional gastrostomy should be planed.

Coelioscopy

With the animal positioned in dorsal recumbency, the surgical field is prepared aseptically by gently wiping the surgical site with sterile cotton-tipped applicators

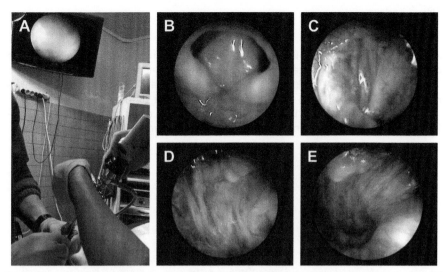

Fig. 2. Stomatoscopy and esophagoscopy in a 2-colored leaf frog (*Phyllomedusa bicolor*). (*A*) The animal is held by an assistant during the procedure. (*B*) Normal view of the choana. (*C*) The strong upper esophageal sphincter. (*D*) Normal esophageal mucosa. (*E*) Lower esophageal sphincter. (*Courtesy of* Norin Chai, DVM, MSc, PhD, Paris, France.)

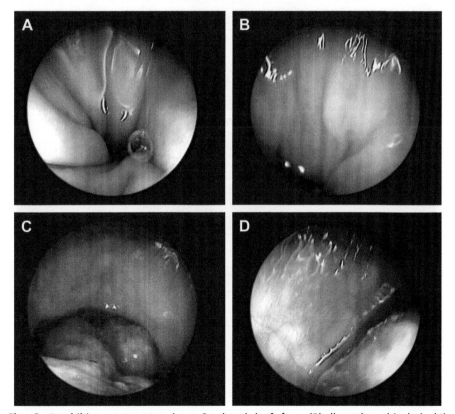

Fig. 3. Amphibian gastroscopy in a 2-colored leaf frog (*Phyllomedusa bicolor*). (*A*) Visualization of the cardia. (*B*) Normal gastric mucosa. (*C*) Normal stomach with food content. (*D*) Transmural visualization of the ovarian follicles. (*Courtesy of* Norin Chai, DVM, MSc, PhD, Paris, France.)

soaked in diluted povidone-iodine solution (1/10) in sterile saline.[10] An alternative is to place a moist sterile gauze with the diluted povidone-iodine solution, left for 10 to 15 seconds (**Fig. 4**A). It is also possible to use sterile gauze soaked in 0.75% chlorhexidine solution and left on the surgical site for at least 10 minutes before surgery.[9]

A 3-mm paramedian skin incision is made in the mid coelom (between the shoulders and the cloaca). Care must be taken not to damage the macroscopic glands,

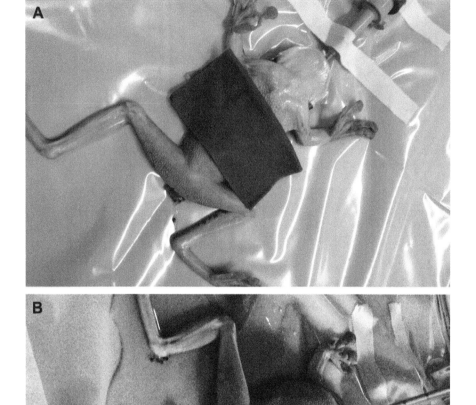

Fig. 4. Coelioscopy in a milk frog (*Trachycephalus resinifictrix*). (*A*) The animal is anesthetized, intubated, and aseptically prepared. (*B*) The rigid telescope-sheath system with insufflation tube is inserted into the pleuroperitoneal cavity. (*Courtesy of* Norin Chai, DVM, MSc, PhD, Paris, France.)

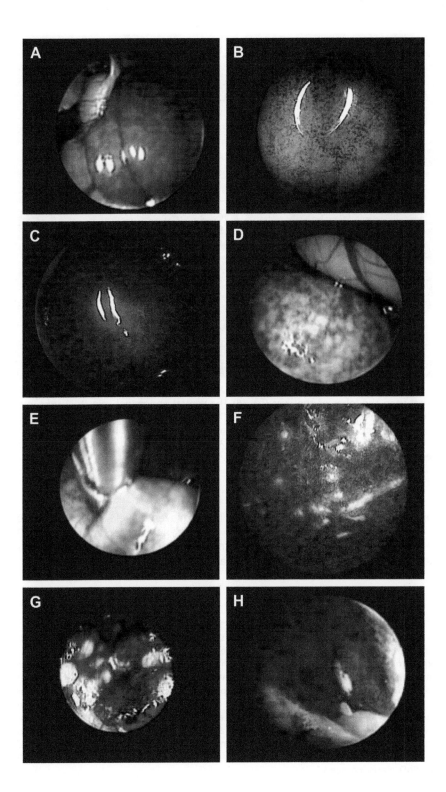

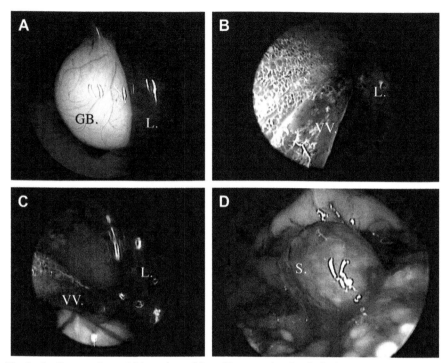

Fig. 6. Coelioscopy in an African clawed frog (*Xenopus laevis; A*) The large gallbladder (*GB.*) lies between the lobes of the liver (*L.*). (*B*) The ventral abdominal vein (*VV.*) runs in the midline inside the ventral coelomic wall. (*C*) The ventral vein travels cranially between the lobes of the liver, to further divide with a branch entering each lobe. (*D*) Spleen (*S.*) with multiple abscesses in an African clawed frog (*X laevis*) caused by *Mycobacterium gordonae* infection. (*Courtesy of* Norin Chai, DVM, MSc, PhD, Paris, France.)

lymph hearts, and blood vessels, especially the midventral vein. After skin incision, the abdominal membrane is elevated, incised, and dissected carefully. The telescope-sheath system is inserted into the pleuroperitoneal cavity, which is insufflated (see **Fig. 4**B). Typically, CO_2 insufflation pressures of 0.5 to 2 mm Hg with a

Fig. 5. Amphibian coelioscopy with emphasis on hepatic evaluation and biopsy. (*A*) The liver of anurans consists in 2 completely separated lobes, here in an African clawed frog (*Xenopus laevis*). (*B, C*) The normal hepatic gross appearance varies from pale gray, pink brown, to black in the African clawed frogs. Note the normal dark pigmentation owing to the presence of melanomacrophages. This is common in most amphibians. (*D*) Hepatic lipidosis in a wide-mouth frog (*Lepidobatrachus laevis*). (*E*) Biopsy of the same liver. (*F*) Focal hepatic discoloration in an African clawed frog caused by *Mycobacterium liflandii* infection. (*G*) Several hepatic abscesses in a western clawed frog (*Xenopus tropicalis*) caused by *Mycobactrium szulgaï* infection. (*H*) Hepatic cystic lesion in an African clawed frog (*X laevis*) caused by *Contracaecum sp.* (*Courtesy of* Norin Chai, DVM, MSc, PhD, Paris, France.)

flow rate not exceeding 0.5 L/min are used. In some situations, especially in very small animals, saline infusion may be preferred over gas. Amphibians have an undivided pleuroperitoneal cavity. The only separated compartment is the pericardial sac.[11] This common coelom permits the visualization of liver, gall bladder, heart,

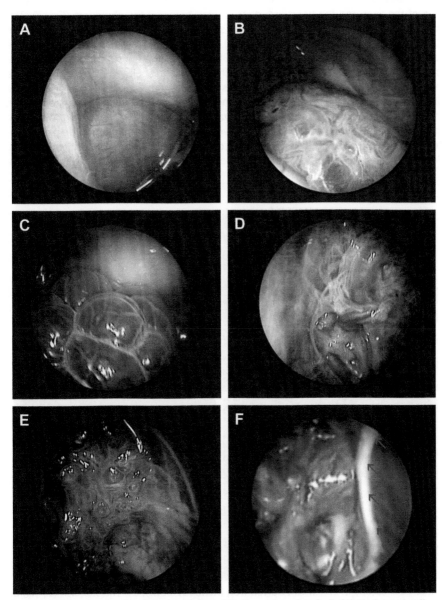

Fig. 7. Coelioscopy in a 2-colored leaf frog (*Phyllomedusa bicolor*). (*A*) Endoscopy allows examination of the pericardium, cardiac surface, and subjective assessment of cardiac activity. (*B–E*) Several states of inflated and deflated lungs. (*F*) A filarial worm parasite near the lungs enclosed in subcutaneous fat (see the *red arrows*). (*Courtesy of* Norin Chai, DVM, MSc, PhD, Paris, France.)

lungs, digestive tract, gonads, kidneys, bladder, and fat body from only a single entry point.

In general, the liver of anurans consists of 2 completely separated lobes (**Fig. 5**).[12] The liver of caudates, such as the axolotl (*Ambystoma mexicanum*), is a single elongated organ that may be partially subdivided. A large gallbladder lies on the midline in the interlobular connective tissue of the liver (**Fig. 6**). The lungs lie dorsal to each lobe of the liver and the heart is further cranial, between the shoulders (**Fig. 7**). The stomach is situated dorsally within the left side of the coelom (**Fig. 8A**). The intestines fill the contralateral right side (see **Fig. 8B**). The intestine may be subdivided into the narrow, coiled small intestine (see **Fig. 8B**) followed by a short, wide large intestine (see **Fig. 8C**) that leads to the cloaca. Each gonad is associated with a conspicuous fat body that is subdivided into numerous digitiform lobes, pressed up against the pleuroperitoneal cavity (see **Fig. 8A, D**). The size of the fat bodies varies greatly with the stage of reproductive cycle.[11] The ovaries vary in size, depending on stage of the reproductive cycle, and may be massive, occupying a large part of the pleuroperitoneal cavity (**Figs. 9A, B, D–F**). The small, ovoid testes are less apparent, located in a dorsal position, and thus covered by other viscera (see **Fig. 8B** and **Fig. 9C**). The

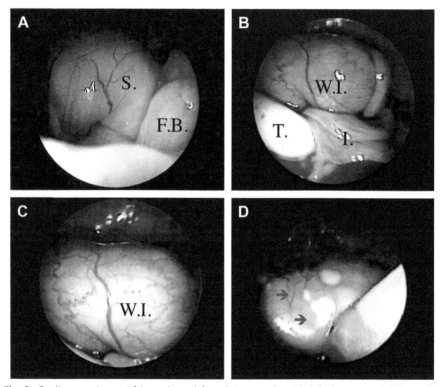

Fig. 8. Coelioscopy in an African clawed frog (*Xenopus laevis*). (*A*) The stomach (*S.*) can be found caudal to the liver varying in size and shape depending on the species and nature of the prey. Note the normal fat bodies (*F.B.*; *B*) and (*C*) Coelomic organs, including the small intestine (*I.*), wide large intestine (*W.I.*), and testis (*T.*). (*D*) Parasitic cysts on stomach of African clawed frog caused by *Contracaecum sp.* (*red arrows*). (*Courtesy of* Norin Chai, DVM, MSc, PhD, Paris, France.)

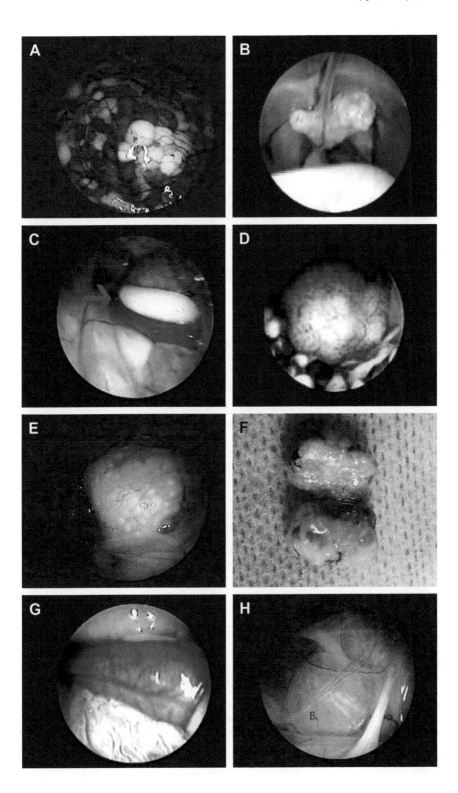

kidneys, paired, dark, flattened, with ovoid structures, are also located dorsocaudally (see **Fig. 9**G).[13] Urinary bladder is large and thin walled in anurans (see **Fig. 9**H).[11]

Biopsy

Endoscopic biopsy of parenchymatous organs or intracoelomic masses may be performed using the 1- or 1.7-mm endoscopic biopsy forceps through the working channel (see **Fig. 5**E). In all cases, samples collected should be submitted for further diagnostic tests (eg, culture and histopathology). Hepatic or renal samplings submitted for culture and histology may be used for ante mortem or post mortem diagnosis.[13]

Carbon Dioxide Removal, Closure of the Coelom, and Postoperative Care

Once the scope is removed, the animal deflates, immediately removing the CO_2 naturally. The coelomic membrane and the skin are closed in 1 layer with simple interrupted sutures. Monofilament nylon seems to be the most appropriate suture in amphibian skin and should be removed in 4 to 8 weeks.[14] The animal should be rinsed copiously with fresh, well-oxygenated water and transferred to a warm, anesthetic-free bath.

BENEFITS OF ENDOSCOPY

The benefits of endoscopy are numerous, but most useful is the ability to collect samples for a definitive diagnosis, accurate prognosis, and direct therapy.

COMPLICATIONS AND POTENTIAL ADVERSE OUTCOMES

Complications resulting from a properly performed endoscopy procedure are rare. However, iatrogenic endoscope trauma can adversely affect organs and biopsy results, as well as result in hemorrhage. The most dramatic complication occurs when the ventral abdominal vein is damaged. This may happen on very small animals, even from a paramedian approach. If sufficient CO_2 is left behind in an aquatic amphibian, buoyancy problems may occur and the animal may be unable to submerge or swim properly.

CURRENT CONTROVERSIES AND FUTURE CONSIDERATIONS

Previous experience and training, especially with reptile endoscopy, is necessary to perform endoscopy in amphibians. However, the benefits of endoscopy are numerous and the development of new techniques and procedures should be encouraged.

Fig. 9. Amphibian coelioscopy. (*A*) In mature females, the ova extend cranially, cover the parietal surface and may occupy large parts of the coelom as showed here in an African clawed frog (*Xenopus laevis*). (*B*) Gender identification in immature great crested newt (*Triturus cristatus*). Note the immature ovaries that are dorsally located. (*C*) Testis (*red arrow*) of an adult 2-colored leaf frog (*Phyllomedusa bicolor*). (*D*) Ovarian abscess in a western clawed frog (*Xenopus tropicalis*) caused by *Mycobaterium szulgai*. (*E*) Ovarian neoplasia in a 2-colored leaf frog (*Phyllomedusa bicolor*). (*F*) The ovary of the frog in **Fig. 9**E cut after surgery. (*G*) Kidney of a 2-colored leaf frog (*P bicolor*). The kidneys are dark red, cigar-shaped cylinders located caudal, lateral to the spine. (*H*) The bladder (*B.*) of a 2-colored leaf frog (*P bicolor*). (*Courtesy of* Norin Chai, DVM, MSc, PhD, Paris, France.)

SUMMARY

The majority of endoscopy procedures described in reptiles (mainly lizards) can be undertaken in most amphibians, if equipment can be matched to patient size. Coelioscopy has been shown to be a successful technique to directly visualize visceral organs and collect tissue samples, and it is a valuable complement to radiography and ultrasonography. The large number of amphibian species requires special knowledge of anatomic differences.

REFERENCES

1. AmphibiaWeb: Information on amphibian biology and conservation, Berkeley (CA). Available at: http://amphibiaweb.org. Accessed December 15, 2014.
2. Kramer L, Dresser BL, Maruska EJ. Sexing aquatic salamanders by laparoscopy. Proceedings Am Assoc Zoo Vet Ann Meeting. San Diego, CA. 1983. p. 193–194.
3. Wright KM. Surgical techniques. In: Wright KM, Whitaker BR, editors. Amphibian medicine and captive husbandry. Malabar (FL): Krieger; 2001. p. 274–83.
4. Boggs L, Theisen S. Endoscopic removal of gastric foreign bodies in an African bullfrog, Pyxicephalus adspersus. Newsl Assoc Reptilian Amphib Vet 1997;7(2):7–8.
5. Murray MJ, Schildger B, Taylor M. Endoscopy in birds, reptiles, amphibians and fish. Tuttlingen (Germany): Endo-Press; 1998. p. 31–54.
6. Carpenter JW, Mashima TY, Rupiper DJ. Exotic animal formulary. 3rd edition. Philadelphia: Saunders; 2005.
7. Mitchell MA. Anesthetic considerations for amphibians. Journal of Exotic Pet Medicine 2009;18(1):40–9.
8. Olsen ID. Digestion and nutrition. In: Kluge AG, editor. Chordate structure and function. 2nd edition. New York: Macmillan; 1977. p. 270–305.
9. Gentz EJ. Medicine and surgery of amphibians. ILAR J 2007;48(3):255–9.
10. Chai N. Anurans. In: Fowler M, Miller R, editors. Zoo and wild animal medicine. 8th edition. St Louis (MO): WB Saunders; 2014. p. 1–13.
11. De Iuliis G, Pulerà D. The dissection of vertebrates. A laboratory manual. First edition. Burlington (MA): Academic Press; Elsevier; 2007. p. 113–30.
12. Crawshaw GJ, Weinkle TK. Clinical and pathological aspects of the amphibian liver. Seminars in Avian and Exotic Pet Medicine 2000;9(3):165–73.
13. Cecil TR. Amphibian renal disease. Vet Clin Exot Anim Anim Pract 2006;9: 175–88.
14. Tuttle AD, Law JM, Harms CA, et al. Evaluation of the gross and histologic reactions to five commonly used suture materials in the skin of the African clawed frog (Xenopus laevis). J Am Assoc Lab Anim Sci 2006;45(6):22–6.

Pulmonoscopy of Snakes

Zdenek Knotek, DVM, PhD, Dip ECZM (Herpetology)*,
Vladimir Jekl, DVM, PhD, Dip ECZM (Small Mammal)

KEYWORDS

- Pulmonoscopy • Endoscopy • Respiratory tract • Air sac • Pathology • Imaging
- Snakes • Reptiles

KEY POINTS

- Pulmonoscopy is a practical ancillary diagnostic tool for the investigation of respiratory disease in snakes.
- Two different approaches exist for pulmonoscopy in snakes: tracheal and transcutaneous.
- Tracheal and transcutaneous methods are safe, and specific contraindications for pulmonoscopy in snakes are not known except for any anesthesia contraindication.
- Pulmonoscopy in snakes requires general anesthesia. Analgesia should be evaluated case by case, but it is strongly recommended with the transcutaneous approach, as soft tissue incision is required.

INTRODUCTION

Pneumonia and various forms of lower respiratory tract disease (LRTD) are common in snakes.[1] The ability of snakes to withstand long periods (weeks or even months) of limited respiratory activity means that respiratory diseases are often well advanced before any clinical signs are seen. Bacterial disease is the most common cause of LRTD in captive snakes, but parasites (lungworms, pentastomids) and viruses have also been identified. Endoscopic examination of the lung is a practical ancillary diagnostic tool for the investigation of respiratory diseases in snakes.[2-4] The body size and length of snakes and anatomic differences between ophidian species necessitate the application of different approaches, which can affect the complexity and effectiveness of examinations.[5] Two different approaches exist for pulmonoscopy in snakes, the tracheal and the transcutaneous approach, and both have been described in detail.[3,6-8]

Topography of the Serpentine Respiratory System

The dorsal tracheal membrane (dorsal ligament), which connects the tips of the tracheal rings, is small (1/4) in the proximal part of the snake respiratory tract

The authors have nothing to disclose.
Faculty of Veterinary Medicine, Avian and Exotic Animal Clinic, University of Veterinary and Pharmaceutical Sciences Brno, 1-3 Palackeho Street, Brno 612 42, Czech Republic
* Corresponding author.
E-mail address: knotekz@vfu.cz

(head and neck) where the main part of trachea (3/4) is the ventral canal made by tracheal cartilaginous rings. Compared with similar-sized mammals, the lung volume of snakes is large, but they only have about 10% to 20% of the lung surface area.[5,9,10] The lung(s) of most snakes occupy a major portion of the body cavity. The lungs vary in relative width and relative length from 8% to 94% snout-to-vent length (SVL).[11] Some species of elapid and viperid snakes have a tracheal lung, which is a proliferation of the dorsal ligament emanating from the dorsal aspect of the trachea, which often functions as the main respiratory organ when lung is compressed.[11] Most snakes (eg, viperids, elapids, and colubrids) have only one functional respiratory lung (right), with the left being vestigial or absent.[5,11] The lung is divided into a functional lung and a relatively avascular saccular lung (air sac), which is a direct continuation of the functional lung and can stretch as far as the second third of the coelom. In some aquatic snakes, the air sac can extend caudally to the cloaca. In some snakes (eg, boids), 2 lungs are present and can be comparable in size, although the left is typically smaller. The length of the tracheal lung ranges from 3% to 44% SVL, the length of the right lung from 8% to 82% SVL, and the length of the right bronchus from 0.5% to 54% SVL.[11]

Snake's Lung Anatomy

All snakes have a right lung (boas and pythons also have a left) located dorsal to the liver and lateral to the stomach on the right side of the visceral cavity. The snake lung is divided into the proximal part (functioning vascular lung) and the distal avascular part—the air sac. Snakes in the families *Anomalepididae, Typhlopidae*, and *Acrochordidae* have multichambered lungs. In other snakes, lungs are single chambered. The snake lung is unicameral.

The trachea may enter the right lung in several ways. The most common condition of tracheal entry is terminal. The trachea enters the most cranial portion of the lung (and the cranial lobe is absent) and the trachea becomes a bronchus on entrance into the lung. Normally, the moderate bronchus terminates around the level of the transition from the vascularized lung to avascular air sac, but the long bronchus may continue into the air sac (in snakes of the family *Bitis*).[11] The subterminal entry means that the trachea enters the mesial side of the right lung ventrally and caudally of its anterior tip. The small cranial lobe projects freely laterally of the trachea (**Fig. 1**).[11]

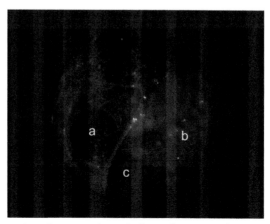

Fig. 1. Pulmonoscopy in a *Boa constrictor*. Endoscopic retrograde view of the cranial lung lobe (a), bronchus (b), and the distal part of the trachea (c).

In snakes, a major portion of the respiratory tract volume is made up of the nonrespiratory air sac. This air sac may act as a reservoir for oxygen during periods of apnea. In aquatic snakes, it may also act as a buoyancy organ.[11] Three different types of reptilian lung parenchyma have been described: (1) trabecular parenchyma consisting of a single layer of low-relief branching muscular structures (*trabeculae*), (2) edicular parenchyma composed of a single layer of trabeculae with raised walls or septa that form cubicles (*ediculae*) that are wider than they are deep, and (3) single- or multiple-layered faviform parenchyma, the compartments (faveoli) of which are deeper than wide and often present a honeycomb appearance. The distribution of parenchyma in snake lungs is heterogeneous.[11] Compared with faveolar lung, the air sac is only poorly vascularized. The air sac wall appears as a semitransparent membrane devoid of muscular tissue or blood vessels (**Fig. 2**).

INDICATIONS/CONTRAINDICATIONS

- Pulmonoscopy is indicated for the evaluation of snakes with clinical signs of respiratory disease, including tachypnea, dyspnea, or tracheal discharge.
- Pulmonoscopy by either technique allows minimally invasive and yet detailed visual examination of the mucosa of lung and air sac.

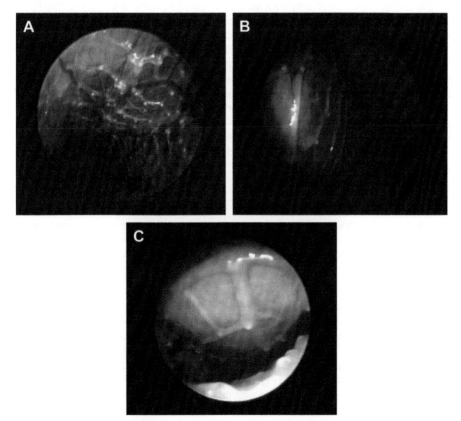

Fig. 2. Endoscopic view of the air sac in a Burmese python (*Python molurus bivittatus*). Note the gradual reduction in a vascular supply from the proximal (*A*) to distal parts (*B, C*) of the air sac.

- The first method of pulmonoscopy in snakes is the traditional direct tracheo-scopy–pulmonoscopy, the second is the pulmonoscopy via the air sac (transcutaneous pulmonoscopy).
- The approach through the air sac provides a feasible method for examining the distal segment of the respiratory system and indirect evaluation of the color of liver, large vessels, and some other organs of the snake coelom.
- Both of the methods are safe; no changes in the respiratory function or the general health of snakes have been observed after endoscopy.
- The only known contraindication is associated with anesthesia.

TECHNIQUE
Instrumentation

The snakes' lung and air sacs can be examined with rigid endoscopes or flexible bronchoscopes of various diameters, depending on the length and diameter of the trachea.[4–8] In small or young snakes, the Hopkins Forward-Oblique Telescope (diameter, 2.7 mm; length, 18 cm; 30°; Karl Storz Endoscope, Tuttlingen, Germany); the Hopkins Slender Telescope (diameter, 1.9 mm to 2.1 mm; length, 18 cm; 30°; Karl Storz Endoscope); and the Semi-rigid Miniature Straight Forward Telescope (diameter, 1.0 mm, length, 20 cm; 0°; Karl Storz Endoscope) have been used with or without an operating sheaths. Rigid telescopes such as the 2.7-mm telescope with the 4.8-mm operating sheath or the 1.9-mm rigid telescope with the 3.3-mm integrated operating sheath enable introduction of flexible endoscopic instruments (1.7 mm or 1.0 mm, respectively). Flexible biopsy forceps, remote injection/aspiration needle, and a small flexible brush are used for biopsy, cytology, and culture. For large snakes, the Wide Angle Forward-Oblique Telescope (diameter, 4.0 mm; length, 30 cm; 30°; Karl Storz Endoscope) or flexible bronchoscopes with small diameter (ø 2.5–5.9 mm) can be used.[8]

Endoscopic images presented in this report were taken with the use of a rigid endoscope (Hopkins Documentation Forward-Oblique Telescope; diameter, 2.7 mm; length,18 cm; 30°; Karl Storz Endoscope) with 4.8-mm diagnostic sheath, xenon light (Xenon Nova, 400–750 nm; Karl Storz Endoscope) and endoscopic camera (Endovision Telekam; Karl Storz Endoscope).

Patient Preparation

Preoperative care
Before the endoscopic examination, routine considerations for general anesthesia, including physical examination, hematology, plasma biochemistry, and fasting should be undertaken. The snake should fast for one food cycle but should have unlimited access to water.

Anesthesia, analgesia
Pulmonoscopy via the trachea is a short painless procedure. Therefore, the use of analgesics is not compulsory, and short-term anesthesia can be achieved with intravenous propofol or alphaxalone.[12] However, if painful procedures are required (eg, biopsy), analgesia is important.[13] For longer procedures, the combination of α-2 adrenergic agonist (eg, [dex]medetomidine) with dissociative anesthetic (eg, ketamine or tiletamine) and benzodiazepine (eg, midazolam or zolazepam) can be used.[8,12–18] It is also possible to induce anesthesia with intravenous propofol or alphaxalone, intubate, and ventilate with isoflurane (or sevoflurane) for 5 to 10 minutes before starting the procedure. For transcutaneous pulmonoscopy via the air sac, the use of analgesics is recommended (eg, opioids and nonsteroidal anti-inflammatory drugs). The use of local anesthesia is also an option.[13,18]

Pulmonoscopy Techniques

Tracheal approach

With the animal properly anesthetized and positioned in ventral recumbency, the endoscope is carefully inserted through the glottis, advanced caudally through the trachea and, if of sufficient length, into the bronchi and lumen of the lung(s). In smaller snakes, the use of rigid scopes might be appropriate for complete pulmonoscopy, as long as the length of the scope is sufficient to reach the distal lung, and the trachea can accommodate the diameter of the equipment. For larger snakes, the use of flexible bronchoscopes will be necessary, as rigid scopes will only permit examination of the anterior trachea.[4] After endoscopy, the animal should recover following standard anesthesia protocols.[18]

Transcutaneous approach

The transcutaneous approach to the air sac and lungs is performed using a rigid telescope, with the animal in left lateral recumbency (for examination of right lung) or right lateral recumbency (for examination of left lung). After aseptic preparation, a small (1–2.5 cm) skin incision is made approximately 35% to 45% SVL between the second and third rows of lateral scales (**Fig. 3**). The subcutaneous, coelomic muscle and coelomic membrane are bluntly perforated. When the wall of the air sac (transparent avascular membrane) is reached, 2 fine stay sutures are placed to elevate it to the level of the skin incision (**Fig. 4**). After perforation of the air sac, the endoscope (rigid with or without the operating sheath, or even a flexible for giant boids) is introduced through the incision and directed cranially into the lower respiratory tract (**Fig. 5**). By directing the endoscope caudally, various visceral organs can be viewed through the transparent air sac (**Fig. 6**).

If there are pathologic changes, the affected part of the lungs can be sampled for further tests (cytology, culture, histology).[4,6–8] The tip of the flexible biopsy forceps is directed near the lung mucosa, and a sample is collected for laboratory investigation (**Fig. 7**). After examination/biopsy, the air sac membrane is closed with a single simple interrupted suture using absorbable suture material. Muscle and skin are closed routinely. This technique has been performed in pythons and boas with good to

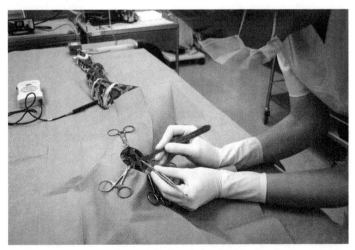

Fig. 3. Short skin incision on the right side of the body of a Burmese python (*Python molurus bivittatus*) to allow transcutaneous pulmonoscopy.

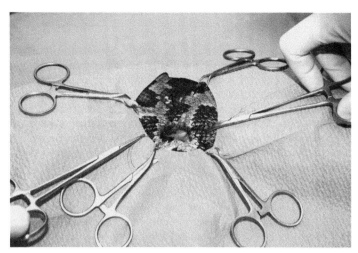

Fig. 4. Transcutaneous pulmonoscopy on a Burmese python (*Python molurus bivittatus*). Two fine stay sutures are placed to elevate the wall of the air sac to the skin incision.

excellent results depending on quality of sample handling.[4,6–8] Specimens that were gently shaken from biopsy forceps into saline solution before fixation in 2% glutaral-dehyde or 10% formalin had good to excellent diagnostic quality.[7,8] Re-evaluation of snakes investigated by this method months or a year later confirmed complete healing of the previous entry and the biopsy sites.[6–8]

COMPLICATIONS AND MANAGEMENT

The authors have not experienced any negative consequences associated with pulmonoscopy in snakes. However, excessive hemorrhage would be considered a complication of the transcutaneous method if the vascular wall of the lung is incised.

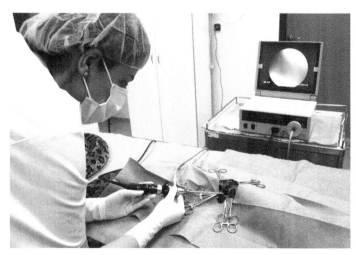

Fig. 5. Transcutaneous pulmonoscopy on a Burmese python (*Python molurus bivittatus*). The rigid endoscope with the operating sheath connected to an endoscopic camera is directed into the air sac.

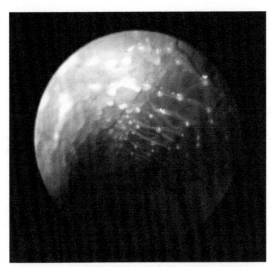

Fig. 6. Transcutaneous pulmonoscopy on a Burmese python (*Python molurus bivittatus*). Endoscopic indirect view of the liver surface (*arrowhead*) through the transparent air sac.

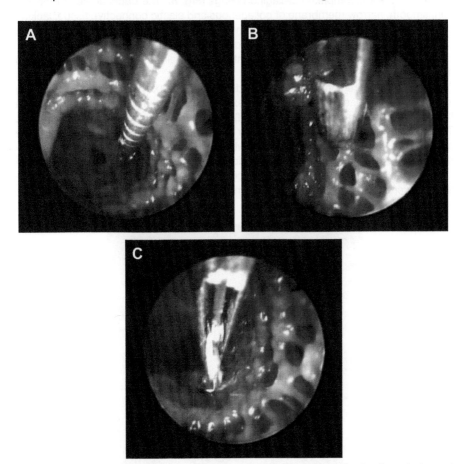

Fig. 7. The practical use of transcutaneous pulmonoscopy for sample collection from the lung of a Burmese python (*Python molurus bivittatus*). The tip of the flexible biopsy forceps is directed to the purulent exudate (*A*), and a sample is collected (*B, C*) for laboratory investigation.

POSTOPERATIVE CARE

No specific postoperative practices are required after pulmonoscopy.

CLINICAL IMPLICATIONS

The tracheal approach is mostly used to image the upper respiratory tract (trachea, primary bronchus). Depending on the size of the snake and equipment available, evaluation of the primary/intrapulmonary bronchus, faveolar lung, transitional zone, and distal air sac is possible. However, the transcutaneous approach is for examination of the lung(s) and air sac(s). Pulmonoscopy via the transcutaneous approach will likely minimize contamination, and samples can be taken aseptically. The transcutaneous approach enables observation of some coelomic organs through the air sac membrane.

NORMAL TRACHEAL, LUNG, AND AIR SAC APPEARANCE

The trachea has incomplete cartilaginous rings (**Fig. 8**). The tracheal membrane is a thin, smooth, narrow membrane of collagenous and elastic connective tissue, lacking muscle fibers. The tracheal membrane increases and gradually transforms into the main part of the respiratory tract in the distal part of the trachea. In many snakes, the vascular portion of the lung extends anteriorly dorsally in the distal trachea forming a tracheal lung.[19]

The respiratory region of the lung is divided and subdivided by interconnecting septae or trabeculae into terminal gas exchange chambers. This gives the lung a honeycomb appearance when opened, flattened, and viewed from above (**Fig. 9**). The heavily perfused lungs are red color and can easily be distinguished from the grey-white air sac, the vascularization of which is much poorer or absent. The 2 clearly defined regions are separated by a transitional zone of varying magnitude in which the parenchyma gradually becomes less concentrated and the faveoli exhibit larger diameters, lower and thinner walls, and fewer horizontal tiers.[4,8,11] In some snake species

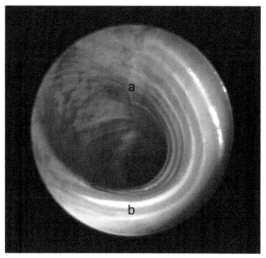

Fig. 8. Tracheoscopy in a Boa constrictor. Tracheal membrane (a) and ventral canal composed of incomplete tracheal cartilaginous rings (b).

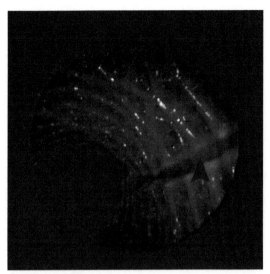

Fig. 9. Tracheoscopy in a Boa constrictor. Note the main bronchus (*arrowhead*) on the ventral aspect of the right lung.

(*Gonyosoma* sp, *Naja* sp, *Boiga* sp, and other arboreal colubrids) the transition from the vascular lung to the avascular air sac is abrupt.

When the endoscope is oriented in the caudal direction, the shape, size and external surface of the liver, spleen, and gallbladder can be seen (see **Fig. 6**). The liver lies behind the external wall of the lungs, and the air sac and appears grey-brown to red-brown. Normally, the caudal part of the air sac is not observed with the endoscope. A peculiar feature of the air sac is an abruptly tapered caudal portion. The air sac constricts to 10% to 20% of its cranial diameter and continues to its tip as a very slender tail. The position of the air sac tip is sexually dimorphic in most species of snakes, with the tip more caudally placed in males than in females.[5,11,20]

COMMON DISEASES OF LUNGS IN SNAKES

Chronic bacterial pneumonia is a major cause of morbidity and mortality in captive snakes, especially imported animals kept under low-quality husbandry practices (eg, suboptimal temperature, very low/high air humidity, and substrate of terrarium contaminated with urine and feces). The major symptom of LRTD in snakes is dyspnea, characterized by open-mouth breathing.[1,19,21–25]

Snakes with LRTD are usually weak and lethargic. Because of long-term anorexia, weight loss may be seen in snake patients with LRTD. Snakes with severe mouth lesions aspirate necrotic debris into the lower respiratory tract. Bacterial pneumonia may easily result from previous stomatitis and trachea infections may result from minimal self-cleaning property of the snake respiratory tract (**Fig. 10**). The lining of the snake respiratory tract has a primitive mucociliary apparatus, resulting in poor clearing of inflammatory exudates from their lungs.[23–25]

Trachea and bronchi are lined with ciliated, nonciliated secretory, and basal epithelial cells. These cells continue into the lung of those reptiles having intrapulmonary bronchi. Infection in the lung leads to the accumulation of exudate within the airways and eventual consolidation of one or more segments of the lung.[21,24] The

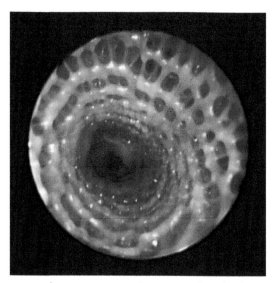

Fig. 10. Transcutaneous pulmonoscopy on a Burmese python (*Python molurus bivittatus*). Note the edematous mucosa and accumulation of purulent exudate caused by chronic bacterial pneumonia by (*Pseudomonas sp*).

exudate is thick and tenacious, and a frothy or purulent exudate may be visualized in the glottis, trachea, lung, and air sac.[24]

Bacterial infections of lungs are common but are generally secondary diseases in immunologically compromised snake patients. Most of the bacteria isolated are from the gram-negative group (eg, *Aeromonas*, *Citrobacter*, *Escherichia*, *Klebsiella*, *Morganella*, *Pasteurella*, *Proteus*, *Providentia*, *Pseudomonas*, and many others). These bacteria are invasive especially after a primary viral infection, such as para-myxovirus pneumonia.[21,25] Infection of lungs with *Mycobacterium haemophilum* and *Mycobacterium marinum* were identified in a python, but *Mycobacteriaceae* are not commonly present in airway mucosa of healthy snakes.[26] Lung mycoses caused with *Aspergillus* or *Paecilomyces* remain confined to the lungs or disseminated to other organ systems.[27] In such clinical cases of LRTD, the endoscopy with pulmonary wash and harvesting the biopsy material for cytology and bacterial culture with sensitivity test are recommended (see **Fig. 7**; **Figs. 11** and **12**).

OUTCOMES

Table 1 compares outcomes with pulmonoscopy methods in snakes between the tracheal and transcutaneous approaches.

CURRENT CONTROVERSIES/FUTURE CONSIDERATIONS

Evaluation of the transcutaneous approach for examination and biopsy of the lungs in boid snakes has been published.[4,6–8] In addition, the direct access to the lung(s) and air sac(s) also facilitates therapy.[6] Indwelling pulmonary catheters can be placed under endoscopic guidance for antibiotic delivery.[28,29] The collection of liver biopsies (and some other organs) through the air sac wall may also be of value in clinical practice (SJ Divers, personal communication, 2013).

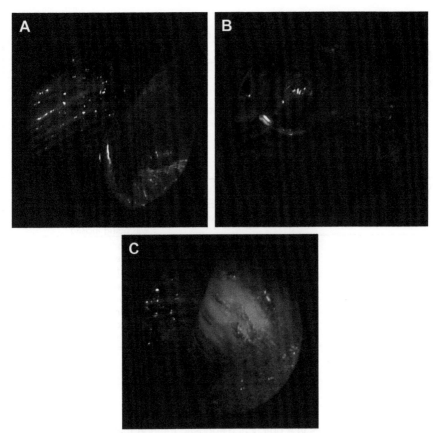

Fig. 11. Endoscopy-assisted air sac catheterization in a Burmese python (*Python molurus bivittatus*). Direct pulmonary wash with sterile saline solution (*A, B*) is followed with aspiration of the sample for laboratory investigation (*C*).

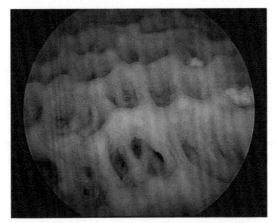

Fig. 12. Transcutaneous pulmonoscopy in a Burmese python (*Python molurus bivittatus*). Note the microscopic yellow particles of purulent exudate in the faveolar mucosa.

Table 1
Pulmonoscopy in snakes—comparison between tracheal and transcutaneous approaches

Pulmonoscopy Method	Tracheal Approach	Transcutaneous Approach
Indications Clinical implications	Tracheoscopy Bronchoscopy Pulmonoscopy Air sac endoscopy (mostly the proximal part of air sac) Bronchial lavage	Endoscopy of air sac Pulmonoscopy Endoscopy of the distal part of trachea Bronchial and lung lavage Air sac lavage Catheter insertion Indirect view on liver and some other organs in coelom
Contraindications	In cases in which anesthesia would be an unacceptable risk.	In cases in which anesthesia would be an unacceptable risk
Complications	Iatrogenic trauma of trachea	Bleeding if the wall of the lung was being incised
Anesthesia, analgesia	Mandatory although may be performed under deep sedation	Mandatory Analgesia: opiods, nonsteroidal anti-inflammatory drugs
Postoperative care	Special treatment not necessary	Closing separately the air sac wall, the muscle layer, and the skin Analgesics should be administered for 5–7 d

SUMMARY

Pulmonoscopy in snakes is a practical diagnostic method that allows detailed visualization and magnification of the lower respiratory tract and facilitates the collection of samples for laboratory tests. The method is indicated for the evaluation of snakes with clinical signs of respiratory disease, including dyspnea or tracheal discharge. Two standard methods of endoscopic examination of the snake lung exist. Noninvasive tracheobronchoscopy using rigid endoscopes allows examination of the trachea, the lung, and air sac in small specimens. In medium to large snakes this method depends on the use of longer rigid or flexible endoscopes of appropriate diameter.

The approach through the air sac allows thorough evaluation of the air sac, transitional zone, faveolar lung, primary/intrapulmonary bronchus, and even the distal part of the trachea. When the endoscope is oriented in the distal direction, the shape, size and external surface of the liver, spleen and gallbladder can be viewed. The air sac endoscopy allows the introduction and placement of an air sac catheter for drug delivery directly in the lung.

Both pulmonoscopy methods are safe, and contraindications for pulmonoscopy in snakes have not been documented. The only known contraindication is associated with anesthesia.

ACKNOWLEDGMENTS

The authors thank Dr A. Musilova, Dr S.M. Rusu, and E. Knotkova for their kind assistance in production of the pictures.

REFERENCES

1. Knotek Z, Kley N, Hess C, et al. Treatment of Chronic Pneumonia in a Burmese Python using the Air Sac Tube Placement Technique. Proc 7th Congres international sur les Animaux Sauvages et Exotique YABOUMBA, Muséum national d'Histoire Naturelle. Paris, March 26–28, 2010. p. 207.
2. Mc Cracken HE. Organ location in snakes for diagnostic and surgical evaluation. In: Fowler ME, Miller RE, editors. Zoo and wild animal medicine: current therapy. 4th.edition. Philadelphia: WB Saunders; 1999. p. 243–9.
3. Taylor M. Endoscopy in birds and reptiles. In: Tams TR, editor. Small animal endoscopy. 2nd edition. , St Louis (MO): Mosby; 1999. p. 433–46.
4. Divers SJ. Endoscopic evaluation of the reptilian respiratory system. Exotic DVM 2001;3(3):61–4.
5. Jekl V, Knotek Z. Endoscopic examination of snakes by access through an air sac. Vet Rec 2006;158:407–10.
6. Knotek Z, Jekl V. Advances in exotic animal endoscopy. Proc. 31st WSAVA/12th FECAVA/14th CSAVA Wold Congress. Prague (Czech Republic), October 11–14, 2006. p. 337–9.
7. Stahl SJ, Hernandez-Divers SJ, Cooper TL, et al. Evaluation of transcutaneous pulmonoscopy for examination and biopsy of the lungs of ball pythons and determination of preferred biopsy specimen handling and fixation procedures. J Am Vet Med Assoc 2008;233:440–5.
8. Divers SJ. Diagnostic endoscopy. In: Mader DR, Divers SJ, editors. Current therapy in reptile medicine and surgery. St Louis (MO): Elsevier Saunders; 2014. p. 154–78.
9. Diethelm G, Stauber E, Tillson M, et al. Tracheal resection and anastomosis for an intratracheal chordoma in a ball python. J Am Vet Med Assoc 1996;209:786–8.
10. Wood SC, Lefant CJ. Respiration: mechanics, control and gas exchange. In: Gans C, Dawson WR, editors. Biology of the Reptilia, vol. 5. London: Academic Press; 1976. p. 225–74.
11. Wallach V. The lung of snakes. Morphology G. In: Gans C, Gaunt AS, editors. Biology of the reptilia. Visceral organs, vol. 19. St Louis (MO): Society for the Study of Amphibians and Reptiles; 1998. p. 93–173.
12. Knotek Z. Reptiles – advances in anaesthesia. Proc. 8th Annual Conference Unusual and Exotic Pet (UEP) Veterinarians. Alice Springs (Australia), October 7–9, 2011. p. 17–31.
13. Sladky K. Analgesia. In: Mader DR, Divers SJ, editors. Current therapy in reptile medicine and surgery. St Louis (MO): Elsevier Saunders; 2014. p. 217–28.
14. Redrobe S. Anesthesia and analgesia. In: Girling SJ, Raiti P, editors. BSAVA manual of reptiles. Gloucester (United Kingdom): BSAVA; 2004. p. 131–46.
15. Knotek Z, Jekl V, Knotkova Z, et al. Tiletamine-zolazepam anaesthesia in reptiles. Proc. BVZS Autumn Meeting. November 11–13, 2005. Royal Veterinary College Hatfield. p. 103–4.
16. Schumacher J, Yelen T. Anesthesia and analgesia. In: Mader DR, editor. Reptile medicine and surgery. St. Louis (MO): Elsevier; 2006. p. 442–52.
17. Bertelsen MF. Squamates (lizards and snakes). In: West G, Heard D, Caulkett N, editors. Zoo animal and wildlife immobilization and anaesthesia. Blackwell (OK): Aimes; 2007. p. 233–44.
18. Schumacher J, Mans C. Anesthesia. In: Mader DR, Divers SJ, editors. Current therapy in reptile medicine and surgery. St. Louis (MO): Elsevier Saunders; 2014. p. 134–228.

19. Schumacher J. Reptile respiratory medicine. Vet Clin North Am Exot Anim Pract 2003;6:213–31.

20. Keogh JS, Wallach V. Allometry and sexual dimorphism in the lung morphology of prairie rattlesnakes, Crotalus viridis viridis. Amphib-reptil 1999;20:377–89.

21. Jacobson ER. Bacterial diseases of reptiles. In: Jacobson E, editor. Infectious diseases and pathology of reptiles. Boca Raton (FL): CRC Press; 2007. p. 461–526.

22. Chitty J. Respiratory system. In: Girling SJ, Raiti P, editors. BSAVA manual of reptiles. 2nd edition. Quedgeley (United Kingdom): BSAVA; 2004. p. 230–42.

23. Stoakes LC. Respiratory system. In: Beynon PH, Lawton MP, Cooper JE, editors. BSAVA manual of reptiles. 1st edition. Cheltenham (United Kingdom): BSAVA; 1992. p. 88–100.

24. Jacobson ER. Overview of reptile biology, anatomy and histology. In: Jacobson E, editor. Infectious diseases and pathology of reptiles. Boca Raton (FL): CRC Press; 2007. p. 1–130.

25. Murray MJ. Pneumonia and normal respiratory function. In: Mader DR, editor. Reptile medicine and surgery. Philadelphia: WB Saunders; 1996. p. 396–405.

26. Hernandez-Divers SJ, Shearer D. Pulmonary mycobacteriosis caused by Mycobacterium haemophilum and Mycobacterium marinum in a royal python. J Am Vet Med Assoc 2002;220:1661–3.

27. Paré JA, Jacobson ER. Mycotic diseases of reptiles. In: Jacobson E, editor. Infectious diseases and pathology of reptiles. Boca Raton (FL): CRC Press; 2007. p. 527–70.

28. Myers DA, Wellehan JF, Isaza R, et al. Air sac tube placement in a ball python (Python regius) to treat respiratory obstruction secondary to pneumonia. Proc. 15th ARAV Annual Conference. Los Angeles (CA), 2008. p. 23.

29. Knotek Z, Kley N, Hess C, et al. Treatment of chronic pneumonia in a Burmese python using the air sac tube placemement Technique. Proc 7th Congres international sur les Animaux Sauvages et Exotique YABOUMBA. Paris, March 26–28, 2010. p. 207.

Clinical Applications of Cystoscopy in Chelonians

Nicola Di Girolamo, DMV, MSc (EBHC),
Paolo Selleri, DMV, PhD, DipECZM (Herpetology & Small Mammals)*

KEYWORDS

- Cystoscopy • Chelonians • Turtles • Tortoises • Liver • Celioscopy

KEY POINTS

- Cystoscopy with rigid and flexible endoscopes is feasible in chelonians.
- The transparency of the urinary bladder wall can be used to visualize the coelom.
- Altered morphology of organs may indicate a diseased system.
- Cystoscopic visualization of the coelom may assist clinicians in achieving owner consensus for further examinations.

INTRODUCTION

The urinary bladder is one of the most unusual organs of chelonians, intriguing scientists for several centuries.[1-3] Historically, cloacoscopy and cystoscopy have been used for evaluation of intrinsic disorders of the cloaca, urinary bladder, and accessory bladders.[4] More recently, a novel diagnostic application of cystoscopy has been described using the transparency of the organ to visualize the coelom.[5]

The value of cystoscopy as a diagnostic tool relies on 2 main features of the chelonian urinary bladder: morphology and size.

Morphology

The bladder wall is composed of mucosa and serosa. The first consists of an epithelial cell layer and subepithelial connective tissue layer (with a few small bundles of smooth muscle cells), whereas the latter (serosa) consists of smooth muscle bundles and connective tissues (**Fig. 1**).[6] Given this structure, the urinary bladder wall has a thin and transparent surface when distended.

Conflicts of interest: The authors declare that they have no financial or nonfinancial competing interests in relation to this article.
Clinica per Animali Esotici, Centro Veterinario Specialistico, Via Sandro Giovannini 53, Roma 00137, Italy
* Corresponding author.
E-mail address: paolsell@gmail.com

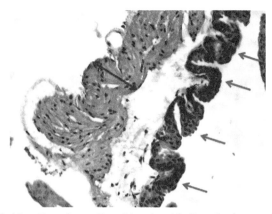

Fig. 1. Urinary bladder, *Testudo* sp. Transitional epithelium (*red arrows*). Smooth muscle layer (*blue arrows*) (original magnification 20×, hematoxylin-eosin stain). (*Courtesy of* Raffaele Melidone, DVM, Dipl ACVP, Irvine, CA.)

Size

The bladder is a greatly distensible organ that can accommodate large quantities of fluids (ie, up to 30% of the total body weight of the chelonian).[1,2,7,8] Therefore, once distended, the urinary bladder comes in contact with most coelomic viscera, including kidneys, gonads, adrenals, small and large intestine, stomach, pancreas, liver, lungs, and heart (**Fig. 2**).

Results of our clinical experience and current research[5,9] show that presence of the urinary bladder wall between the endoscope and the coelomic cavity does not

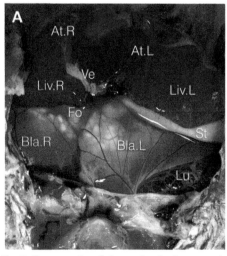
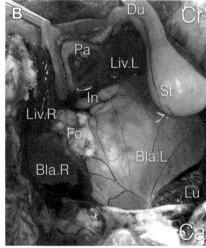

Fig. 2. Topography of the coelomic viscera and anatomic relationships with a fully distended urinary bladder. Adult female red-eared slider turtle (*Trachemys scripta elegans*). (*A*) Topography after plastron removal. (*B*) The stomach and the duodenum were reflected. At.L, left atrium; At.R, right atrium; Bla.L, urinary bladder, left lobe; Bla.R, urinary bladder, right lobe; Ca, caudal; Cr, cranial; Du, duodenum; Fo, follicles; In, intestine; Liv.L, liver, left lobe; Liv.R, liver, right lobe; Lu, lungs; Pa, pancreas; St, stomach; Ve, ventricle.

preclude the visualization of coelomic organs in chelonians and that this technique may be valuable to reptile clinicians.

INDICATIONS

Chelonian cystoscopy is indicated for:

- Chelonians with a nonspecific illness, as an initial screening technique to identify the diseased organ
- Chelonians with dystocia, potentially to screen for ectopic eggs in the bladder
- Chelonians with uroliths, for diagnosis and possible treatment
- Chelonians that underwent trauma, to evaluate bladder integrity
- Severely debilitated chelonians, in which more invasive diagnostic procedure may be dangerous
- Selected species of chelonians lacking sexual dimorphism or for selected immature chelonians, in order to identify the sex

Cystoscopy is contraindicated for:

- Selected species/size of chelonians because of the risk of iatrogenic bladder rupture
- Chelonians that have previously been diagnosed with cystitis or bladder opacity

TECHNIQUE
Chelonian Positioning

Chelonians may be positioned in dorsal or ventral recumbency for cloacoscopy.[5,10–12] In the authors' experience, placing the chelonian in ventral recumbency provides easier access to the urinary bladder. The following are instructions for replicating the authors' technique:

- Small chelonians (<100 g): the operator holds the turtle in ventral recumbency with the left hand, while the right hand maneuvers the rigid endoscope (**Fig. 3A**).[5]
- Medium-sized chelonians (100–2000 g): an assistant elevates the turtle away from the table to expose the cloaca (see **Fig. 3B**). The assistant is responsible for coordinating with the operator, tilting the animal if necessary for improved visibility as needed. The operator may also gain stability by placing the elbows on the surgical table.

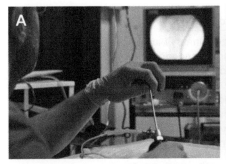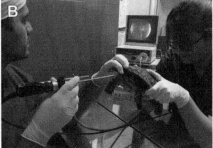

Fig. 3. Positioning of small chelonian for cystoscopy. (*A*) Single-operator technique. This is the authors' favorite approach for small chelonians (<100 g).[5] (*B*) Two-operators technique. Note that the assistant leans the elbows on the work-top and is opposite to the operator, who faces the monitor. Fluid infusion was interrupted as cystoscopy was terminated.

- Large-sized (>2000 g) and instrumented chelonians: if the chelonian is too big for proper handling, it is positioned on an elevated surface, to allow the hind limbs and tail to hang.[12] This position is also used for chelonians of all sizes that require general anesthesia and are therefore connected to medical equipment (eg, intubated, catheterized). Most of these animals require longer anesthesia and additional procedures (eg, ectopic egg retrieval, urolith removal, celioscopy).

Special equipment
In the authors' experience cystoscopy has been performed successfully in small to medium-sized chelonians (eg, 20–4000 g) with a 2.7-mm diameter, 18-cm length, 30° viewing rigid endoscope housed within a 3.5-mm protective sheath (64019 BA, Storz, Karl Storz Gmbh and Co, Tuttlingen, Germany) or with a 9.5-French, 14-cm length, 30° viewing rigid telescope with working channel (Storz, Karl Storz Gmbh and Co, Tuttlingen, Germany). In smaller chelonians (eg, *Testudo* sp, *Cuora* sp, *Trachemys* sp, *Graptemys* sp, <20 g) we suggest the use of smaller equipment, such as a 1.9-mm rigid endoscope with a separated or integrated operating sheath (Storz, Karl Storz Gmbh and Co, Tuttlingen, Germany) or integrated 8-French cystourethroscope (27030 KA, Storz, Karl Storz Gmbh and Co, Tuttlingen, Germany).[13] In larger chelonians or in certain terrestrial species (eg, *Geochelone* sp) the use of flexible endoscopes should be considered,[11] because the prominence of the caudal carapacial scutes may impede appropriate maneuvering of a rigid endoscope.

ENDOSCOPY PROCEDURES
Cystoscopy

The endoscope is gently inserted in the vent and directed cranially (**Fig. 4**A) in order to reach the cloaca. The cloaca is a saclike cavity into which the ureters, gonadal ducts, colon, and bladders empty.[14] In some aquatic turtles, paired saclike structures, the accessory bladders, open into the cloaca dorsal to the colon (see **Fig. 4**B). The endoscope, once in the cloaca, is directed toward the urethral opening, which is located ventral to the rectum (see **Fig. 4**C and D). Access to the urethral sphincter is gained by gentle ventral pressure. Warm (30°C) fluids are infused (1 drop every 3–4 seconds) during the procedure to allow distension of the urethral opening. Careful attention should be paid to avoid overdistension of the bladder in small chelonians. Gentle pressure and fluid infusion are usually sufficient to gain access to the urinary bladder.

Identification of Coelomic Organs via Cystoscopy

Chelonians have a large, bilobed, vascularized urinary bladder (see **Fig. 2**; **Fig. 5**B and C).[3,15] The empty bladder is not transparent and does not allow visualization of coelomic viscera (see **Fig. 5**A). Infusion of fluids should be interrupted when the bladder is distended enough to permit visualization of coelomic viscera. This technique is identical to the one described for visualization of gonads in immature Hermann's tortoises (*Testudo hermanni*), marginated tortoises (*Testudo marginata*), and yellow-bellied slider turtles (*Trachemys scripta*),[5] except that, once access to the urinary bladder is gained, the endoscope is directed:

1. Cranially to visualize liver, intestine, stomach, heart, pancreas
2. Dorsally to visualize lungs
3. Dorsolaterally to visualize left and right kidneys, gonads, and left and right adrenal glands

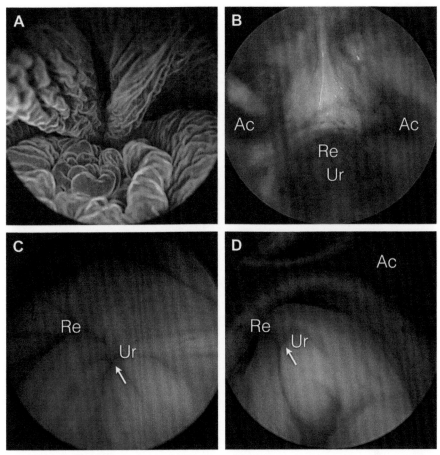

Fig. 4. Cloacoscopy and cystoscopy in red-eared sliders (*T scripta elegans*) and Hermann's tortoises (*Testudo hermanni*). (*A*) Normal, melanistic aspect of the mucosa preceding the cloaca. (*B*) Representative image of the cloaca in a freshwater turtle. Note the presence of accessory bladders (Ac) lateral to the rectum (Re). The access to the bladder is reached by inserting the endoscope in the urethral opening (Ur) under fluid instillation. (*C* and *D*) Comparative appearance of the urethral opening (*arrows*) in turtles (*C*) and tortoises (*D*) and its relationship to the rectum.

Adjustments to the described directions are required when cystoscopy is performed with the animal in dorsal recumbency. In some instances (eg, when the gastrointestinal [GI] tract is distended), tilting the animal into dorsal recumbency may aid in the visualization of obscured organs.

Uric acid accumulations are commonly found in the urinary bladder (see **Fig. 5**D), and should not be considered pathologic. In some neonate/juvenile animals, the caudal vena cava (dorsal to the urinary bladder) and the yolk sac (cranial to the urinary bladder) may also be identified.

Identification of the gastrointestinal tract via cystoscopy
The distended urinary bladder comes into contact with various sections of the GI tract, including stomach and small and large intestines. With the animal in ventral

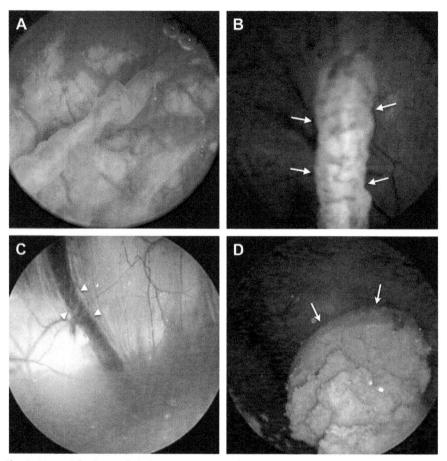

Fig. 5. Normal findings of chelonian cystoscopy (*Testudo* sp, *Trachemys* sp). (*A*) The urinary bladder is not distended and lacks transparency, therefore not allowing visualization of the coelomic organs. (*B*) Incomplete septum dividing the 2 lobes of the urinary bladder (*arrows*). (*C*) Normal vasculature of the urinary bladder wall (*arrowheads*). (*D*) Small quantities of uric acids in the urinary bladder are normal (*arrows*).

recumbency during cystoscopy, the stomach is located in the left midcoelom and may be distinguished from the intestine by its shape and size. In young chelonians, some sections of the GI tract are transparent and allow visualization of the ingesta (**Fig. 6**A). The large intestine may present with a longitudinal striped pattern (see **Fig. 6**B).

In chelonians with severe distension of the intestinal tract (see **Fig. 6**C, F) the external morphology of the intestine may be altered, with blood vessels prominent on the serosal surface (see **Fig. 6**E). In the authors' experience, this abnormal pattern is easily identified during cystoscopy (see **Fig. 6**D) and in association with other diagnostic tests (eg, radiography) may aid in establishing the diagnosis.

Identification of liver, pancreas, and spleen via cystoscopy

In chelonians, the liver is large and occupies most of the ventrocranial coelom (see **Fig. 2**A). The left lobe is connected to the stomach by the gastrohepatic ligament, whereas the right lobe is connected to the duodenum by the hepatoduodenal ligament

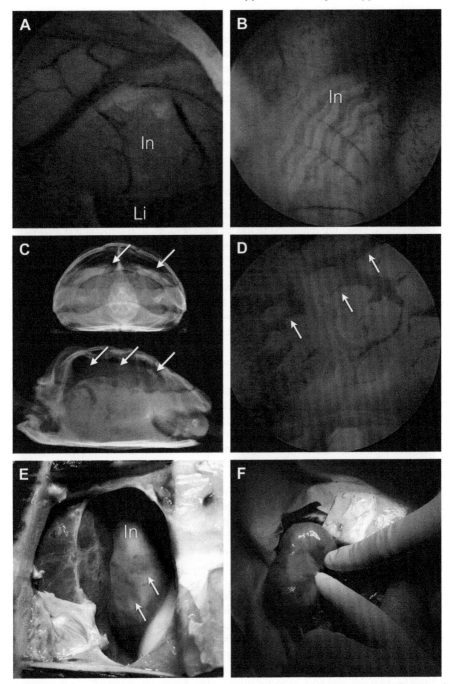

Fig. 6. Clinical application of cystoscopy for visualization of the GI tract. (*A* and *B*) Normal intestine in hatchling and juvenile turtles (*Trachemys scripta scripta, Cuora trifasciata*). (*C*) Anteroposterior and lateral radiographs of a Russian tortoise (*Agrionemys horsfieldii*) showing severe enlargement of the GI tract (*arrows*). (*D*) On cystoscopy the intestine appeared dilated with several hemorrhages on the serosa (*arrows*). (*E*) Intraoperative plastronotomy confirmed the dilatation and the hemorrhages (*arrows*) on the serosa. (*F*) Note that the whole GI tract was dilated because of ingested bark. Li, liver.

(see **Fig. 2**B).[14] During cystoscopy, the dorsal surface and caudal edges of the liver are visualized when the urinary bladder is moderately to maximally distended. The liver in healthy chelonians (except breeding females) is brown to dark red, with sharp edges and homogeneous texture (**Fig. 7**A). In the authors' experience, visualization of the liver allows identification of focal, multifocal, and diffuse morphologic alterations of the liver (see **Fig. 7**B–F). Biopsy and hence diagnosis is not possible through cystoscopy. During cystoscopic examination the following characteristics should be evaluated for abnormalities:

- Color (see **Fig. 7**B, E, F)
- Texture (see **Fig. 7**C, D)
- Edges (eg, rounded edges may indicate hepatomegaly) (see **Fig. 7**E)

Pancreas, spleen, and gallbladder are visualized through cystoscopy, depending on the interposition and the dilatation of the GI tract (**Fig. 8**). The pancreas is visualized from the left lobe of the urinary bladder, and is in contact with the stomach, duodenum, and liver (see **Fig. 8**A). Alterations in the shape and morphology of the pancreas can potentially be visualized. The spleen is difficult to locate and is sometimes visible from the left lobe of the urinary bladder, close to the pancreas. The gallbladder is located on the caudal surface of the right liver lobe. During cystoscopy, the distal portion of the gallbladder is visible (see **Fig. 8**B). In the authors' experience, the biliary ducts are not easily visualized because of the interposition of the intestine.

Identification of heart and lungs via cystoscopy

The heart is located in the cranioventral coelom (see **Fig. 2**A). With the bladder fully distended, a view of the beating heart is usually possible (**Fig. 9**A, B). Only disorders that result in visible changes in the external aspects of the heart may be identified (but not definitively diagnosed) through cystoscopy, including cardiomegaly, atrial and/or ventricular distension, pericardial effusion with or without cardiac tamponade, macroscopic pericardial changes (eg, changes that may be caused by fibrotic pericarditis, suppurative pericarditis), forms of myocarditis with macroscopic changes (eg, granulomatous myocarditis), and neoplasms.

A moderate distension of the bladder permits visualization of the lungs dorsally. The lungs are easily recognizable because of the characteristic edicular tissue (see **Fig. 9**C, D). With cystoscopy, only a limited portion of the lungs (ie, their ventral aspect) may be visualized. Lesions that can be observed through this window are those in which accumulation of fluids (eg, suppurative pneumonia, edema) or nodular changes (eg, fungal or mycobacterial granulomatous pneumonia, neoplasms) develop.

Identification of the kidneys and reproductive tract via cystoscopy

The kidneys are paired structures located in the caudodorsal retrocoelom and are in close association with the gonads. To visualize the kidneys and gonads, the endoscope is directed dorsally and laterally. On endoscopy, the kidneys are visualized as brown to pink, lobulated, flat to elliptical structures (**Fig. 10**A). Because of their retrocoelomic location, 2 transparent structures lie between the endoscope and the kidneys (ie, bladder wall and coelomic membrane), limiting their visualization. In immature chelonians the ovaries are elongated, yellow/white to translucent, slightly convoluted organs characterized by rounded, whitish follicles. The oviduct is a straight, flat, transparent to white band located immediately lateral and parallel to the ovary. In mature chelonians the ovaries are characterized by variably sized, yellowish to orange follicles and the oviducts are pinkish to white, well-developed, hollow organs. The testes are usually superimposed on the kidneys and are elongated to oval/round in

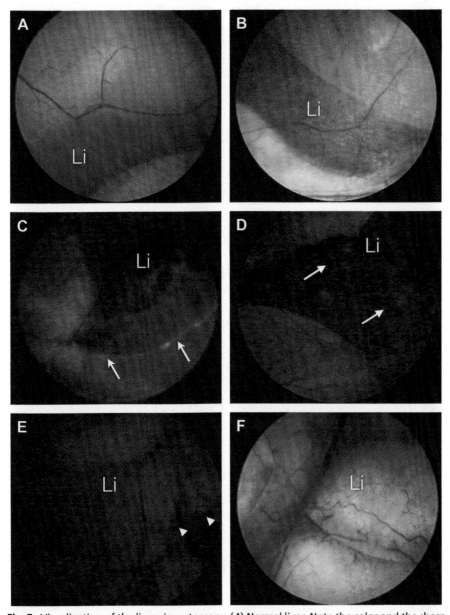

Fig. 7. Visualization of the liver via cystoscopy. (*A*) Normal liver. Note the color and the sharp edges. (*B*) Liver, discolored. The turtle was confirmed to have moderate hepatic lipidosis by celioscopic biopsy. (*C*) Liver with whitish diffuse surface alterations. Note the scalloped margins (*arrows*). (*D*) Liver with multifocal, irregularly shaped, white-tan, and roughly round areas of discoloration on the capsular surface (*arrows*). Granulomatous hepatitis was subsequently diagnosed by celioscopic biopsy. (*E*) Liver, discolored. The rounded margins (*arrowheads*) suggest hepatomegaly. (*F*) Liver, discolored.

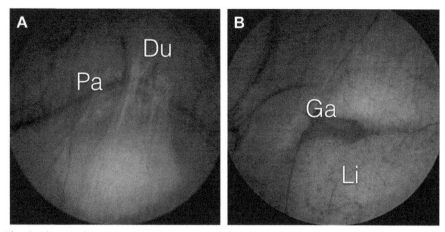

Fig. 8. Liver and pancreas visualization. (*A*) Visualization of the pancreas via cystoscopy. Note the proximity with the duodenum. (*B*) Visualization of the gallbladder through the right lobe of the urinary bladder. Ga, gallbladder.

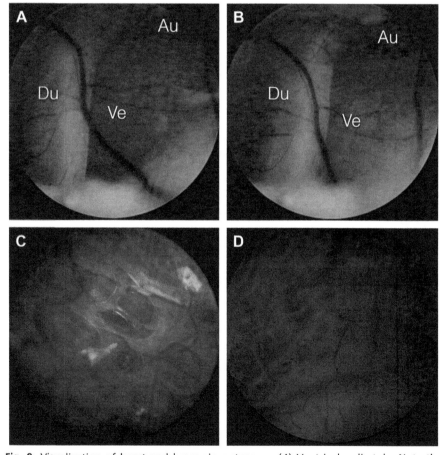

Fig. 9. Visualization of heart and lungs via cystoscopy. (*A*) Ventricular diastole. Note the dilation of the ventricle. (*B*) Ventricular systole. (*C* and *D*) Ventral aspect of the lungs. The edicular structures are easily identified. Au, auricle.

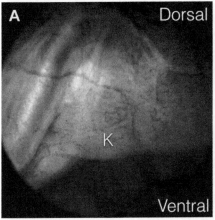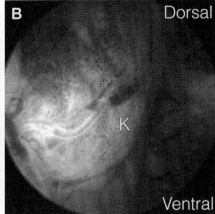

Fig. 10. Kidney visualization through cystoscopy in a red-eared slider (*T scripta elegans*). (*A*) Urinary bladder cystoscopy. (*B*) Right accessory bladder cystoscopy. The accessory bladder view shows the lateral aspect of the kidney, whereas the urinary bladder view shows its ventral aspect. K, kidney.

shape, tan to yellow in color, and have a smooth surface characterized by a tight net of superficial blood vessels.[5] Note that both feminine and masculine organs may have significant changes according to species and seasonality. More detailed information on the use of endoscopy for evaluation of the reproductive tract in chelonians is provided elsewhere in this issue.

Identification and Treatment of Bladder Disorders via Cystoscopy

Urinary bladder calculi
Urinary bladder calculi are a common occurrence in chelonians and are easily diagnosed by means of plain radiography.[7] Cystoscopy may confirm the diagnosis and aid in urolith removal. The authors have successfully removed small calculi using a purposefully designed endoscopic basket (Stone Extractor, 4-wire basket, outer diameter 0.4 mm, Storz, Karl Storz Gmbh and Co, Tuttlingen, Germany) through the working sheath of the telescope in chelonians as small as 27 g (**Fig. 11**A and B). Large uroliths have been fragmented into smaller parts using holmium laser (holmium:yttrium-aluminum-garnet [Ho:YAG], Quanta System, Italy) (see **Fig. 11**C). In a yellow-bellied slider turtle (*T scripta scripta*), a 2100-μm Ho:YAG laser (QuantaSystem Q1, Quanta System S.p.A., Solbiate Olona, VA, Italy) with a 365-μm fiber probe was used through the operating sheath of the telescope for lithotripsy.[16] The laser was first set at 12 W/1.2 J/10 Hz to fragment the calculus into several parts, and then at 8 W/0.7 J/12 Hz to pulverize the material into tiny fragments. Large fragments were removed using an endoscope basket, and small fragments were flushed out with irrigation.[16]

Ectopic eggs in the urinary bladder
Ectopic eggs in the urinary bladder are frequently diagnosed.[11,12,17,18] Oxytocin therapy may be a predisposing factor for the presence of ectopic egg in the organ.[12] In the authors' experience, ectopic eggs have been observed in conjunction with metabolic bone disease and a lack of appropriate digging substrate.

Plain radiography does not allow the identification of the exact location of the eggs and may lead to misinterpretations (eg, salpinges vs bladder).[11] Cystoscopy may allow localization of the egg by indirect or direct visualization (ectopic eggs in the bladder)

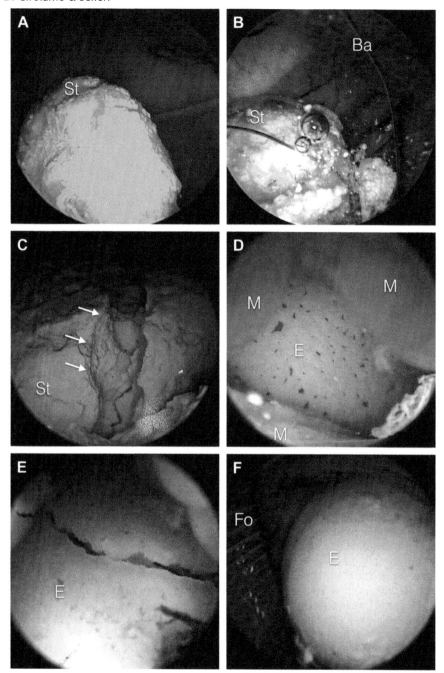

Fig. 11. Diagnosis and management of urinary bladder disorders in chelonians. (*A*) Visualization of a urolith via cystoscopy in a Hermann's tortoise (*T hermanni*). (*B*) Removal of the urolith with a 4-wire basket. (*C*) Destruction of a urolith by use of a holmium laser (*arrows*) in a yellow-bellied slider turtle (*T scripta scripta*). (*D*) An ectopic egg in the urinary bladder of a Hermann's tortoise. (*E*) An ectopic, broken egg in the urinary bladder of a Hermann's tortoise. (*F*) Destruction of the ectopic egg in (*D*) with a forceps. Ba, basket; E, egg; Fo, forceps; M, bladder neck mucus; St, bladder stone. ([*C*] *Courtesy of* Giordano Nardini, DMV, PhD, Dipl ECZM (Herpetology), Modena, Italy.)

(see **Fig. 11**D, E). Techniques of varying degrees of invasiveness may be used to treat this condition:

1. Plastron osteotomy followed by cystotomy
2. Prefemoral incision followed by cystotomy
3. Cystoscopic approaches, including removal of the entire egg with a snare,[11,12] or destruction of the egg and removal of the fragments followed by lavage (see **Fig. 11**F)[18]

Bladder rupture and urocoelom

Cystoscopy may be useful to evaluate bladder integrity in traumatized chelonians or in chelonians with chronic cystitis caused by ectopic eggs and uroliths (**Figs. 12 and 13**).

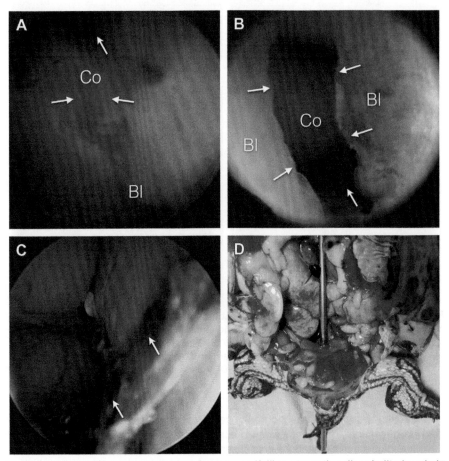

Fig. 12. Rupture of the urinary bladder after trauma (fall) in a juvenile yellow-bellied turtle (*T scripta scripta*). (*A*) The urinary bladder (Bl) does not distend during cystoscopy. Arrows indicate the rim of the tear on the urinary bladder wall. The coelom (Co) is visible through the lesion. (*B*) Close-up view of the tear under saline infusion. (*C*) The endoscope is passed through the lesion. Coelomic viscera are visible as in celioscopy. Note the lack of interposition of the bladder between the telescope and the viscera, and the presence of blood clots in the coelom (*arrows*). (*D*) Necropsy. A rod is passed through the cloaca, the urethra, and the lesion on the urinary bladder and reaches the coelom.

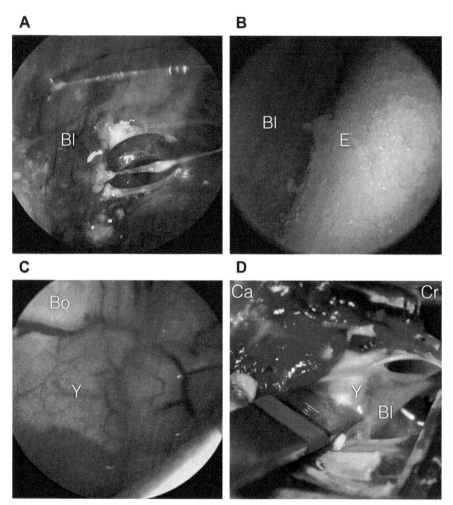

Fig. 13. Rupture of the urinary bladder in an adult female Hermann's tortoise with a broken ectopic egg in the bladder. (*A*) Cystoscopy showing altered internal aspect of the urinary bladder with presence of fibrinous material. (*B*) The shell of the broken egg (E) in the bladder. (*C*) Celioscopy through the ruptured urinary bladder and visualization of the yolk (Y) on the surface of the bowel (Bo). (*D*) Intraoperative plastronotomy. Removal of the egg from the urinary bladder.

In mammals, abdominal ultrasonography, retrograde contrast radiography, and retrograde contrast computed tomography are used for evaluation of bladder integrity.[19,20] Such techniques have limitations in chelonians because of their anatomy. Ultrasonography is limited by the presence of the shell, whereas retrograde cystography is limited by the need for cystoscopic guided catheterization of the urinary bladder. In chelonians, cystoscopy may be a more practical tool to evaluate bladder integrity, although fluid infusion and the risks of distributing contaminated material throughout the coelom must be considered.

During cystoscopy, rupture of the urinary bladder can be determined by:

1. Lack of distension following fluid infusion (see **Fig. 12**A, B)

2. Direct visualization of the coelomic viscera (ie, view is not obscured by bladder wall) (see **Figs. 12**C and **13**C)
3. Presence of fibrinous material inside the bladder (**Fig. 13**A)

Other findings

Cystoscopy may be useful to evaluate the macroscopic aspect and obtain biopsy of the bladder (**Fig. 14**A). Cystitis has been reported in chelonians[12] and its diagnosis may be confirmed through cystoscopy (see **Fig. 14**B). Parasites (eg, Polystomatidae) are occasionally found in the urinary bladder (see **Fig. 14**C, D).[21] Their significance is unclear, but they are presumed to be clinically unimportant.[22]

Accessory Bladder Cystoscopy

Accessory bladders, sometimes called bursae[23] or cloacal bladders,[15] are 2 saclike structures that open into the cloaca. Accessory bladders have been described in several aquatic and semiaquatic chelonians, but have not been described in terrestrial

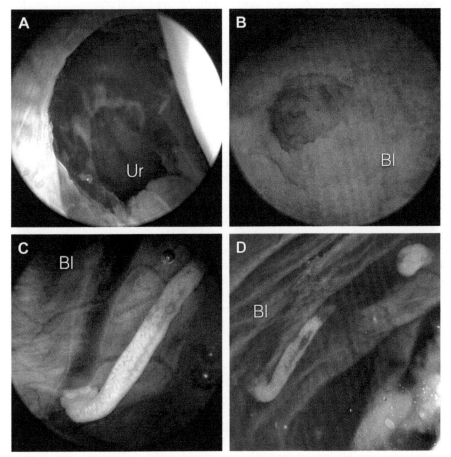

Fig. 14. Additional findings. (A) Cloacitis in a red-eared slider turtle. Note the inflammation of the mucous membranes. (B) Cystitis in a yellow-bellied slider turtle. Thickening of the urinary bladder wall (Ur). In this case the bladder was not transparent even after distension. Cystitis was confirmed by necropsy. (C) Endoscopic view of Polystomatidae in the urinary bladder of a red-eared slider turtle. (D) The Polystomatidae in (C).

chelonians.[2,23,24] The biological role of the accessory bladders is still unclear. The most widely accepted theory is that the accessory bladders function in aquatic respiration, buoyancy control, and/or as a water reservoir on land.[15]

Gaining access to the accessory bladders is usually easier and faster than gaining access to the urinary bladder,[25] because there is no sphincter or urethra (or bladder neck). Depending on the species, the accessory bladders may be as thin and transparent as the urinary bladder. Compared with the urinary bladder, these more lateral accessory structures are small in size, and are in topographic contact with:

- Respective kidney (see **Fig. 10**B)
- Respective lung
- Small intestine
- Large intestine
- Respective testis (male)
- Ovaries and oviduct (female)

Accessory bladder cystoscopy is rapid and may provide additional insights into the evaluation of the coelom.

LIMITATIONS

The main limitation of cystoscopic coelom evaluation is that it does not allow for biopsy or sample collection of the visceral organs. Therefore histopathologic, cytologic, and microbiological analyses cannot be performed, and a definitive diagnosis cannot be made.

Sterility

Despite the use of sterile technique, sterile cystoscopy cannot be achieved because the entrance of the endoscope into the urinary bladder is preceded by the passage through the proctodeum.[4] The passage of the endoscope through the proctodeum could cause the transfer of microorganisms into the urinary bladder. However, presence of bacteria in the urine of chelonians has also been shown in samples obtained by cystocentesis[26] and is considered to be normal.[26,27] In humans undergoing cystoscopy, the incidence of urinary tract infections was not significantly different whether sterile or clean techniques were used.[28] This may be important to consider when diagnostic cystoscopy is performed in the field, where sterility is rarely possible, or in conservation programs, where time required to sterilize the instruments between different animals and costs related to the sterilization procedures are main concerns. Although sterility may not be possible, we suggest the use of aseptic techniques to prevent disease transmission between animals.

Species-specific Differences

The order Testudines contains more than 300 species.[29] Although the published literature describes visualization of viscera through the urinary bladder in only 4 chelonian species,[5,9] we suggest that this technique, with proper execution, could be adapted to most terrestrial and semiaquatic chelonians because of their anatomic similarities. At present the only contraindication seems to be in yellow-bellied sliders (*T scripta scripta*), in which bladder rupture was a common problem (Proenca, unpublished data, 2015). Therefore, species-specific trials may be needed before applying this technique broadly, especially in species with peculiar adaptive morphology, such as pancake tortoises (*Malacochersus tornieri*), or large differences in size, such as Galápagos tortoises (*Chelonoidis nigra*).

COMPLICATIONS AND POTENTIAL ADVERSE OUTCOMES

Emesis

In a previous report of diagnostic cystoscopy, emesis was the only adverse reaction observed in 4 out of 25 tortoises.[5] Because 2 of the tortoises vomited during cystoscopy and 2 following administration of reversal agents, no clear cause of emesis was able to be determined. Emesis in chelonians was not reported in studies in which medetomidine,[30] medetomidine-ketamine,[31–35] or morphine were administered.[36] Seven percent of the hatchling turtles undergoing celioscopy given a combination of medetomidine-ketamine-morphine vomited after naloxone and atipamezole administration.[13]

In another study, 2 out of 12 leopard tortoises (Geochelone pardalis) vomited after intravenous injection of atipamezole.[37] We hypothesize that stomach compression, secondary to bladder distension, may possibly have a role in these emetic episodes. The bladder in chelonians is in strict topographic relationship with the GI tract, and the coelomic cavity in chelonians is not distensible. During cystoscopy, a certain amount of bladder distension is necessary to achieve adequate coelom visualization. At present, it is unclear whether starving before cystoscopy is needed in order to avoid emesis.

Bladder Rupture

Although rupture of the bladder is a concern, our experience suggests that, if proper technique is used, cystoscopy is safe, and overdistension or rupture of the urinary bladder does not occur in the following species/genera: Centrochelys sulcata, Chelonoidis sp, Chrysemys sp, Cuora sp, Emys sp, Graptemys sp, Kinosternon sp, Heosemys sp, Pseudemys sp, Siebenrockiella sp, Sternotherus sp, Stygmochelis pardalis, Terrapene sp, Testudo sp, and Trachemys sp.

Recently, in a comparative report between endoscopic and cystoscopic gender identification in yellow-bellied sliders (T scripta scripta), bladder rupture during cystoscopy occurred in 8 out of 30 individuals.[38]

Other Complications

Other complications were not reported during diagnostic cystoscopy or therapeutic cystoscopy, with the exception of 1 out of 3 Florida cooter turtles (Pseudemys floridana floridana) that underwent cystoscopic removal of ectopic eggs.[12] The turtle died within several days of the cystoscopy, and necropsy revealed granulomatous bacterial cystitis. The investigators hypothesized that the prolonged presence of the egg in the urinary bladder may have induced cystitis and predisposed this turtle to infection and mucosal injury.[12]

POSTOPERATIVE CARE

Postoperative care of chelonians undergoing cystoscopy depends on:

- The anesthetic plan reached during the procedure
- The aim and the consequent invasiveness of the procedure (removal of ectopic egg is more invasive, diagnostic cystoscopy is less invasive)
- The general status of the animal

In the authors' experience there is no need to administer systemic antibiotics after diagnostic cystoscopy, whereas antimicrobial therapy is recommended when operative cystoscopy is performed (eg, urolith removal, egg removal) on culture and sensitivity.

PRACTICE MANAGEMENT

The authors offer cystoscopic coelomic visualization mainly for 2 purposes and with 2 distinct fees:

- In diseased chelonians this procedure is offered as a first-line diagnostic (ie, in combination with appropriate diagnostic imaging and laboratory testing). Medical approach to chelonians is often frustrating, with localization of the diseased organ often difficult. By showing the client the morphologic alterations of organs, compliance is achieved for further, definitive, procedures (eg, celioscopy and biopsy).
- In immature chelonians this procedure is proposed for early gender identification. In the authors' practice, owners are motivated to perform early gender identification for chelonians of high commercial value in order to sell known sexes and facilitate pair formation.

The fees are different for these procedures, with the diagnostic cystoscopy costing approximately 5 times the sexing cystoscopy fee (ie, around 150 to 200 Euros [≈US$180–250) versus 30 to 40 Euros (≈US$35–50) per animal. In the case of operative cystoscopy, the fees vary depending on the aim and the duration of the procedures.

SUMMARY

Cystoscopy may be useful to evaluate morphologic changes in viscera without surgical access to the coelom. In these cases, although a definitive, causal diagnosis cannot be achieved, a clear identification of the diseased system through cystoscopy may be possible.

Considering the challenge of the medical approach to chelonians, a technique allowing fast and minimally invasive visualization of coelomic organs is extremely valuable.

ACKNOWLEDGMENTS

The authors appreciate the assistance provided by Dr Raffaele Melidone, Dr Giordano Nardini, and Kate Moore during the drafting of this article.

REFERENCES

1. Perrault C. Description anatomique d'une grande Tortue des Indes. Mem Acad Roy Sci Paris 1676;3:395–422 (reprinted 1733).
2. Lesueur CA. Vessies auxiliares dans les Tortues du genre Émyde. Compt Rend Acad Sci 1839;10:456–7.
3. Grant C. The southwestern desert tortoise, *Gopherus agassizii*. Zoologica 1936; 21:225–9.
4. Coppoolse KJ, Zwart P. Cloacoscopy in reptiles. Vet Q 1985;7:243–5.
5. Selleri P, Di Girolamo N, Melidone R. Cystoscopic sex identification of posthatchling chelonians. J Am Vet Med Assoc 2013;242:1744–50.
6. LeFevre ME, Gennaro JF, Brodsky WA. Properties of isolated mucosal and serosal fractions of turtle bladder. Am J Physiol 1970;219:716–23.
7. Frye FL. 2nd edition. Biomedical and surgical aspects of captive reptile husbandry, vol. II. Melbourne (Australia): Krieger Publishing; 1991.
8. Kolle P. Urinalysis in tortoises. In: Proceedings of the 7th Annual Conference Association of Reptilian and Amphibian Veterinarians. Reno (NV): 2000. p. 111–3.

9. Di Girolamo N, Melidone R, Catania S, et al. Use of cystoscopy to visualize morphological alteration of liver in a posthatchling turtle (*Cuora trifasciata*). J Am Anim Hosp Assoc, in press.

10. Divers SJ. Reptile diagnostic endoscopy and endosurgery. Vet Clin North Am Exot Anim Pract 2010;13:217–42.

11. Mans C, Foster JD. Endoscopy-guided ectopic egg removal from the urinary bladder in a leopard tortoise (*Stigmochelys pardalis*). Can Vet J 2014;55:569–72.

12. Minter LJ, Wood MW, Hill TL, et al. Cystoscopic guided removal of ectopic eggs from the urinary bladder of the Florida cooter turtle (*Pseudemys floridana floridana*). J Zoo Wildl Med 2010;41:503–9.

13. Hernandez-Divers SJ, Stahl SJ, Farrell R. An endoscopic method for identifying sex of hatchling Chinese box turtles and comparison of general versus local anesthesia for coelioscopy. J Am Vet Med Assoc 2009;234:800–4.

14. Hyman LH. Comparative vertebrate anatomy. 2nd edition. Chicago: University of Chicago Press; 1942.

15. Jørgensen CB. Role of urinary and cloacal bladders in chelonian water economy: historical and comparative perspectives. Biol Rev Camb Philos Soc 1998;73: 347–66.

16. Nardini G, Leopardi S, Di Girolamo N. Endoscopic laser lithotripsy in a freshwater turtle. In: Proceedings of the 20th Annual Conference Association of Reptilian and Amphibian Veterinarians. Indianapolis (IN): 2013. p. 23.

17. Thomas HL, Willer CJ, Wosar MA, et al. Egg-retention in the urinary bladder of a Florida cooter turtle, *Pseudemys floridana floridana*. J Herpetol Med Surg 2002; 12:4–6.

18. Knotek Z, Jekl V, Knotkova Z, et al. Eggs in chelonian urinary bladder: is coeliotomy necessary? In: Proceedings of the 16th Annual Conference Association of Reptilian and Amphibian Veterinarians. Milwaukee (WI): 2009. p. 118–21.

19. Chan DP, Abujudeh HH, Cushing GL Jr, et al. CT cystography with multiplanar reformation for suspected bladder rupture: experience in 234 cases. Am J Roentgenol 2006;187:1296–302.

20. Boysen SR, Rozanski EA, Tidwell AS, et al. Evaluation of a focused assessment with sonography for trauma protocol to detect free abdominal fluid in dogs involved in motor vehicle accidents. J Am Vet Med Assoc 2004;225: 1198–204.

21. Platt TR. Helminth parasites of the western painted turtle, *Chrysemys picta belli* (Gray), including *Neopolystoma elizabethae* n. sp. (Monogenea: Polystomatidae), a parasite of the conjunctival sac. J Parasitol 2000;86:815–8.

22. Wilkinson R. Clinical pathology. In: McArthur S, Wilkinson R, Meyer J, editors. Medicine and surgery of tortoises and turtles. Oxford (United Kingdom): Blackwell Publishing; 2004. p. 141–86.

23. Smith HM, James LF. The taxonomic significance of cloacal bursae in turtles. Trans Kans Acad Sci 1958;61:86–96.

24. Anderson J. On the cloacal bladders and peritoneal canals in Chelonia. J Linean Soc Zool 1876;12:434–44.

25. Di Girolamo N, Insacco G, Selleri P, et al. Comparison of urinary and accessory bladder approach during cloacoscopy of chelonians. In: Proceedings of the 19th Annual Conference Association of Reptilian and Amphibian Veterinarians. Oakland (CA): 2012. p. 74.

26. Innis CJ. Observations on urinalyses of clinically normal captive tortoises. In: Proceedings of the 4th Annual Conference Association of Reptilian and Amphibian Veterinarians. Houston (TX): 1997. p. 109–12.

27. Gibbons PM, Horton SJ, Brandl SR. Urinalysis in box turtles, *Terrapene* spp. In: Proceedings of the 7th Annual Conference Association of Reptilian and Amphibian Veterinarians. Reno (NV): 2000. p. 161–8.

28. Fozard JB, Green DF, Harrison GS, et al. Asepsis and out-patient cystoscopy. Br J Urol 1983;55:680–3.

29. Fritz U, Havaš P. Checklist of chelonians of the world. Vertebrate zoology, vol. 57. Dresden (Germany): Museum für Tierkunde; 2007. p. 149–368.

30. Sleeman JM, Gaynor J. Sedative and cardiopulmonary effects of medetomidine and reversal with atipamezole in desert tortoises (*Gopherus agassizii*). J Zoo Wildl Med 2000;31:28–35.

31. Greer LL, Jenne KJ, Diggs HE. Medetomidine-ketamine anesthesia in red-eared slider turtles (*Trachemys scripta elegans*). Contemp Top Lab Anim Sci 2001;40: 9–11.

32. Chittick EJ, Stamper MA, Beasley JF, et al. Medetomidine, ketamine, and sevo-flurane for anesthesia of injured loggerhead sea turtles: 13 cases (1996–2000). J Am Vet Med Assoc 2002;221:1019–25.

33. Dennis PM, Heard DJ. Cardiopulmonary effects of a medetomidine-ketamine combination administered intravenously in gopher tortoises. J Am Vet Med Assoc 2002;220:1516–9.

34. Harms CA, Eckert SA, Kubis SA, et al. Field anaesthesia of leatherback sea tur-tles (*Dermochelys coriacea*). Vet Rec 2007;161:15–21.

35. Knafo SE, Divers SJ, Rivera S, et al. Sterilisation of hybrid Galapagos tortoises (*Geochelone nigra*) for island restoration. Part 1: endoscopic oophorectomy of fe-males under ketamine-medetomidine anaesthesia. Vet Rec 2011;168:47.

36. Sladky KK, Miletic V, Paul-Murphy J, et al. Analgesic efficacy and respiratory ef-fects of butorphanol and morphine in turtles. J Am Vet Med Assoc 2007;230: 1356–62.

37. Lock BA, Heard DJ, Dennis P. Preliminary evaluation of medetomidine/ketamine combinations for immobilization and reversal with atipamezole in three tortoise species. Bull Assoc Reptilian Amphibian Vet 1998;8:6–8.

38. Proenca L, Divers SJ. Comparison between coelioscopy versus cloacoscopy for gender identification in immature turtles (*Trachemys scripta*). In: 2nd International Conference on Avian, Herpetological and Exotic mammal medicine. Paris (France). p. 356.

Gender Identification by Cloacoscopy and Cystoscopy in Juvenile Chelonians

Albert Martínez-Silvestre, DVM, MSc, PhD, Acred AVEPA (Exotic Animals), Dipl ECZM (Herpetology)[a],[*], Ferran Bargalló, DVM[b], Jordi Grífols, DVM, MSc[b]

KEYWORDS

- Cloacoscopy • Cystoscopy • Gender identification • Chelonian • Tortoise • Turtle
- Reproductive

KEY POINTS

- Sexual dimorphism is apparent in most adult chelonians, but appears at, and not before, maturation.
- The primary method of classifying sex in hatchlings and juvenile chelonians is the direct observation of gonads through celioscopy.
- Cloacoscopic gender identification of external genitalia is not reliable because of the high degree of misinterpretation between phallus and clitoris, especially in juveniles.
- Cystoscopy is an alternative noninvasive technique (performed through natural openings) for gender identification and is often effective for the visualization of gonads.
- Further studies are necessary to verify safety and efficacy of cystoscopic gender identification in different species of chelonians.

 Videos of endoscopic evaluation and cystoscopy evaluation accompany this article at http://www.vetexotic.theclinics.com/

INTRODUCTION

In recent years, breeding of chelonians has become more common because of the popularity of tortoises and turtles as pets as well as their inclusion in recovery plans of endangered species.[1] Because of these circumstances, there is not only special interest in knowing the sex of subadults but also of newborn animals.

Disclosure: The authors have nothing to disclose.
[a] CRARC (Catalonian Reptile and Amphibian Rescue Center), C/Santa Clara, s/n Masquefa 08783, Spain; [b] Zoologic Badalona Veterinary Clinics, C/Conquista, 74, Badalona 08912, Spain
* Corresponding author.
E-mail address: albertmarsil@outlook.com

Sexual dimorphism is apparent in most adult chelonians. As a general guideline, males have longer tails with distal cloaca openings, plastron concavity, differences in size and weight, and distinctive behaviors. In some species, males have different toenail lengths; bones or scales; eye, skin, or nose color; submandibular glands; and even an ability to vocalize. However, all these items are secondary sexual characteristics that appear at, and not before, maturation.[2]

The sex of hatchlings can be identified by numerous methods. In several studies with wild tortoises or sea turtles, some investigators have used indirect estimates of nest sex ratios. However, because of gender differences associated with variable thermal conditions, these indirect methods are considered imprecise.[3,4] The radioimmunoassay of testosterone and/or estrogen is another indirect method for sex classification, but it must be validated for each species to which it is applied. To date, this method has been successfully used for sex identification of the Arrau River turtle (*Podocnemis expansa*), loggerhead sea turtle (*Caretta caretta*), and green sea turtle (*Chelonia mydas*).[5,6]

Therefore, the primary method of classifying sex remains the direct observation of gonads in hatchlings and juveniles. Immature ovarian follicles and nonactive testes are visible inside the coelomic cavity of even young turtles.[7]

Endoscopy has been shown to be one of the main techniques for gender identification by direct visualization of gonads.[7] Celioscopy is a minimally invasive technique performed through the prefemoral fossa, requiring an adequate anesthetic plane.[7] In addition to gender identification, some surgical operations, such as orchiectomy or ovarian biopsies, can be performed using this system.[7] Cystoscopy is an alternative noninvasive technique (performed through natural openings) for gender identification that can provide excellent visualization, without surgery, and results in a rapid recovery time.

INDICATION AND CONTRAINDICATIONS FOR GENDER IDENTIFICATION BY CLOACOSCOPY AND CYSTOSCOPY IN JUVENILE CHELONIANS

The indications and contraindications for gender identification by cloacoscopy and cystoscopy in juvenile chelonians are presented in **Table 1**.

APPROACH

The technique of cloacoscopy/cystoscopy is the same for all species. Each species, genus, or family can have particular anatomy that must be appreciated.[8] Gender identification by cloacoscopy/cystoscopy consists of indirect observation of the gonads via a natural anatomic opening, the cloaca, and through the bladder wall.[9] For these procedures clinicians take advantage of the transparency of membranes forming

Table 1
The most common indications and contraindications for gender identification by cloacoscopy and cystoscopy in juvenile chelonians

Indications	Contraindications
Gender identification by indirect gonad visualization in juveniles weighing >150 g	Presence of yolk sac (it might hinder indirect gonad visualization in hatchlings)
—	Risk of mucosa damage, bladder (including accessory bladders) and cloaca rupture
—	Some species have no accessory vesicles

both urinary bladder and accessory vesicles (also known as cloacal bursae or accessory bladders) (**Fig. 1**).[8,10] Only some species of turtles have accessory vesicles. As a general rule, many aquatic turtles have accessory vesicles, whereas they are not present in terrestrial species.[8] Some details on the differences between species are provided in **Table 2**.

Thus, in species without cloacal bursae, observation of gonads must be done by entering the bladder. The main disadvantage of cystoscopy is the presence of uric acid crystals and sediments that can hinder visualization.

Accessory vesicles are always close to the proctodeum and, in many species, they are highly vascularized. Their basic functions are to provide buoyancy control and store water that is used on land for softening the ground for nest excavation. They are also used in stress situations (to create repulsion from predators).[8,10] They usually consist of a transparent membrane in which no urine is stored. Accessory vesicles can be filled and emptied quickly through the cloaca, and may therefore be used to effect short-term changes in lung volume and, hence, buoyancy.[10] In some species the accessory vesicular membrane lacks papillae. In the big-headed turtle (*Platisternon megacephala*), although the membrane is transparent, the density of highly vascularized papillae hinders the vision of gonads (**Fig. 2A**). In the Hilaire's side-necked turtle (*Phrynops hilarii*) accessory vesicles have a thin membrane covered with vascularized folds (plicae) (see **Fig. 2B**). Other species such as the Central America wood turtle (*Rhinoclemmys pulcherrima*) have a dark pigmented mucosa around the proctodeum that makes visualization difficult or impossible.

TECHNIQUE/PROCEDURE
Preparation/Patient Positioning

Turtles are placed in ventral recumbency, and the cloaca is flushed using warmed saline. This procedure allows filling of the accessory vesicles, and removes urates and fecal material.

Cloacal lavage can be performed in conscious animals because stress urination can be helpful for emptying the urinary bladder and accessory vesicles. In box turtles

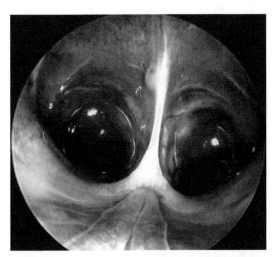

Fig. 1. Cloacoscopic view of the entrance to the accessory vesicles using insufflation of air in a male European pond turtle (*Emys orbicularis*). The transparent membrane cannot be appreciated on this picture.

Table 2
Special features of the main families of continental tortoises and turtles at the time of the cloacoscopy, as well as some internal peculiarities specific to certain species

Family	Accessory Vesicles Present	Accessory Vesicles Absent	Common Name	Details of Interest
Carettochelyidae	Carettochelis insculpta	—	Pig-nosed turtle	Multilobulated clitoris
Chelydridae	Chelydra serpentina	—	Snapping turtle	—
	Macrochelys temminckii	—	Alligator turtle	—
Emydidae	Emys orbicularis/Emys trinacris	—	European pond turtle	Two big accessory vesicles
	Graptemys pseudogeographica	—	Common map turtle	—
	Trachemys scripta	—	Red-eared slider	—
	Trachemys emolli	—	Nicaraguan slider	—
	Pseudemys floridana	—	Coastal plain cooter	—
	Chrysemys picta	—	Painted turtle	—
	Mauremys leprosa	—	Mediterranean turtle	Two big accessory vesicles
	Mauremys mutica	—	Asian yellow pond turtle	—
	Mauremys sinensis	—	Chinese stripe-necked turtle	—
	Mauremys anamensis	—	Annam pond turtle	—
	Malaclemys terrapin	—	Diamondback terrapin	—
	Cuora amboinensis	—	Malayan box turtle	One small accessory vesicle
	Cuora flavomarginata	—	Yellow-margined box turtle	One small accessory vesicle
	Cyclemys dentata	—	Asian leaf turtle	—
	Terrapene carolina	—	Common box turtle	—
	—	Rhinoclemmys pulcherrima	Central America wood turtle	Dark pigmented mucosa
Kinosternidae	—	Sternotherus odoratus	Musk turtle	—
	Kinosternon scorpioides	—	Scorpion mud turtle	—
Platysternidae	Platysternon megacephalum	—	Big-headed turtle	Papillae sieved accessory vesicles

Family	Species	Common name	Notes
Testudinidae	Testudo hermanni	Herman's tortoise	—
	Testudo graeca	Moorish tortoise	—
	Testudo marginata	Greek tortoise	—
	Testudo kleinmanni	Egyptian tortoise	—
	Gopherus berlandieri	Texas tortoise	—
	Geochelone elegans	Indian star tortoise	—
	Chelonoidis carbonaria	Red footed tortoise	Large clitoris
	Chelonoidis denticulata	Yellow footed tortoise	Large clitoris
	Stigmochelys pardalis	Leopard tortoise	—
	Centrochelys sulcata	African spur thigh tortoise	—
	Astrochelys radiata	Radiated tortoise	—
	Aldabrachelys gigantea	Aldabra giant tortoise	—
	Geochelone chilensis	Chaco tortoise	—
	Manouria emys	Asian giant tortoise	—
Trionychidae	Apalone ferox	Florida softshell turtle	—
	Pelodiscus sinensis	Chinese softshell turtle	—
Chelidae	Phrynops hilarii	Hilaire's side-necked turtle	Accessory vesicle with plicae
Pelomedusidae	Pelusios subniger	East African mud turtle	Two small accessory vesicles
	Pelomedusa subrufa	African helmeted turtle	One small accessory vesicle
	Emydura subglobosa	Red-bellied short-necked turtle	—
Podocnemididae	Podocnemis unifilis	Yellow-spotted Amazon river turtle	One small accessory vesicle

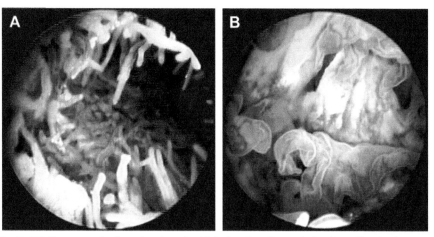

Fig. 2. (*A*) Cloacoscopic view showing the high density of vascularized papillae in the proctodeum of a big-headed turtle (*P megacephala*). (*B*) Cloacoscopic view of vascularized folds or plicae on the proctodeum in a side-necked turtle of the genus *Phrinops*.

(*Terrapene* or *Cuora*), a Farabeuf abdominal retractor can be used to prevent closure of the carapace during examination (**Fig. 3**).

Surgical anesthesia using inhalants is rarely required, but analgesia and tranquilization are beneficial.[11] Anesthesia time rarely, if ever, exceeds 20 minutes. Drugs recommended for this purpose are propofol, alfaxalone, or a combination of (dex) medetomidine, ketamine, and an opiate (eg, morphine or hydromorphone).[9,11–13] Normally, both loss of consciousness and recovery from anesthesia are rapid and uneventful.[13] In hatchlings, intravenous administration of anesthesia is impractical, so the intramuscular route is used. Intrathecal anesthesia using lidocaine can also be useful[14] and facilitates relaxation of hind limbs, tail, and cloaca, thereby facilitating cloacoscopy, especially in larger species. Postoperative analgesics, like meloxicam or tramadol, should also be considered.[12,13,15]

Basic Equipment

Rigid telescope: 2.7 mm, 30°, 18 cm with a 3.5-mm protective sheath
Xenon light source with light cable
Endovideo camera
Monitor
Fluid set for lactated Ringer solution infusion (1 drop every 3–4 seconds)

Special Equipment

Portable battery endoscope
Direct light source

Different diameter endoscopes can be used for this technique depending on the size of the turtle and the cloaca opening. However, diameters of 1.9 mm to 4 mm are generally preferred for most animals. In turtles weighing more than 200 g, the diameter of the cloacal sphincter and the diameter of the bladder or accessory vesicle entrance usually do not represent a physical limitation for this procedure. In very small chelonians (eg, <20 g), the use of a small telescope (eg, 1.9-mm, rigid 30°-viewing endoscope) should be used to avoid possible size-related trauma. The endoscopic

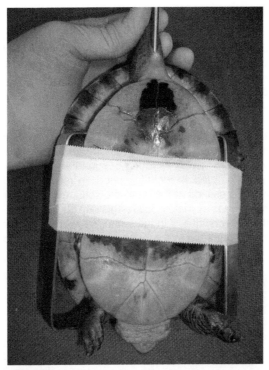

Fig. 3. Positioning of an Amboina box turtle (*Cuora amboinensis*) for cloacoscopy using the Farabeuf abdominal retractor. The instrument is used to prevent natural closure of the caudal plastron hinge.

equipment can be cleaned and disinfected by immersion in 2.4% glutaraldehyde solution for 15 minutes and rinsed with sterile distilled or deionized water between each procedure.

TECHNIQUE/PROCEDURE
Cloacoscopy

The patient is placed in ventral recumbency. The endoscope is inserted through the cloaca, progressing cranially. One finger and thumb are placed around the vent to act as a valve in order to control the fluid infusion and avoid the outflow of lactated Ringer solution. With the animal in ventral recumbency, 4 structures can be seen within the proctodeum: genitalia (ventral), urodeal folds, coprodeal entrance, and entrances to accessory vesicles (see **Figs. 1** and **5**A). If cloacoscopic accessory vesicular examination is performed, the endoscope easily enters the wide, natural openings.

Sometimes air insufflation into the proctodeum allows easy access to the accessory vesicles (Video 1) without the use of lactated Ringer solution. When air is used for the expansion of the vesicles, urate or digestive remnants do not remain floating in front of the endoscope, which can improve the overall image.

Access to the accessory vesicles is simple and decreases the possibility of forcing or damaging the urethral opening. In species in which these structures exist, examining them before resorting to examination from within the urinary bladder is advisable.

PHALLUS/CLITORIS IDENTIFICATION

The first image that is seen when the endoscope enters in the cloaca is the phallus or clitoris. In females, the clitoris consists of a small structure similar in shape to a phallus (**Fig. 4**A, see Video 1). In adult males, the phallus is bent anteriorly, has a differentiated longitudinal groove (see **Fig. 4**B), glans (see **Fig. 4**C), and its color is normally bright pink to black. In the Sicilian pond turtle (*Emys trinacris*) young tortoises can have a gray phallus, more similar to a female clitoris.[16] Unlike squamates (phallic erection by eversion), chelonian erection is caused by tumescence of 2 spongy bodies: the corpus spongiosum/cavernosum and corpus fibrosum.[17,18] Therefore, differentiation of phallus and clitoris can be difficult when the organ is flaccid within the cloaca, and is almost impossible to identify in young or subadult individuals (see **Fig. 4**D).[17]

In one study that attempted to identify gender in red-eared sliders (*Trachemys scripta elegans*) by the presence of the phallus/clitoris, males were misdiagnosed as females (100%) and females as males (38%). This rate clearly shows the degree of error associated with this technique.[19] In the author's experience, in some species, the clitoris is almost nonexistent, as in the big-headed turtle (*P megacephala*). In other

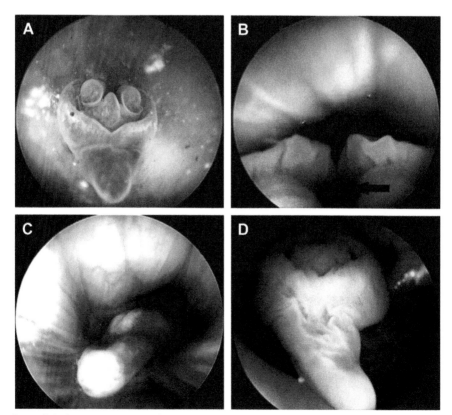

Fig. 4. (*A*) Cloacoscopic view of the clitoris of a mature Moorish tortoise (*Testudo graeca*). Note the small structure similar to a phallus. (*B*) Cloacoscopic view of the longitudinal groove (*arrow*) of the phallus in a male immature Moorish tortoise (*T graeca*). (*C*) Close endoscopic view of a glans in an immature male Moorish tortoise (*T graeca*). (*D*) Cloacoscopic view of the phallus in a subadult male marginated tortoise (*Testudo marginata*). Note the similarity with the clitoris in **Fig. 4**A.

species, such as the red footed tortoise (*Chelonoidis carbonaria*), the clitoris is highly variable in size and degree of differentiation. Endocrine disruption can result in females with a pseudophallus (with groove, glans, and corpus cavernosum), increasing the possibilities of inaccurate assignment of gender.[20]

CYSTOSCOPY

Insufflation of air can be performed in accessory vesicles but not in the urinary bladder, for which warm (30°C) lactated Ringer solution is preferred. If the urinary bladder is not naturally distended with transparent urine, the operator needs to expand and distend the bladder with fluid.

For access to the urinary bladder, the endoscope is directed toward the urethral opening, which is located ventral to the entrance of the colon (see **Fig. 4**B). In a few cases, the urethral opening is not clearly identified and the colon can be used as an anatomic landmark (Video 2). The urethral opening is usually seen in a horizontal plane in land tortoises (**Fig. 5**B), whereas it is seen in a vertical plane in terrapins and aquatic turtles (see **Fig. 5**A). Once the endoscope is in the proximity of the colonic orifice, a gentle caudal retraction of the endoscope allows visualization of the urethral opening.[9]

Lactated Ringer solution (1 drop every 3 to 4 seconds) permits distension of the urethral opening and aids entry into the bladder. Once access to the urinary bladder is gained, the endoscope is guided dorsolaterally until the gonads can be seen. The urinary bladder is a greatly distensible organ that can contain large quantities of fluid.

GONAD IDENTIFICATION

Chelonian gonads are located in the dorsocaudal coelom, lying cranioventrally to the retrocoelomic kidneys. They are usually found in close association with the caudal lungs and colon.[9] In juvenile turtles the immature testis is elongated to round/oval, smooth, yellowish, with a smooth surface with superficial blood vessels, and attached dorsally by a short mesorchium (**Fig. 6**). The epididymis is cream in color, convoluted, and continues caudally as the ductus deferens.

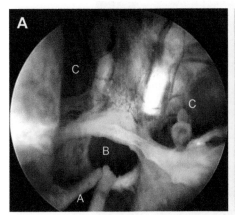 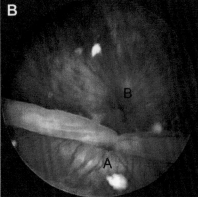

Fig. 5. (*A*) Cloacoscopic view of the entrance to the accessory vesicles after sterile fluid infusion in a male European pond turtle (*E orbicularis*). A, Urodeal folds; B, distal colon sphincter (or entrance); C, accessory vesicles. (*B*) Cloacoscopic view of proctodeum and urodeum in a Herman's tortoise (*Testudo hermanni*) using sterile fluid infusion. A, Urodeum; B, distal colon sphincter. Note the absence of accessory vesicles.

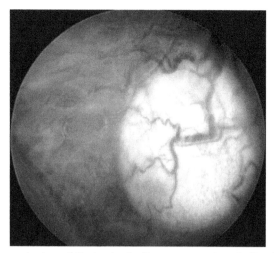

Fig. 6. Close endoscopic view of the testis of a European pond turtle (*E orbicularis*) through the transparent accessory vesicle membrane. Note the yellowish organ with small blood vessels. The bigger blood vessels belong to the vesicle membrane.

The immature oviduct is a straight, flat, transparent to white band located immediately dorsal and parallel to the ovary. The immature ovaries are long, irregular, semi-transparent organs. Round and white to yellow follicles can be seen developing throughout the organ. Previtellogenic follicles are separated from each other and do not completely fill the parenchyma of the organ (**Fig. 7**).[19]

In general, the identification of the gonad by indirect visualization through cystoscopy is reliable, but sometimes is difficult and not safe (discussed later). This technique is easier in young terrestrial or giant tortoises (>150 g weight) than in young

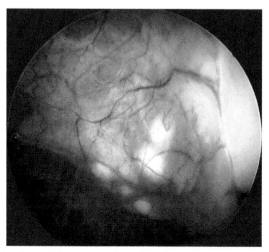

Fig. 7. Cloacoscopic view of the ovary of a subadult European pond turtle (*E orbicularis*) through the transparent accessory vesicle membrane. Note the white to yellow follicles within the ovary.

turtles weighing less than 100 g. In hatchling land tortoises (*Testudo hermanni*) gender identification by cystoscopy was accurate compared with gonadal histology.[9]

COMPLICATIONS AND MANAGEMENT

In the author's experience, there are several factors that can affect the reliability of gender identification by cloacoscopy/cystoscopy:

1. Obesity. Fat tissue may cover and hide the gonads.
2. In offspring less than 6 months old, the presence of the internalized yolk sac greatly complicates the identification of other coelomic structures, which makes this technique less helpful.
3. The presence of distended intestinal loops can hinder the identification of the gonads. Thus, 3 days of starving can be helpful.
4. Infectious diseases that cause inflammation and loss of transparency of bladder membranes can negatively affect visualization.
5. Emesis has been reported as an adverse reaction in 16% of anesthetized hatchling Herman's tortoises (*T hermanni*) undergoing cystoscopy.[9]

POSTOPERATIVE CARE

Postoperative care is simple and usually does not require the use medication, with few exceptions (eg, use of antiinflammatories because of mucosa damage). Usually, tortoises are eating and behaving normally after 24 hours.

CURRENT CONTROVERSIES/FUTURE CONSIDERATIONS

The order Testudines contains more than 300 species. This article shows that cystoscopic gender identification can be performed in the turtle families shown in **Table 2**. However, a recent study performed in 30 clinically healthy immature (36–90 g) *Trachemys scripta* shows that only 10% (3 of 30) of the animals had their gender accurately identified by cystoscopy and 7 of 30 animals experienced bladder or cloacal rupture.[21] Therefore, more studies are necessary to verify safety and efficacy of cystoscopic gender identification in different species. In addition, the gonads of chelonians may vary in size and aspect seasonally, and this may complicate their identification, especially in turtles that hibernate.[22,23] Further studies focusing on seasonal fluctuations of gonadal morphology in chelonians are needed.

SUMMARY

Identifying sex in young chelonians by cloacoscopy or cystoscopy is an alternative noninvasive technique (performed through natural openings) that is often effective for the visualization of gonads. Moreover, some important anatomic differences exist between different chelonians and further studies are necessary to verify safety and efficacy of the procedures.

ACKNOWLEDGMENTS

To the veterinary technicians at the Zoologic Badalona Veterinaria, especially Simon Lopez, as well as the technicians in the CRARC center, especially Isabel Verdaguer, Silvia Merchan, Juan Miguel Cano, and Joaquim Soler.

SUPPLEMENTARY DATA

Supplementary data related to this article can be found online at http://dx.doi.org/10.1016/j.cvex.2015.04.009.

REFERENCES

1. Ballasina D, Vandepitte V, Mochi E, et al. The necessity of reintroductions of captive bred *Geochelone sulcata*. Strategies for management and set up of captive breeding groups. International Congress on Chelonian Conservation, II. Dakar, Senegal; 2003. 12.
2. Blanvillain G, Owens D, Kuchling G. Hormones and reproductive cycles in turtles. In: Norris D, Lopez KH, editors. Hormones and reproduction in reptiles. London: Academic Press; 2011. p. 277–303.
3. Hulin V, Girondot M, Godfrey MH, et al. Mixed and uniform brood sex ratio strategy in turtles. In: Wyneken J, Godfrey MH, Bels V, editors. The facts, the theory and their consequences (biology of turtles). Boca Raton (FL): CRC Press; 2008. p. 279–90.
4. Lance VA, Valenzuela N. A hormonal method to determine the sex of hatchling giant river turtles, *Podocnemis expansa*. Application to endangered species research. Am Zool 1992;32:16.
5. Gross TS, Crain DA, Bjomdal KA, et al. Identification of sex in hatchling loggerhead turtles (*Caretta caretta*) by analysis of steroid concentrations in chorioallantoic/amniotic fluid. Gen Comp Endocrinol 1995;99:204–10.
6. Xia ZR, Li PP, Gu HX, et al. Evaluating non invasive methods of sex identification in Green sea turtle (*Chelonia mydas*) hatchlings. Chelonian Conservation and Biology 2011;10:117–23.
7. Hernandez-Divers SJ, Stahl SJ, Farrell R. An endoscopic method for identifying sex of hatchling Chinese box turtles and comparison of general versus local anesthesia for coelioscopy. J Am Vet Med Assoc 2009;234:800–3.
8. Pickel FW. The accessory bladders of the testudinata. Zoological Bulletin 1899;2(6):291–302.
9. Selleri P, Di Girolamo N, Melidone R. Cytoscopic sex identification of posthatchling chelonians. J Am Vet Med Assoc 2013;242:1744–50.
10. Peterson CC, Gomez D. Buoyancy regulation in two species of freshwater turtle. Herpetologica 2008;64:141–8.
11. Divers SJ, Innis CJ, Stah SJ, et al. Coelioscopic orchidectomy in red-eared terrapins (*Trachemys scripta elegans*): a model for chelonian endosurgery. ICARE 2013;1:125–6.
12. Innis CJ. Endoscopy and endosurgery of the chelonian reproductive tract. Vet Clin North Am Exot Anim Pract 2010;13:243–54.
13. Divers SJ. Reptile diagnostic endoscopy and endosurgery. Vet Clin North Am Exot Anim Pract 2010;13:217–42.
14. Mans C, Lahner LL, Steagall P, et al. Feasibility, efficacy and inter-operator variability of spinal anaesthesia in female red-eared slider turtles (*Trachemys scripta elegans*). ICARE 2013;1:162–3.
15. Greenace CB, Paul-Murphy J, Sladky KK, et al. Reptile and amphibian analgesia. J Herp Med Surg 2005;15:24–9.
16. Spadola F, Insaccoi G. Endoscopy of cloaca in 51 *Emys trinacris* (Frist et al, 2005): morphological and diagnostic study. Acta Herpetologica 2009;4:73–81.
17. Larkins CE, Cohn MJ. Phallus development in the turtle *Trachemys scripta*. Sex Develop 2014;1–9. http://dx.doi.org/10.1159/000363631.

18. DeSolla SR, Portelli MJ, Spiro H, et al. Penis displays of snapping turtles (*Chelydra serpentina*) in response to handling: defensive or displacement behavior? Chelonian Conservation and Biology 2001;4:187–9.
19. Perpiñan D, Costa T, Bargallo, et al. Correlation between gonad histology and endoscopic sex determination in juvenile red-eared turtles (*Trachemys scripta elegans*). ICARE 2013;1:126–7.
20. Guix JC, Fedullo DL, Molina FB. Masculinization of captive females of *Chelonoidis carbonaria* (Testudinidae). Rev Esp Herpetol 2001;15:67–77.
21. Proença L. Comparison between coelioscopy versus cloacoscopy for gender identification in immature turtles (Trachemys scripta). ICARE, II, Paris, France. 142–43.
22. Carvalho D, Cesar dos Santos A, Fernandes L, et al. Body and testicular biometric parameters of the scorpion mud turtle (*Kinosternon scorpioides*). Acta Scientiarium 2014;36:477–81.
23. Casares M, Rübel A, Honegger RE. Observations on the female reproductive cycle of captive giant tortoises (*Geochelone* spp.) using ultrasound scanning. J Zoo Wildl Med 1997;28(3):267–73.

Endoscopic Sex Identification in Chelonians and Birds (Psittacines, Passerines, and Raptors)

CrossMark

Stephen J. Divers, BSc(Hons), BVetMed, DZooMed,
DipECZM (Herpetology, Zoo Health Management), DACZM, FRCVS

KEYWORDS

• Bird • Psittacine • Reptile • Chelonian • Endoscopy • Sex identification

KEY POINTS

• Most birds and juvenile chelonians are sexually monomorphic, and sex identification through other means is often necessary.
• Endoscopy is a minimally invasive system to identify sex, and, unlike DNA techniques, is immediate and also evaluates for maturity and abnormalities.
• Endoscopic sex identification is safe and rapid, and few complications have been reported.

INTRODUCTION

Avian endoscopy dates back several decades, and the first published report that the author is aware of appeared in 1978 and described the evaluation of gonads in conscious birds.[1] Since that time, continued progress and refinement of human pediatric cystoscopy equipment has resulted in the development of a dedicated avian endoscopy system.[2] Indeed, it is this human cystoscopy system that was later used for reptiles, small mammals, and fish.[3–5] Despite the advent of DNA probes for sex identification of many avian and some reptile species, clinicians involved with zoos, conservation projects, or breeders may still be asked to perform "surgical sexing" because of the immediate results, and the added ability to identify maturity and abnormalities.

The author has nothing to disclose.
Department of Small Animal Medicine and Surgery, College of Veterinary Medicine, University of Georgia, 2200 College Station Road, Athens, GA 30602, USA
E-mail address: sdivers@uga.edu

vetexotic.theclinics.com

EQUIPMENT

For most practices, the 2.7-mm telescope system (with the usual camera, monitor, and light source) can be used for sex identification purposes in animals down to 100 g or even smaller. For birds, by virtue of their air sac system, insufflation or irrigation is contraindicated, and therefore only a 3.5-mm protection sheath is required. However, for reptiles CO_2 insufflation or saline irrigation is necessary and the protection sheath may provide inadequate flow, necessitating the use of the 4.8-mm operating sheath. In smaller animals weighing less than 100 g the 1.9-mm telescope with integrated sheath is preferred; in animals heavier than 10 kg, larger telescopes may be more suitable (**Fig. 1**).

As stated, birds require no insufflation; however, for small juvenile chelonians (and indeed other reptiles), sterile fluid infusion (often lactated ringers) is used to create the telescope-gonad space necessary for visualization. Fluid seems to be more effective than gas for animals weighing less than 200 g, and provides greater clarity for tiny structures in comparison with gas insufflation. The bag of warm sterile fluids is suspended above the patient and connected via an intravenous fluid line to one of the ports of the sheath. A second egress line, although rarely required, can be connected to the second port, with the other end placed into a collection bucket under the table (**Fig. 2**). The addition of 500 mg of ceftazidime to a liter bag provides a concentration of 0.5 mg/mL and can be used to provide intraoperative antibiosis if necessary. For larger animals, for which large volumes of saline would be required, a dedicated endoflator and CO_2 insufflation to 3 to 5 mm Hg provides good visualization.

Typically, endoscopic sex identification is usually performed for a group of animals rather than an individual, with limited time for equipment sterilization between animals. Therefore, it is important to restrict such a group procedure to a single source or breeder (to prevent cross infection), and to perform high-level disinfection, rather than true sterilization of equipment between animals. In practical terms equipment may be wiped, placed in glutaraldehyde for 5 to 30 minutes, and rinsed with sterile water between animals. At the University of Georgia, the fee structure for sex identification was (as of January 2015) $500 for initial setup and $51.06 per animal; however, such fees may be expected to vary considerably depending on geographic location

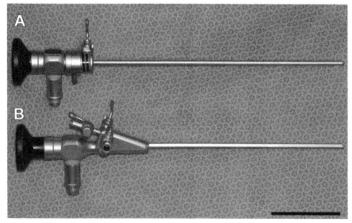

Fig. 1. (*A*) A 2.7-mm × 18-cm telescope housed within a 3.5-mm protection sheath. (*B*) A 1.9-mm telescope with integrated sheath. Scale bar: 5 cm.

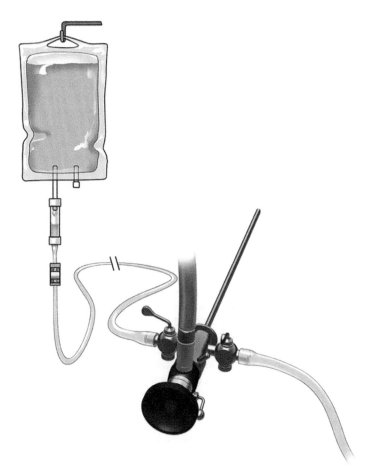

Fig. 2. Fluid infusion system for coelioscopic sex identification in small juvenile chelonians. (*Courtesy of* Kip Carter, Educational Resources, University of Georgia.)

and practices expenses. Nevertheless, a sliding scale (with the cost per animal decreasing as the numbers increase) is useful to encourage batch processing.

BIRDS

Unlike most animals, birds are blessed with an air sac system that essentially provides the endoscopist with a preinsufflated patient. Thanks to this unique anatomy and the pioneering work of Greg Harrison, Michael Taylor, Lorenzo Crosta, Michael Lierz, and other avian veterinarians, rigid endoscopy has enjoyed considerable popularity in avian practice over the past 3 decades.[2,6]

Patient Preparation and Anesthesia

Most young birds presented for routine sex identification are typically healthy. Nonetheless, knowledge of avian anatomy and physiology, species-specific husbandry, and nutritional and breeding practices are vital. Preanesthetic evaluations should include physical examination (including accurate measurement of body weight), and consideration given to routine hematology and plasma biochemistry testing. Fasting should be in accordance with body size and feeding strategy, and concentrate on emptying the crop (if present), proventriculus and ventriculus. For example, the smallest birds (eg, finches, budgerigars) should be fasted for no more than 30 to 60 minutes; small to medium-sized birds (eg, lovebirds, cockatiels) for 1 to 2 hours, medium to large birds (eg, African grays, amazons, cockatoos, macaws) for 3 to 6 hours, and most large raptors (eg, red-tailed hawk, great-horned owl) for 12 hours.

General anesthesia is recommended for all endoscopy procedures to avoid risking damage to equipment, patient, or staff. Previous suggestions that endoscopic "sexing" can be performed in conscious birds are no longer acceptable.[1] Premedication (eg, midazolam and butorphanol for psittacines) should be considered. Most birds are easily induced using isoflurane or sevoflurane by face mask. The disadvantages of intubation (eg, tracheal stricture) may exceed the benefits because of the short duration of the procedure that is often measured in seconds rather than minutes. Respiratory rate, heart rate, pulse oximetry, and Doppler ultrasound are monitored. Vascular access for intraoperative fluid therapy is rarely indicated for basic reproductive evaluation and sex identification, as the procedure is typically rapid.

Endoscopic Procedure

The most commonly used procedure involves a left approach into the air sac system because male and female reproductive organs can always be seen (only a few species have bilateral ovaries). The bird is positioned in right lateral recumbency with wings secured dorsad over the bird's back using self-adhesive tape. The left pelvic limb is pulled craniad and secured to the neck, again using self-adhesive bandage, to expose the left flank. The entry site is located immediately behind the last rib, and just ventral to the flexor cruris medialis muscle as it courses from caudal stifle to ischium (**Fig. 3**). Alternatively, a cranial to the pelvic limb approach can be used. Very few feathers need to be plucked before aseptic preparation of the area. Following a 2- to 4-mm skin incision, straight hemostats, directed in a slight craniodorsal direction, are used to bluntly dissect between the thin subcutaneous tissues and enter the left caudal thoracic (or abdominal) air sac. The hemostats are replaced by the sheathed telescope, and

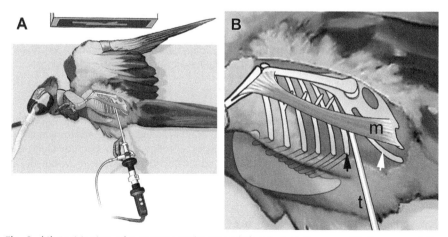

Fig. 3. (A) Positioning of a macaw undergoing left-sided coelioscopy. (B) Close-up of the telescope (t) entry site just behind the last rib (*black arrow*), ventral to the flexor cruris medialis muscle (m), and well cranial of the pubis (*white arrow*). (*Courtesy of* Educational Resources, University of Georgia.)

correct position within the caudal thoracic air sac is confirmed by the identification of lung (straight ahead), cranial thoracic air sac (left), abdominal air sac (right), caudal edge of liver and proventriculus (ventral), and ribs and intercostal muscles (dorsal).

Perforation into, and exploration of, the left abdominal air sac is accomplished by pressing the tip of the telescope against the air sac membrane, and advancing the telescope in a sweeping motion until the membranes are breached. Normal membranes are transparent, and tissues in the adjacent air sac can be visualized and avoided. Great care is required when breaking through thickened, opaque air sacs because vision is impaired and visceral trauma can occur if the telescope is blindly advanced. On entry into the left abdominal air sac, the cranial division of the left kidney is identified and, in close association, the left adrenal gland and gonad.

The mature testes of most birds are oblong and smooth, with visible blood vessels coursing across the surface. The convoluted vas deferens can be traced from gonad to cloaca. Testicular size increases dramatically during the breeding season (**Fig. 4**).

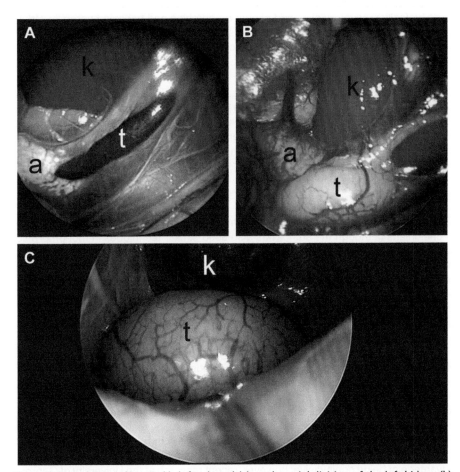

Fig. 4. (*A*) Immature left testis (t), left adrenal (a), and cranial division of the left kidney (k) in a juvenile Moluccan cockatoo (*Cacatua moluccensis*). (*B*) Adult (nonbreeding) left testis (t), left adrenal (a), and cranial division of the left kidney (k) in a yellow-fronted amazon (*Amazona ocrocephala*). (*C*) Large active left testis (t) and cranial division of the left kidney (k) in a breeding pigeon (*Columba livia*).

The mature ovary is suspended by an obvious mesovarium that courses across the cranial division of the left kidney, and resembles a cluster of follicles. The oviduct can be traced from caudal to the gonad to the cloaca. The oviduct of immature females is small and straight, whereas in adults that have previously produced eggs it can be large and convoluted. Sex identification is seldom difficult in adults. In juveniles, the gonads are much smaller and less well differentiated (**Fig. 5**). However, the testis will generally be smooth while the ovary is more irregular, and the mesovarium can still be identified.

If an abnormal testis is identified in an adult male, biopsy can be undertaken but is seldom, if ever, indicated in juveniles.[7] There is no need to repair the small holes punctured in the air sac membranes, as they generally heal within 5 to 10 days. A single absorbable (eg, poliglecaprone 25) suture that incorporates both muscle and skin (or a 2-layer closure) is recommended for closure.

Postoperative Care

Birds typically recover quickly, and should be perching and behaving normally within minutes of recovery. There is still controversy concerning the use of opiates and other analgesics in birds, and taxa-specific effects have been documented; however, the author uses meloxicam routinely.[8,9]

Complications

Complications are rare because most birds are young and healthy. Minor hemorrhage following entry can occur, which although clinically insignificant can cause delay. Most endoscopy issues are related to operator error until experience and ability have been gained. Postoperative subcutaneous emphysema may occur rarely, but typically resolves spontaneously within a few days.

REPTILES

Sex identification of reptiles is a more recent development and has been most utilized in chelonians (although the author has also used similar techniques in monomorphic lizards). Sex determination in most chelonians is temperature dependent, and private breeders, curators, researchers, and conservationists often need to identify sex in rare or endangered species, especially when precise incubation parameters have not been elucidated. To address these concerns, several methodologies including sex hormone measurements, identification of specific gene expression, and endoscopy have been developed; however, only endoscopy can provide an immediate answer and determine the normality of the internal reproductive organs.[10–17]

Most techniques rely on the insertion of a rigid endoscope into the coelom to directly view the gonads, and as chelonians lack a true abdominal cavity, the term coelioscopy is more appropriate than laparoscopy.[18,19] Some reports have not described any form of insufflation (and have suffered from restricted visualization) while others have failed to use any form of general anesthesia (which has been shown to be inadequate).[14,20,21] More recently, cloacoscopy and cystoscopy techniques that identified the gonads of Hermann's tortoises (*Testudo hermanni*) through the transparent wall of the fluid-distended bladder have been described.[22] This approach has the distinct advantage of being noninvasive; however, recent research at the University of Georgia concluded that the technique was unsafe in sliders (*Trachemys scripta*) (Proenca and colleagues, unpublished data, 2014). There is also some concern regarding the accuracy of transmembranous visualization in comparison with direct coelioscopic examination when evaluating very immature and poorly differentiated gonads (**Fig. 6**).

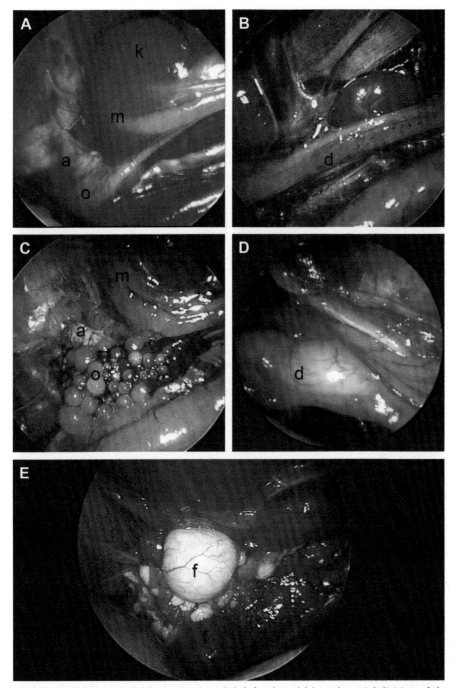

Fig. 5. (*A*) Immature ovary (o), mesovarium (m), left adrenal (a), and cranial division of the left kidney (k) in a juvenile yellow-fronted amazon (*A ocrocephala*). (*B*) Thin, straight oviduct (d) in an immature umbrella cockatoo (*Cacatua alba*). (*C*) Adult (nonbreeding) ovary (o), ovarian ligament (m) and left adrenal gland (a) in an adult umbrella cockatoo. (*D*) Large, wide oviduct (d) in a breeding pigeon (*C livia*). (*E*) Large active ovary with 2 preovulatory follicles (f) in a breeding pigeon (*C livia*).

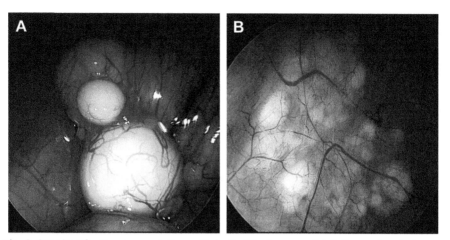

Fig. 6. Sex identification in an adult aquatic turtle (*Trachemys scripta*). Comparison between direct coelioscopic examination (*A*) and transmembranous cloacoscopic/cystoscopic examination (*B*). While the differences are obvious in these adult turtles, their presence may become significant when examining smaller, poorly differentiated gonads.

What initially started as a research and conservation tool has now developed into a regular clinical service offered to breeders and zoo curators.[3,21] To date, sex in more than 300 juveniles (as small as 10 g) have been confirmed endoscopically from several species, including radiated tortoises (*Astrochelys radiata*), Aldabra tortoises (*Aldabrachelys gigantea*), Galapagos tortoises (*Chelonoidis nigra*), Hermann's tortoises (*T hermanni*), Asian box turtles (*Cuora flavomarginata*), and sliders (*T scripta*). The following description represents the current approach to providing this service at the University of Georgia.

Patient Preparation and Anesthesia

Whereas most reptiles presented for diagnostic coelioscopy are ill, most juveniles presented for sex identification are healthy. However, because of their small size, other challenges often exist. Animals should be at least 4 to 6 months of age to ensure that internalized yolk sacs have been completely absorbed. Each animal must be uniquely and permanently identified. When dealing with juveniles weighing less than 100 g, physical examination is often limited but must include an accurate body weight (eg, to the nearest 0.1 g for animals <25 g). Routine blood sampling can be performed if animal size and finances permit.

Although conscious endoscopy under local anesthesia may be legally permitted under a scientific research license, visceral discomfort and compromised welfare would seem largely avoidable given recent developments in reversible injectable anesthetics.[23–26] Some investigators have reported using only local anesthesia for chelonian coelioscopy, but this provides inadequate restraint and analgesia.[20] In a recent comparison of local versus general anesthesia for chelonian coelioscopy, objective anesthetic scores were significantly better for procedures conducted with general (injectable) anesthesia compared with local lidocaine alone.[27] Certainly in clinical practice, general anesthesia (or deep sedation combined with local anesthesia) is required for any coelioscopic sex identification.[27,28]

The inability to gain intravenous access and the impracticality of endotracheal intubation dictates the choice of injectable anesthesia. For practical purposes, it may be necessary to dilute drugs using sterile water to achieve a measurable volume. The creation of an Excel spreadsheet with each animal's identification, weight, and calculated drug doses simplifies the process. Ketamine-dexmedetomidine-hydromorphone (or morphine) combinations have been consistently successful. Aquatic and semiaquatic species seem more sensitive, and dose rates of 10 to 20 mg/kg ketamine and 0.05 mg/kg dexmedetomidine are effective, whereas for terrestrial tortoises higher doses are often needed in the range of 20 to 40 mg/kg ketamine and 0.1 mg/kg dexmedetomidine. This dissociative-α2 combination is augmented with an opiate analgesic, and hydromorphone (0.5 mg/kg) is preferred over morphine (1.5 mg/kg) because the latter frequently results in respiratory depression.[23] All anesthetics are combined into a single syringe and injected intramuscularly into the left forelimb. Animals are then placed in a warm, quiet incubator (80°–85°F/26.7°–29.4°C) for 30 to 40 minutes. Once adequately induced, the pelvic limbs are taped caudad to expose the prefemoral fossae. Local lidocaine (42 mg/kg) is injected into the left prefemoral fossa (or the right prefemoral fossa if the surgeon is left-handed and prefers to enter through the right side). Right lateral positioning is easily accomplished by placing the animal between 2 rolled and taped towels (**Fig. 7**). Small patient size and short procedural time tend to prevent instrumentation for anesthetic monitoring purposes. However, withdrawal reflexes should be lost but corneal reflexes retained.

Following the procedure, meloxicam 0.2 mg/kg is injected intramuscularly or subcutaneously into the right forelimb. Atipamezole at 10 times the dexmedetomidine milligram dose is injected intramuscularly into the right pelvic limb, and results in rapid recovery within 20 minutes. If opiate-induced respiratory depression persists despite reversal, naloxone 0.2 mg/kg intramuscularly is effective.

Endoscopic Procedure

With the animal positioned appropriately and following aseptic preparation, a 2- to 3-mm craniocaudal skin incision is made into the center of the left prefemoral fossa (or right prefemoral fossa if left-handed). Small straight hemostats are inserted through the incision, directed craniad, and used to bluntly enter the coelom. The hemostats are opened slightly before being replaced by the telescope connected to sterile, warm fluid infusion (lactated ringers). Unlike CO_2 insufflation, there is no need to attempt an airtight seal between the sheathed telescope and the skin. Indeed, a slightly larger incision allows excess fluid to drain freely from the coelom. Only sufficient fluid to enable visualization should be instilled. The addition of excess fluid

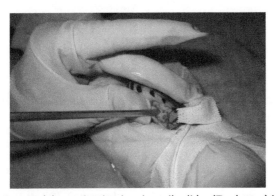

Fig. 7. Coelioscopic gonadal examination in a juvenile slider (*Trachemys*) in right lateral recumbency and supported between 2 rolled and taped towels.

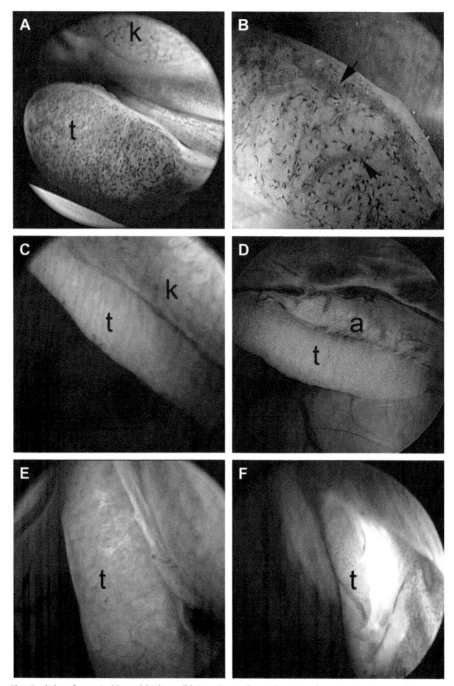

Fig. 8. (*A*) Left testis (t) and kidney (k) in a juvenile male Asian box turtle (*Cuora flavomarginata*). (*B*) Close-up of the left testis demonstrating the superficial blood vessels (*arrows*) and pigmentation. This unusual morphology exemplifies the need to gain species-specific experience and sex comparisons. (*C*) Poorly differentiated left testis (t) and kidney (k) in a 50-g juvenile male radiated tortoise (*Astrochelys radiata*). (*D*) Well-differentiated left testis (t) and closely associated adrenal (a) in a 150-g juvenile male radiated tortoise. (*E*) Left testis (t) in a juvenile male Hermann's tortoise (*Testudo hermanni*). (*F*) Left testis (t) in a juvenile male Aldabra tortoise (*Aldabrachelys gigantea*).

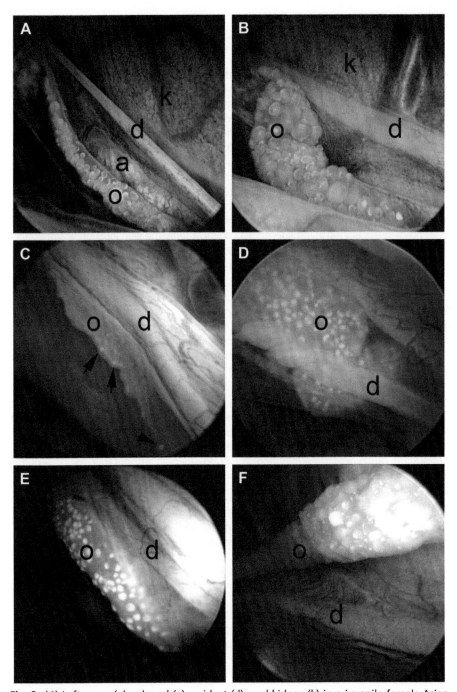

Fig. 9. (A) Left ovary (o), adrenal (a), oviduct (d), and kidney (k) in a juvenile female Asian box turtle (*Cuora flavomarginata*). (B) Close-up of the left ovary (o), oviduct (d), and kidney (k) of a 20-g Asian box turtle. Note the numerous visible follicles throughout the ovarian parenchyma; such early differentiation is uncommon in most species. (C) Poorly differentiated left ovary (o) with few follicles (*arrows*) and oviduct (d) in a 50-g juvenile female radiated tortoise (*A radiata*). (D) Well-differentiated left ovary (o) with many follicles and oviduct (d) in a 150-g juvenile female radiated tortoise. (E) Left ovary (o) and oviduct (d) in a juvenile Galapagos tortoise (*Chelonoidis nigra*). (F) Left ovary (o) and oviduct (d) in a juvenile Hermann's tortoise (*T hermanni*).

(especially if unable to freely drain through the incision) can cause visceral displacement including bladder prolapse through the surgical site. The liver, gastrointestinal tract, and lung are usually obvious, and the lung is followed caudally. At the caudal edge of the lung, the left gonad and kidney are encountered. The immature male testis is usually elongated to round, and may be white to darkly pigmented. However, almost invariably the testis is smooth with superficial blood vessels (**Fig. 8**). The immature ovary is elongated and may be white to yellow with a more irregular, often granulomatous appearance, but only a few follicles may be evident within the parenchyma (**Fig. 9**). In very young animals, the gonads may be poorly differentiated; however, the immature oviduct if usually a much more substantial structure than the pronephric duct of males. Once the sex has been identified, a clear photograph of the gonad is recorded. Fluid may be aspirated via the sheath, or simply allowed to drain by temporarily holding the animal in left lateral recumbency. Only the skin incision is closed using absorbable material (eg, poliglecaprone 25) and a single everting mattress suture. For aquatic species the incision should also be sealed using tissue adhesive.

Postoperative Care

Reptiles are typically ambulatory within 20 minutes of reversal. Chelonians are bathed in shallow water, taking precautions to ensure that the surgical sites are above the water line. Normal feeding commences the following day. Clients are provided with an Adobe document (color) that identifies each animal's sex with a photograph of the gonad.

Complications

Coelioscopic sex identification has been proved to be safe, effective, and essentially 100% accurate in several chelonian species.[14,21,29,30] Errors and complications, although rare, can be associated with preexisting disease/sepsis, iatrogenic bladder perforation, equivocal determination in young animals attributable to inadequate gonadal differentiation, and misidentification resulting from inexperience with a particular species, poor equipment, or poor technique.[29,31,32] To minimize such issues:

1. Start with juveniles at least 12 to 18 months of age to develop competence with a particular species before proceeding with smaller and younger animals.
2. Plan in advance and develop an efficient system with staffed induction, surgery, and recovery areas.
3. Use a quality, small-diameter telescope with color monitor and photodocumentation for later review. If the animal is equivocal, it often helps to review all the images together.
4. Use a consistent, injectable, anesthetic regime.
5. Start with the largest animal in the group and work toward the smallest.
6. Use sterile fluids (eg, lactated ringers) to improve visualization.

REFERENCES

1. Harrison GJ. Endoscopic examination of avian gonadal tissues. Vet Med Small Anim Clin 1978;73(4):479–84.
2. Taylor M. Endoscopic examination and biopsy techniques. In: Ritchie BW, Harrison GJ, Harrison LR, editors. Avian medicine: principles and application. Fort Worth (FL): Harrison Bird Diets International; 1994. p. 327–54.
3. Divers SJ. Diagnostic endoscopy. In: Mader DR, Divers SJ, editors. Current therapy in reptile medicine and surgery. St Louis (MO): Elsevier; 2014. p. 154–78.

4. Divers SJ. Exotic mammal diagnostic and surgical endoscopy. In: Quesenberry KE, Carpenter JW, editors. Rabbits, ferrets and rodents—clinical medicine and surgery. 3rd edition. Philadelphia: Elsevier; 2012. p. 485–501.
5. Stetter M. Minimally invasive surgical techniques in bony fish (Osteichthyes). Vet Clin North Am Exot Anim Pract 2010;13(2):291–9.
6. Divers SJ. Avian diagnostic endoscopy. Vet Clin North Am 2010;13(2):187–202.
7. Crosta L, Gerlach H, Bürkle M, et al. Endoscopic testicular biopsy technique in psittaciformes. J Avian Med Surg 2002;16:106–10.
8. Sladky KK, Krugner-Higby L, Meek-Walker E, et al. Serum concentrations and analgesic effects of liposome-encapsulated and standard butorphanol tartrate in parrots. Am J Vet Res 2006;67(5):775–81.
9. Paul-Murphy J, Ludders JW. Avian analgesia. Vet Clin North Am Exot Anim Pract 2001;4:35–45.
10. Pieau C, Dorizzi M, Richard-Mercier N. Temperature-dependent sex determination and gonadal differentiation in reptiles. EXS 2001;(91):117–41.
11. Wibbels T, Cowan J, LeBoeuf R. Temperature-dependent sex determination in the red-eared slider turtle, *Trachemys scripta*. J Exp Zool 1998;281(5):409–16.
12. Rhen T, Willingham E, Sakata JT, et al. Incubation temperature influences sex-steroid levels in juvenile red-eared slider turtles, *Trachemys scripta*, a species with temperature-dependent sex determination. Biol Reprod 1999;61(5): 1275–80.
13. Rhen T, Lang JW. Temperature-dependent sex determination in the snapping turtle: manipulation of the embryonic sex steroid environment. Gen Comp Endocrinol 1994;96(2):243–54.
14. Kuchling G. Endoscopic sex determination in juvenile freshwater turtles, *Erymnochelys madagascariensis*: morphology of gonads and accessory ducts. Chelonian Conserv Biol 2006;5(1):67–73.
15. Coppoolse KJ, Zwart P. Cloacoscopy in reptiles. Vet Q 1985;7(3):243–5.
16. Wyneken J, Epperly SP, Crowder LB, et al. Determining sex in posthatchling loggerhead sea turtles using multiple gonadal and accessory duct characteristics. Herpetologica 2007;63(1):19–30.
17. Gross TS, Crain DA, Bjorndal KA, et al. Identification of sex in hatchling loggerhead turtles (*Caretta caretta*) by analysis of steroid concentrations in chorioallantoic/amniotic fluid. Gen Comp Endocrinol 1995;99(2):204–10.
18. Hernandez-Divers SJ. Diagnostic and surgical endoscopy. In: Raiti P, Girling S, editors. Manual of reptiles. 2nd edition. Cheltenham (United Kingdom): British Small Animal Veterinary Association; 2004. p. 103–14.
19. Hernandez-Divers SJ, Hernandez-Divers SM, Wilson GH, et al. A review of reptile diagnostic coelioscopy. J Herp Med Surg 2005;15:16–31.
20. Rostal D, Grumbles J, Lance V, et al. Non-lethal sexing techniques for hatchling and immature desert tortoises (*Gopherus agassizii*). Herp Mono 1994;8:103–16.
21. Hernandez-Divers SJ, Stahl SJ, Farrell R. An endoscopic method for identifying sex of hatchling Chinese box turtles and comparison of general versus local anesthesia for coelioscopy. J Am Vet Med Assoc 2009;234(6):800–4.
22. Selleri P, Di Girolamo N, Melidone R. Cystoscopic sex identification of posthatchling chelonians. J Am Vet Med Assoc 2013;242(12):1744–50.
23. Sladky KK, Miletic V, Paul-Murphy J, et al. Analgesic efficacy and respiratory effects of butorphanol and morphine in turtles. J Am Vet Med Assoc 2007;230: 1356–62.
24. Harms CA, Eckert SA, Kubis SA, et al. Field anaesthesia of leatherback sea turtles (*Dermochelys coriacea*). Vet Rec 2007;161(1):15–21.

25. Dennis PM, Heard DJ. Cardiopulmonary effects of a medetomidine-ketamine combination administered intravenously in gopher tortoises. J Am Vet Med Assoc 2002;220(10):1516–9.

26. Greer LL, Jenne KJ, Diggs HE. Medetomidine-ketamine anesthesia in red-eared slider turtles (*Trachemys scripta elegans*). Contemp Top Lab Anim Sci 2001; 40(3):9–11.

27. Hernandez-Divers SJ, Stahl SJ, Farrell R. Endoscopic gender identification of hatchling Chinese box turtles (*Cuora flavomarginata*) under local and general anesthesia. J Am Vet Med Assoc 2009;234(6):800–4.

28. Schumacher J, Yellen T. Anesthesia and analgesia. In: Mader DR, editor. Reptile medicine and surgery. 2nd edition. St Louis (MO): Saunders-Elsevier; 2006. p. 442–52.

29. Kuchling G, Griffiths O. Endoscopic imaging of gonads, sex ratios, and occurrence of intersexes in juvenile captive-bred Aldabra giant tortoises. Chelonian Conserv Biol 2012;11(1):91–6.

30. Kuchling G, Lopez FJ. Endoscopic sexing of juvenile captive-bred ploughshare tortoises *Geochelone yniphora* at Ampijoroa, Madagascar. Dodo 2000;36:94–5.

31. Innis C. Testes morphology in *Cuora flavomarginata*: a response to Kuchling and Griffiths (2012; Chelonian Conservation and Biology 11[1]). Chelonian Conserv Biol 2012;11(2):273–4.

32. Kuchling G. Reply to the commentary of Charles J. Innis: "Testes Morphology in *Cuora flavomarginata*". Chelonian Conserv Biol 2012;11(2):274–5.

Coelioscopic and Endoscope-Assisted Sterilization of Chelonians

Laila M. Proença, MV, DVM, MS, PhD[a],*,
Stephen J. Divers, BSc(Hons), BVetMed, DZooMed,
DipECZM (Herpetology, Zoo Health Management), DACZM, FRCVS[b]

KEYWORDS

- Chelonia • Orchiectomy • Ovariectomy • Ovariosalpingectomy • Coelioscopy
- Endoscope assisted • Sterilization • Endosurgery

KEY POINTS

- Minimally invasive techniques for chelonian sterilization can be offered for many species, representing a new revenue stream for exotic animal practices and decreasing reproductive disease.
- Prefemoral coeliotomy (soft tissue approach) provides faster recovery, shorter healing times, and reduced pain compared with traditional central plastron coeliotomy.
- Coelioscopic and endoscope-assisted chelonian sterilization offer superior visualization, compared with nonendoscopic prefemoral techniques.
- Orchiectomy of chelonians with elongated testes is only currently possible with the aid of endoscopy and the use of endosurgical instruments.

 Videos on Coelioscopic orchiectomy and Endoscope-assisted oophorectomy accompany this article at http://www.vetexotic.theclinics.com/

INTRODUCTION

Elective sterilization is a safe and well-established surgical procedure performed in dogs and cats worldwide.[1,2] Conversely, chelonian sterilization has been mostly performed as part of the treatment of a reproductive disorder, because of the intricate anatomy and difficult access to the reproductive organs.[3-7]

The authors have nothing to disclose.
[a] VCA Animal Hospitals, 12401 West Olympic Boulevard, Los Angeles, CA 90064, USA;
[b] Department of Small Animal Medicine and Surgery, College of Veterinary Medicine, University of Georgia, 2200 College Station Road, Athens, GA 30602, USA
* Corresponding author.
E-mail address: laila.proenca@vca.com

Previously, in order to gain access to the testes and ovaries, one would have to perform a central plastron coeliotomy, a recognized invasive, traumatic, and long surgical procedure.[3,4] Later, the development of soft tissue prefemoral approach allowed a less-invasive but still limited access to the coelom and reproductive tract. As an example, prefemoral coeliotomy may not provide adequate visualization of the coelomic cavity in chelonians that have relatively small prefemoral fossae. In addition, exteriorization of the ovaries through the prefemoral coeliotomy of immature females is not possible. Nevertheless, the benefits of prefemoral coeliotomy include faster recovery, shorter healing times, and reduced pain when compared with traditional central plastron coeliotomy.[5–8]

With advances in chelonian endoscopy, novel techniques for soft tissue prefemoral coelioscopic and endoscope-assisted sterilization have been published.[5,7,9–11] Such techniques were shown to provide the same benefits as traditional prefemoral approaches, with the advantage of improved visualization of the coelomic cavity and the ability to perform intracorporeal surgery.[7] At present, minimally invasive techniques for chelonian sterilization can be offered for many species, opening a new revenue stream for exotic practitioners.

This article summarizes and describes current coelioscopic and endoscope-assisted chelonian sterilization techniques. An appreciation of the normal chelonian anatomy, physiology, and anesthesia is paramount, and the reader is encouraged to review the previously published literature.

INDICATIONS FOR CHELONIAN STERILIZATION

- Permanent prevention of unwanted breeding (eg, population management, management of inbreeding individuals, contraception of hybridized specimens)[5–7,9–14]
- Management of behavioral problems (eg, male aggression, traumatic courtship)
- Treatment and/or prevention of reproductive diseases and disorders
  - Follicular stasis
  - Dystocia
  - Ovarian/salpingial/oviductal disease (eg, rupture, torsion, impaction, infection, neoplasia)
  - Ectopic egg/follicle and/or egg yolk coelomitis
  - Adjunct treatment of reproduction-related prolapses of the cloaca, oviduct, or phallus
  - Testicular disease (neoplasia, infection)

CONTRAINDICATIONS FOR CHELONIAN STERILIZATION

- Any contraindication for anesthesia and/or surgery.[5,7,14]
- Size of the prefemoral fossa when compared with the target structure (ie, follicle/egg/mass/abscess must be smaller than the prefemoral fossa).
- Lack of appropriate equipment.
- Lack of appropriate training.

ENDOSCOPIC EQUIPMENT

- Telescope: The most versatile telescope used in exotic pet medicine is the 2.7-mm, 30° 18-cm telescope.[7,8,15,16] Protection sheath (3.5 mm) is optional but strongly recommended to avoid damage to the telescope, but a larger operating sheath is not required and may indeed be a hindrance if space is restricted. For larger animals, 5-mm (5–100 kg) or 10-mm (>100 kg) telescopes may be required.
- Endovideo camera.

- Xenon light source and light cable: Depending on the size of the animal, halogen light might be used (animals weighing<2 kg).
- Imaging capture system (optional).
- Monitor: Optionally, 2 monitors might be connected to the camera to permit coelioscopy from either side of the table.
- Ring and elastic stay retractor (eg, Lone star retractor, CooperSurgical Inc, Trumbull, CT, USA).
- 3-mm (<10 kg) to 5-mm (>10 kg) Babcock forceps (Storz, Tuttlingen, Germany) with ratchet handle.
- Appropriately sized stainless-steel vascular clips and applicator (eg, Hemoclips, Teleflex, Morrisville, NC, USA).
- 3-mm (<10 kg) to 5-mm (>10 kg) short curved Metzenbaum scissors (Storz, Tuttlingen, Germany), with a nonracket handle and radiosurgery connector.
- 3-mm (<10 kg) to 5-mm (>10 kg) bipolar endoscopic forceps.
- 3-mm (<10 kg) to 5-mm (>10 kg) atraumatic (or fenestrated) forceps with ratchet handle.
- Radiosurgery preferred for animals less than 10 kg (eg, Surgitron 4.0 MHz, Ellman International, Inc, Hicksville, NY, USA); 5-mm (10–100 kg) or 10-mm (>100 kg) LigaSure (Covidien, Mansfield, MA, USA) preferred for larger animals.
- Mechanical holding arm for the telescope or a surgical assistant (optional).

PATIENT PREPARATION

Routine considerations for preanesthetic evaluation and surgical preparation should be performed. Fasting times depend on the size and species but are typically between 24 and 72 hours. Preoperative coelomic ultrasonography can help confirm the size and nature of the reproductive tract and assist with surgical planning. The animal should be encouraged to defecate and urinate before surgery, in order to reduce the chances of iatrogenic trauma to the bladder or large intestine. Digital stimulation to the cloaca or shallow bathing can be effective. Different anesthesia protocols are available, and the reader is encouraged to review the latest literature.[16–18] Local infiltration with 2 mg/kg lidocaine is generally used at the prefemoral incision site and may be combined with intrathecal lidocaine.[10,14]

ORCHIECTOMY
General Comments

Orchiectomy in chelonians is a challenging procedure, because the testes are located in the dorsocaudal coelomic cavity and intimately associated with the kidney below the carapace. The mesorchium is short, such that the testes cannot be exteriorized from the coelom.[8,11,19] It is important to notice that the surgical technique differs depending on the testicular size and shape, which can change dramatically with age and even season.

Endoscopic orchiectomy was successfully performed in 28 juvenile to adult red-eared sliders and 1 adult eastern painted turtle (*Chrysemys picta picta*), with small, globoid testes (0.5–1 cm in diameter) and mean bodyweight of 436 g.[11] For these species, orchiectomy was possible using a single vascular clip and/or radiosurgical scissors with limited dissection. By contrast, this procedure in the only juvenile Amazon river turtle (*Podocnemis unifilis,* weighing 1.5 kg) in the study was protracted and complicated because of the elongated nature of the gonads (4–5 cm in length).[8] The investigators were able to perform bilateral orchiectomy through a single incision on the left prefemoral fossa (right lateral recumbency) in 22 of the 27 animals in the study. However, the remaining 5 turtles required bilateral incisions, thus right and left lateral recumbency were necessary.

Endoscope-assisted orchiectomy was also successfully performed in 10 Hermann's tortoises (*Testudo hermanni* sp.) with testes of similar shape and size (oval and with 0.8–1 cm diameter) and mean body weight of 796.5 g. In contrast to the species described above, the Herman's tortoise in the study presented an even shorter mesorchium and orchiectomy was only possible through a bilateral prefemoral approach, using one or more vascular clips. The investigators considered that radiosurgery was practical for the tortoises because of the risk of damaging the adjacent tissue.[11]

Feasible and practical technique of endoscopic orchiectomy in chelonians with elongated testis has been described in 7 adult Mojave desert tortoises (testicle length of approximately 6–8 cm and mean weight of 7 kg). Surgery was successfully conducted through a bilateral prefemoral approach via sequential vascular clip ligation and radiosurgery (monopolar/bipolar). Bipolar endoscopic forceps were considered indispensable because of the extensive mesorchial attachments and their close association with the kidney.[7]

Patient Positioning

Once surgical anesthesia has been achieved, the hind limbs should be extended caudal and taped together to expose both prefemoral fossae. On a heated surgery table, the animal should first be positioned in lateral recumbency, with the use of towels or a vacuum bean bag. This lateral position draws organs away from the least dependent fossa and reduces iatrogenic trauma during entry. The prefemoral fossa and surrounding shell are aseptically prepared and draped using standard techniques.[7,8] Right lateral recumbency for an initial left prefemoral approach is preferred by right-handed surgeons; however, if the contralateral gonad cannot be reached, a bilateral approach may be necessary.

Surgical Technique

The craniocaudal skin incision should extend approximately 50% to 75% of the craniocaudal length of the prefemoral fossa (**Fig. 1**A). The subcutaneous tissues are bluntly dissected, and the aponeurosis of the tendinosis parts of the ventral and oblique abdominal muscles are identified and incised exposing the coelomic membrane (see **Fig. 1**B, C). A 3-mm incision is made in the coelomic membrane to permit insertion of the telescope and confirm entry into the coelom (see **Fig. 1**D). The coelomic membrane incision is extended, taking care not to damage the often voluminous and closely associated bladder, large intestine, septum horizontale (postpulmonary septum), or lung. It is wise to cease assisted respiration during entry to reduce the size of the lung. A ring and elastic stay retractor is positioned to improve exposure of the coelom (see **Fig. 1**E). If the urinary bladder is distended and obstructing the surgical view, cystocentesis can be performed. The use of a single prefemoral coeliotomy incision permits the use of multiple instruments without the need for separate ports/cannulae (**Fig. 2**).[5,7] A mechanical arm can be used to hold the telescope, freeing both hands of the surgeon for instrument use (**Fig. 3**); alternatively, a surgical assistant is required to support the scope (**Fig. 4**).[6,11,16]

After endoscopic examination of the coelomic cavity, the left testis is identified and grasped with the Babcock forceps inserted alongside the telescope.[8,16] The testis is elevated, and the mesorchium is exposed (**Figs. 5**A, B and **6**A–C). To free the testis from its mesorchial attachments, 3 techniques have been described.[7,8,16] The first

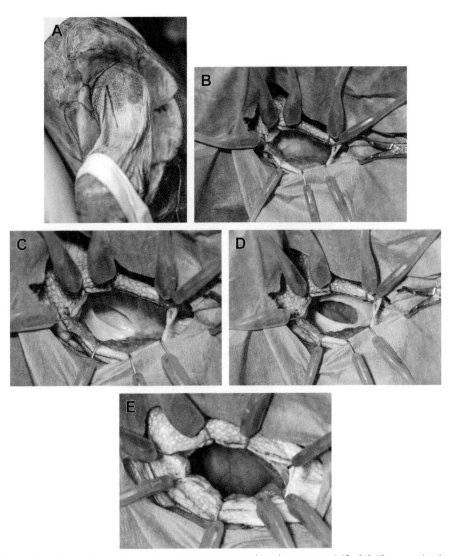

Fig. 1. Prefemoral coeliotomy in a desert tortoise (*Gopherus agassizii*). (*A*) The tortoise is positioned in right lateral recumbency to expose the right prefemoral fossa. The line indicates the length and location of the prefemoral incision. (*B*) After prefemoral skin incision, the subcutaneous tissues are bluntly dissected to expose the aponeurosis of the tendinosis parts of the ventral and oblique abdominal muscles. (*C*) After incision of this aponeurosis, the coelomic membrane is visualized. (*D*) The coelomic membrane is carefully incised to reveal the coelomic organs. (*E*) The coelomic membrane incision is extended, and a ring and elastic stay retractor is positioned to improve exposure of the coelom. (*Copyright* © 2015 The University of Georgia. All Rights Reserved.)

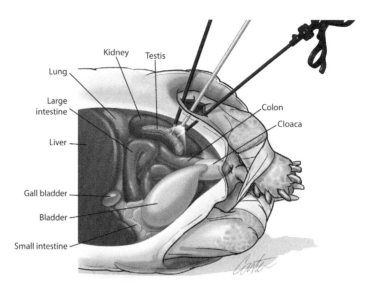

Fig. 2. Regional anatomy and instrument position during prefemoral coelioscopic orchiectomy of a male desert tortoise (*Gopherus agassizii*) in right lateral recumbency. (*Copyright* © 2015 The University of Georgia. All Rights Reserved.)

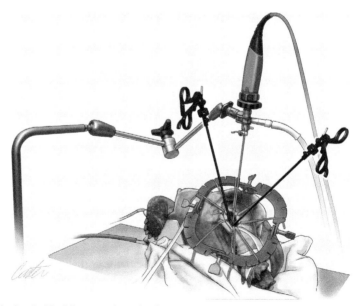

Fig. 3. Mechanical holding arm (MHA) telescope orientation during prefemoral coelioscopic orchiectomy of a male desert tortoise (*Gopherus agassizii*). The optimal position of the MHA telescope is achieved when the telescope is positioned perpendicular to the table, in the middorsal region of the incision. A ring and elastic stay retractor is used to improve exposure of the coelom. (*Copyright* © 2015 The University of Georgia. All Rights Reserved.)

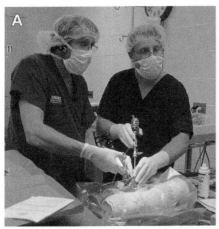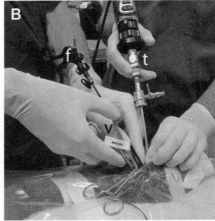

Fig. 4. Orchiectomy in red-eared slider (*Trachemys scripta elegans*). (*A*) One surgeon manipulates the instruments, while the assistant holds the camera. (*B*) Close-up of the instrument manipulation. (*Copyright* © 2015 The University of Georgia. All Rights Reserved.)

is preferred for larger elongated testes, whereas the latter 2 are more suitable for smaller rounded testes;

1. A combination of stainless-steel vascular clips, bipolar coagulation, and dissection using 3-mm scissors (with and without monopolar coagulation) was used to dissect the testes free in a caudal to cranial direction (see **Fig. 5C–F**, Video 1).
2. Ligation of the mesorchium using a stainless-steel vascular clip, followed by transection of the mesorchium distal to the clip using 3-mm curved Metzenbaum scissors (see **Fig. 6D–F**).
3. Monopolar coagulation and incision using 3-mm curved Metzenbaum scissors connected to a radiosurgical unit (see **Fig. 6G–I**).

After complete removal of the left testis, the coelomic cavity is inspected to verify hemostasis. If the right testis cannot be isolated from the left approach, the left prefemoral coeliotomy is closed in a routine manner (**Fig. 7**) and the procedure repeated via the right prefemoral fossa.

OOPHORECTOMY/OVARIECTOMY/OVARIOSALPINGECTOMY
General Comments

Elective and therapeutic prefemoral endoscope-assisted ovariectomy or ovariosalpingectomy have been described in several species of chelonians, including the red-eared slider, Galapagos tortoise (*Geochelone nigra*), box turtle (*Terrapene carolina*), painted turtle (*Chrysemys picta*), 4-eyed turtle (*Sacalia bealei*), and Chinese red-necked pound turtle (*Chinemys kwangtungensis*).[5,9,10,15] Prefemoral endoscope-assisted ovariectomy and ovariosalpingectomy have been successfully used to treat reproductive disorders such as obstructive and nonobstructive dystocia and ectopic eggs.[5,9,10]

Patient Positioning

Dorsal recumbency is generally preferred for mature individuals, but the animal can be placed in lateral recumbency for the coeliotomy approach and subsequently repositioned into dorsal recumbency for the endoscopic procedure. In the authors' experience, identification and exteriorization of the mature ovaries is easier with the

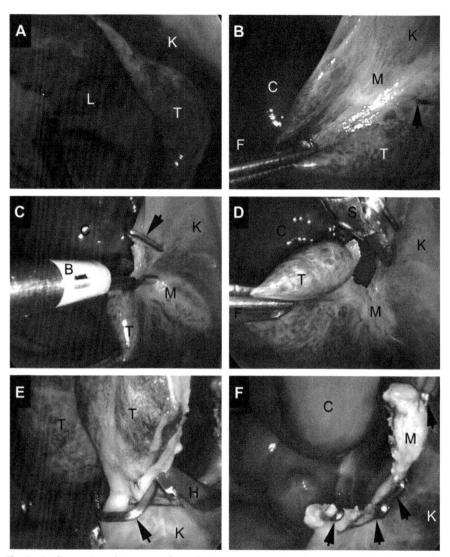

Fig. 5. Coelioscopic orchiectomy of a male desert tortoise (*Gopherus agassizii*) via sequential vascular clip ligation and radiosurgical dissection. (*A*) Telescopic view of the caudal coelom via a left prefemoral approach. (*B*) Atraumatic endoscopic forceps (F) used to expose the mesorchium and associated vasculature (*arrow*). (*C*) Stainless-steel vascular clip (*arrow*) has been placed on the caudal aspect of the mesorchium, close to the kidney, before mesorchial coagulation using bipolar forceps (B). (*D*) Mesorchial dissection using short curved Metzenbaum scissors (S). (*E*) Placement of vascular clip (*arrow*) across the cranial aspect of the mesorchium. (*H*) Vascular clip applicator. (*F*) View of the ligation clips (*arrows*) across the mesorchium remnant after excision of the testis. C, colon; K, kidney; L, Lung; M, mesorchium T, testis. (*From* Proença L, Fowler S, Kleine S, et al. Single surgeon coelioscopic orchiectomy of desert tortoises (*Gopherus agassizii*) for population management. Vet Rec 2014;175:404; with permission.)

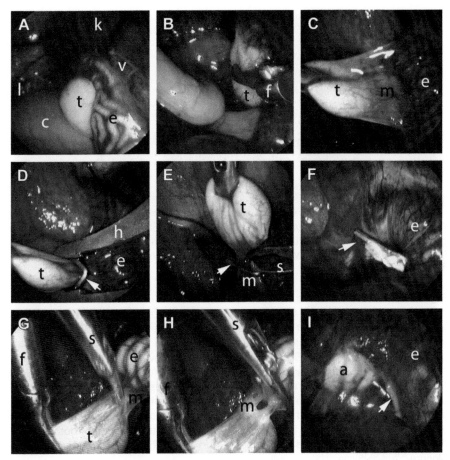

Fig. 6. Endoscopic orchiectomy in the red-eared slider (*Trachemys scripta elegans*) via a unilateral prefemoral incision. (*A*) View of the left testis (t) and epididymis (e) closely associated with the kidney (k) and renal vein (v). The descending colon (c) and caudal lung (l) are also visible. (*B*) 3 mm Kelly forceps (f) are introduced and used to grasp the testis (t). (*C*) The forceps are angled to retract the testis (t) cranially away from the epididymis (e) to expose the mesorchium (V) and associated vascular supply. (*D–F*) Orchiectomy using vascular clips. A vascular clip applicator (v) is introduced, and a single clip (*arrows*) is placed across the mesorchium, between the testis (t) and the epididymis (e), before the testis is dissected free using 3-mm scissors (s). (*G–I*) Orchiectomy using radiosurgery. While retracting the testis (t) away from the epididymis (e), monopolar scissors (s) are used to coagulate the mesorchial vessels, before dissecting the testis free and removing with forceps (f). After orchiectomy, the adrenal gland (a) can be seen. (*Copyright* © 2015 The University of Georgia. All Rights Reserved.)

animal in dorsal recumbency but greater care must be taken to avoid iatrogenic organ trauma. When dealing with immature ovaries, a bilateral approach is typically required with the animal in lateral recumbency.

Mature Chelonian Ovariectomy/Oophorectomy

Following a left prefemoral approach, the left ovary consisting of variably sized follicles is identified using the telescope (**Fig. 8**A, B). The endoscopic atraumatic forceps are used to grasp the interfollicular tissue and gently exteriorize the gonad (see

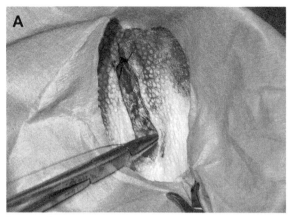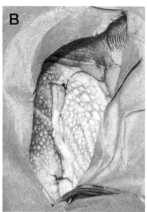

Fig. 7. (*A*) Coelomic closure was accomplished with a simple continuous pattern of the coelomic aponeurosis and subcutaneous tissues with appropriately sized absorbable suture. (*B*) The skin is closed routinely. (*Copyright* © 2015 The University of Georgia. All Rights Reserved.)

Fig. 8C–E). Once the ovary is elevated to the level of the prefemoral incision, delicate manual manipulation is used to exteriorize the organ completely. Care must be taken to assure that the entire left ovary is exteriorized from the cavity. The mesovarial vasculature is identified and ligated using stainless-steel vascular clips and/or coagulation, as necessary (see **Fig. 8**F, Video 2). The left ovary is transected, distal to the ligation, using Metzenbaum scissors and removed before inspection of the coelom to verify hemostasis. In many cases, the right ovary can also be visualized from this left approach and can be removed as previously described. If the ovary cannot be visualized or cannot be exteriorized via the left prefemoral incision, the left side is closed and a right prefemoral approach is performed. After complete resection of both ovaries, the coelomic cavity should be inspected to verify hemostasis, before routine closure.[5,9,10,13,16]

Immature Chelonian Ovariectomy/Oophorectomy

When dealing with immature animals, the mesovarium is short and it is impossible to exteriorize the ovaries using the technique described above. Instead, an intracorporeal technique is required and has been described for the Galapagos tortoise (**Fig. 9**).[12] The paired immature ovaries reside in the caudodorsal coelom, in close association with the retrocoelomic kidney (similar to the position of the testes in males). The technique for ovariectomy is very similar to that described earlier for elongated testes, that is, a progressive dissection through the mesovarium. However, the immaturity and subsequent reduced blood supply to the ovaries does not require vascular clip ligation. Even in a 30-kg juvenile Galapagos tortoise, dissection can be accomplished using scissors with monopolar coagulation (**Fig. 10**).

Ovariosalpingectomy

The ovariosalpingectomy is performed using the endoscopic atraumatic forceps with ratchet handle to grasp the oviduct and carefully exteriorize the organ through the prefomoral incision. The vasculature of the mesovaria and mesosalpinx are ligated using suitably sized vascular clips, before transection. The oviduct is ligated close to the insertion with the cloaca and transected.[5,9,10,13]

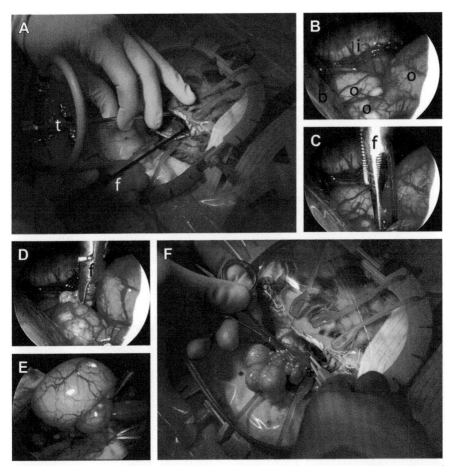

Fig. 8. Endoscope-assisted oophorectomy in an adult red-eared slider (*Trachemys scripta el-egans*). (*A*) Following a prefemoral approach to the coelom, the ipsilateral ovary is located and retracted to the incision using the telescope (t) and 3-mm atraumatic forceps (f). (*B*) Endoscopic view of the caudal coelom demonstrating the ovary and 3 large ova (o), closely associated with the bladder (b) and intestine (i). (*C*) Endoscopic view of 3-mm atraumatic forceps (f) being used to grasp the interfollicular tissue. (*D*) Endoscopic view of the ovary being gently retracted toward the prefemoral incision. (*E*) External view (taken using the telescope) demonstrating the first 2 follicles of the ovary exteriorized through the prefemoral incision. (*F*) Continued manipulation to exteriorize the whole ovary proceeds surgical oophorectomy using radiosurgery. In most animals, the contralateral ovary can also be removed through the same prefemoral incision. (*Copyright* © 2015 The University of Georgia. All Rights Reserved.)

Prefemoral Coeliotomy Closure

Closure is typically routine with the size of the suture material depending on the size of the animal and surgeon preference. For most pet species, the authors have used absorbable poliglecaprone 25 (MONOCRYL Plus; Ethicon, Cornelia, GA), on a tapered needle in a simple continuous pattern to close the coelomic aponeurosis and subcutaneous tissues, and either poliglecaprone 25 or polydioxanone (PDS II; Ethicon) on a cutting needle and in a simple horizontal mattress pattern to close the skin.

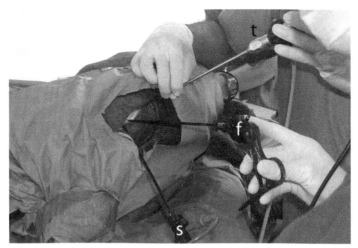

Fig. 9. Ovariectomy in a juvenile Galapagos tortoise. One surgeon manipulates the instrumentation while the second maintains camera and telescope positioning. (*Copyright ©* 2015 The University of Georgia. All Rights Reserved.)

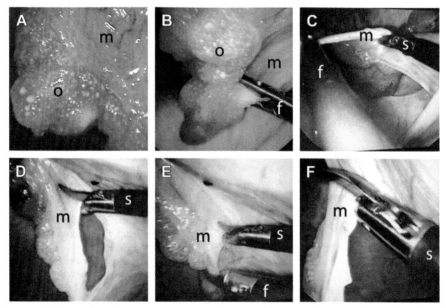

Fig. 10. Endoscopic left oophorectomy in a juvenile Galapagos tortoise (*Geochelone nigra*) with all instrumentation inserted through the right prefemoral fossa. (*A*) Normal, immature, left ovary (o) suspended from the caudodorsal body wall by a short mesovarium ligament (m). (*B*) Grasping forceps (f) are introduced and used to grasp the mesovarium (m) but not the friable ovary (o). (*C*) The mesovarium (m) is stretched by moving the forceps (f) cranially, while radiosurgical scissors (s) are used to incise through the suspensory ligament. (*D–F*) Dissection through the mesovarium (m) continues using forceps (f) and scissors (s) until the ovary is dissected free and can be removed through the prefemoral incision. The incision is closed before the procedure is repeated via the right prefemoral fossa to remove the contralateral ovary. (*Copyright ©* 2015 The University of Georgia. All Rights Reserved.)

Table 1
Complications associated with coelioscopic ovariectomy in chelonians and their management

Complication	Management
Iatrogenic organ perforation during coeliotomy approach (ie, bladder, intestine)	The viscus should be repaired using fine suture material. If severe, a transplastron coeliotomy (osteotomy) may be required. In any case, profuse coelomic lavage and antimicrobial therapy are required
Follicle/egg rupture	The follicle/egg can be removed from the coelom using suction and/or atraumatic forceps (for egg shell). Thorough lavage of the coelom is necessary. Antibiotic therapy may be warranted if the ova was infected
Ectopic follicle/egg	The follicle/egg can be retrieved from the coelom using light suction (directly with the sterile hose) or by using sterile cotton-tipped applicators or a sterile spoon. Thorough lavage is warranted
Hemorrhage	The site of the hemorrhage must be identified and stopped. Radiosurgery, electrocautery, vascular clips, and suture may be useful. If all these attempts fail, local pressure with a sterile cotton-tipped applicator and/or absorbable gelatin sponge (Gelfoam, Baxter, Deerfield, IL, USA) may be used. Assessment of packed cell volume (PCV) is warranted, and blood transfusion may be indicated in extreme cases
Size of the egg/follicle is larger than that of prefemoral fossa incision	The follicles should be measured ultrasonographically before endosurgery Attempt should be made to extend the prefemoral incision to the maximum length. If not enough, aborting the procedure (if elective) or converting to plastron osteotomy should be considered. In some cases, the follicle/egg, when exposed to the level of the prefemoral incision, can be aspirated and then retrieved. However, one should be aware that the weight of the follicle/egg may cause rupturing of the vasculature of the mesovarium, complicating the surgical procedure
Oviductal rupture	Hemiovariohysterectomy or bilateral ovariohysterectomy should be considered
Postoperative coelomitis	Consecutive coelom lavages with warm sterile saline should be performed. Cytology (gram stain), culture, and sensitivity are recommended before starting antibiotic therapy
Iatrogenic organ lesion due to monopolar collateral damage (ie, kidney, intestine, bladder, lung, adrenal)	General clinical health as well as specific organ function should be monitored with blood tests and/or imaging. In case of damage to the intestines or bladder, partial resection should be considered, because subsequent necrosis may lead to perforation postoperatively
Organ prolapse (ie, bladder) through the prefemoral incision	The prolapsed organ should be kept clean and moist until correction. The site and prolapsed organ should be aseptically prepared and lavaged. The incision should be reopened and the organ replaced in the coelomic cavity. Thorough lavage of the coelom with warm sterile saline is required. The incision site must be resutured with caution to avoid recurrent prolapses
Suture dehiscence	Thorough lavage of the coelom with warm sterile saline is needed. The incision site must be resutured with caution to avoid recurrent prolapses. Treatment of the cause of dehiscence is required (ie, infection)

COMPLICATIONS AND MANAGEMENT

The most common complications and management of coelioscopic and endoscope-assisted chelonian sterilization are presented in **Table 1**. Routine standards of care regarding hospitalization, supportive management, and critical care treatment are based on each individual case. It is noteworthy that postsurgical infections are rare, even following field surgeries, because only tissues to be removed are exteriorized and there is no direct exposure of internal viscera (as there would be during a traditional transplastron coeliotomy).

POSTOPERATIVE CARE

General postoperative care should include:

- Pain management (may vary according to the surgical procedure and disease, if present). General pain control might include, but is not limited to, the following:
  - Meloxicam 0.2 mg/kg, administered orally, subcutaneous, intramuscularly (IM), or intravenously every 24 to 48 hours,[20]
  - Hydromorphone 0.5 mg/kg subcutaneously or IM every 24 hours,[21] or
  - Tramadol 5 to 10 mg/kg orally[22]
- Daily monitoring and aseptic care of the surgical wound.
- Daily monitoring of weight, food, and water intake.
- Daily monitoring of urination and defecation (eg, lack of urination might suggest bladder rupture or dehydration).
- Access to bathing should be limited such that the surgical incision is not below the water line for the first 7 days (or sooner if sealed using tissue adhesive).
- Animal should be kept separate from cohabitants until fully recovered.
- Orchiectomized males should be kept separated from fertile females. Chelonian spermatozoa are known to persist within the epididymis for 4 to 6 months,[23] and therefore it may be wise to keep orchiectomized males away from fertile females for at least 6 months.[8]
- Antibiotic therapy is recommended when infection is present and should be based on culture and sensitivity testing. However, oxytetracycline (10 mg/kg, IM) has been used preemptively in case of elective sterilization under suboptimal circumstances or unknown patient history for population management projects.[7,10,14]

CURRENT CONTROVERSIES/FUTURE CONSIDERATIONS

- Owing to the small number of publications involving only selected number of species, further studies involving different species are needed to assess the safety of coelioscopic and endoscope-assisted sterilization more widely. Extrapolations among species should be carefully considered.
- Although the current techniques for chelonian sterilization have been shown to be safe and effective, one should be prepared for complications due to variations in gonadal size and shape (age and seasonal).
- It is hoped that additional experience with a wider variety of species and innovations in endoscopic equipment and techniques will lead to further improvements in chelonian sterilization.

SUMMARY

Minimally invasive techniques for chelonian sterilization can be offered for many species, representing a potentially new revenue stream in exotic pet practice. Soft tissue prefemoral coeliotomy provides faster recovery, shorter healing times, and reduced pain when compared with traditional transplastron coeliotomy. Coelioscopic and endoscope-assisted chelonian sterilization offer superior visualization, compared with nonendoscopic prefemoral techniques. Orchiectomy of chelonians with elongated testes is only currently possible with the aid of endoscopy and the use of endosurgical instruments. Further studies involving different species of chelonians are needed to assess the safety of coelioscopic and endoscope-assisted sterilization more widely. Extrapolations among species should be carefully considered.

SUPPLEMENTARY DATA

Supplementary data related to this article can be found online at http://dx.doi.org/10. 1016/j.cvex.2015.05.004.

REFERENCES

1. DeTora M, McCarthy RJ. Ovariohysterectomy versus ovariectomy for elective sterilization of female dogs and cats: is removal of the uterus necessary? J Am Vet Med Assoc 2011;239:1409–12.
2. Stevens B, Posner L, Jones C, et al. Comparison of the effect of intratesticular lidocaine/bupivacaine vs. saline placebo on pain scores and incision site reactions in dogs undergoing routine castration. Vet J 2013;196:499–503.
3. Lawson GO, Garstka WR. Castration of turtles, *Pseudemys scripta*. J Ala Acad Sci 1985;56:89.
4. Mader DR, Bennett RA, Funk RS, et al. Surgery. In: Mader DR, editor. Reptile medicine and surgery. 2nd edition. St. Louis (MO): Elsevier; 2006. p. 581–630.
5. Innis CJ, Hernandez-Divers S, Martinez-Jimenez D. Coelioscopic-assisted prefemoral oophorectomy in chelonians. J Am Vet Med Assoc 2007;230:1049–52.
6. Innis CJ, Boyer TH. Chelonian reproductive disorders. Vet Clin North Am Exot Anim Pract 2002;5:555–78.
7. Proença L, Fowler S, Kleine S, et al. Single surgeon coelioscopic orchiectomy of desert tortoises (*Gopherus agassizii*) for population management. Vet Rec 2014; 175:404.
8. Innis CJ, Feinsod R, Hanlon J, et al. Coelioscopic orchiectomy can be effectively and safely accomplished in chelonians. Vet Rec 2013;172:526.
9. Mans C, Sladky K. Diagnosis and management of oviductal disease in three red-eared slider turtles (*Trachemys scripta elegans*). J Small Anim Pract 2012;53: 234–9.
10. Knafo SE, Divers SJ, Rivera S, et al. Sterilisation of hybrid Galapagos tortoises (*Geochelone nigra*) for island restoration. Part 1: endoscopic oophorectomy of females under ketamine-medetomidine anaesthesia. Vet Rec 2011;168:47.
11. Paries S, Funcke S, Ziegler L, et al. Endoscopic assisted orchiectomy in Herman's tortoises (*Testudo hermanni* sp.). Tierarztl Prax Ausg K Kleintiere Heimtiere 2014;42:383–9.
12. Frye FL, Dybdal NO, Harshbarger JC. Testicular interstitial cell tumor in a desert tortoise (*Gopherus agassizi*). The Journal of Zoo Animal Medicine 1988;55–8.
13. Minter LJ, Landry MM, Lewbart GA. Prophylactic ovariosalpingectomy using a prefemoral approach in eastern box turtles (*Terrapene carolina carolina*). Vet Rec 2008;163:487.
14. Rivera S, Divers SJ, Knafo SE, et al. Sterilisation of hybrid Galapagos tortoises (*Geochelone nigra*) for island restoration. Part 2: phallectomy of males under intrathecal anaesthesia with lidocaine. Vet Rec 2011;168:78.

15. Divers SJ. Endoscopy equipment and instrumentation for use in exotic animal medicine. Vet Clin North Am Exot Anim Pract 2010;13:171–85.

16. Divers SJ. Endoscope-assisted and endoscopic surgery. In: Mader DR, Divers SJ, editors. Current therapy in reptile medicine and surgery. St Louis (MO): Elsevier Health Sciences; 2014. p. 179–96.

17. Schumacher J, Mans C. Anesthesia. In: Divers SJ, Mader DR, editors. Current therapy in reptile medicine and surgery. St Louis (MO): Elsevier Health Sciences; 2014. p. 134–53.

18. Divers SJ. Reptile diagnostic endoscopy and endosurgery. Vet Clin North Am Exot Anim Pract 2010;13:217–42.

19. O'Malley B. Tortoises and turtles. Clinical anatomy and physiology of exotic species. London: Elsevier Saunders; 2005. p. 41–56.

20. Divers SJ, Papich M, McBride M, et al. Pharmacokinetics of meloxicam following intravenous and oral administration in green iguanas (*Iguana iguana*). Am J Vet Res 2010;71:1277–83.

21. Mans C, Lahner LL, Baker BB, et al. Antinociceptive efficacy of buprenorphine and hydromorphone in red-eared slider turtles (*Trachemys scripta elegans*). J Zoo Wildl Med 2012;43:662–5.

22. Baker BB, Sladky KK, Johnson SM. Evaluation of the analgesic effects of oral and subcutaneous tramadol administration in red-eared slider turtles. J Am Vet Med Assoc 2011;238:220–7.

23. Lofts B, Tsui HW. Histological and histochemical changes in the gonads and epididymides of the male soft-shelled turtle, *Trionyx sinensis*. J Zool 1977;181:57–68.

Video Telescope Operating Microscopy

Stephen J. Divers, BSc(Hons), BVetMed, DZooMed,
DipECZM (Herpetology, Zoo Health Management), DACZM, FRCVS

KEYWORDS

- Endoscopy • VITOM • Operating microscopy • Magnification • Microsurgery

KEY POINTS

- Focused illumination and magnification are requisites for successful microsurgery, which is frequently required for exotic pet surgery.
- Existing endoscopy equipment can be used with a mechanical arm to create an operating microscopy system.
- Veterinarians with existing endoscopy light source and camera equipment should consider the video telescopic operating microscope system as a viable alternative to traditional magnification systems.

INTRODUCTION

According to a 2007 US pet census, there are around 106 million exotic pets in the United States, compared with around 150 million dogs and cats.[1] Of particular interest is that, while the dog and cat population has only grown by 13% since 2001, the exotic pet population has increased by more than 30% during the same period. Most of these exotic species are psttacines, passerines, turtles, snakes, lizards, ferrets, rabbits, rodents, and fish, and owners have come to expect a comparable level of medicine and surgery for these animals as they do for domesticated species. High owner expectations coupled with the fact that most exotic pets weigh less than 2 kg means that the exotic animal surgeon has to face 2 major obstacles:

1. A huge diversity in taxa-specific anatomy, physiology, and disease
2. A heavy reliance on magnification for adequate surgical visualization and microsurgical techniques.

The author has nothing to disclose.
Department of Small Animal Medicine and Surgery, College of Veterinary Medicine, University of Georgia, 2200 College Station Road, Athens, GA 30602, USA
E-mail address: sdivers@uga.edu

Vet Clin Exot Anim 18 (2015) 571–578
http://dx.doi.org/10.1016/j.cvex.2015.05.007
1094-9194/15/$ – see front matter © 2015 Elsevier Inc. All rights reserved.

This need for excellent visualization using a focused light source and magnification has been well documented in many exotic animal texts and has in-part fueled recent developments in minimally invasive endoscopic and endosurgical techniques.[2–5] Nevertheless, we are far from being able to perform all procedures endoscopically, and therefore, the need for traditional, open surgical techniques in small exotic species remains of paramount importance.

ILLUMINATION AND MAGNIFICATION: VIDEO TELESCOPIC OPERATING MICROSCOPE

Traditionally, adequate surgical lighting has been achieved by the use of large, focused overhead light units. Although magnification can be achieved using operating microscopes, their expense and reduced maneuverability have made them less favored by most exotic animal practitioners. Instead, headband or frame-mounted operating loupes with a dedicated light source have gained popularity because they are more affordable, versatile, and simpler to operate.

The recent development of a video telescopic operating microscope (VITOM-25; Karl Storz Veterinary Endoscopy America Inc, Goleta, CA, USA) has provided another option for delivering high-quality focused illumination and magnification. The VITOM uses existing endoscopy equipment, specifically, the light source, camera, and documentation hardware that is commonly used in practice in order to perform extracorporeal visualization of surgical procedures.

The VITOM 25 system is composed of a 11-cm 0° rod-lens telescope that is held 25 to 60 cm above the surgical site by means of a mechanical arm that clamps to the operating table (**Fig. 1**). The system provides a depth of field of 2 to 6 cm and a range of fields of view and magnifications dependent on distance from the surgical site (**Table 1**). The articulated, mechanical arm has a single lock mechanism that controls all 5 joint functions, thereby facilitating easy, rapid positioning. A metal clamp holds the telescope and light guide cable in place. Illumination is controlled at the light source, while the surgeon controls zoom, focus, white balance, and photo/video documentation from the camera. It is noteworthy that the mechanical holding arm can hold any telescope, including the 2.7-mm, and can replace a surgical assistant when performing endoscope-assisted or endosurgery. The VITOM system is autoclavable and typically sterilized before placement and positioning by sterile surgical

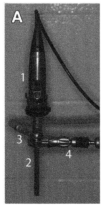
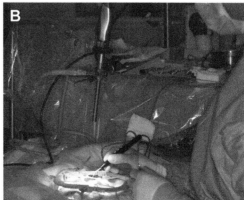

Fig. 1. (*A*) Endoscopy camera (1), VITOM telescope (2), and light guide cable (3), held in place using the clamp and articulated arm (4). (*B*) Intraoperative view of the VITOM system positioned above the surgical site.

Table 1
Specifications of the video telescopic operating microscope system when used with an Image 1 camera, xenon light source, and 26-inch (66 cm) monitor

	Field of View		Reproduction Scale	
Working distance between telescope and surgical site	Camera zoom ×1	Camera zoom ×2	Camera zoom ×1	Camera zoom ×2
25 cm	5 cm	3.5 cm	8×	16×
50 cm	10 cm	7 cm	4×	8×

staff. The array of potential uses is large and includes almost any situation wherein microsurgery would be an advantage; however, just 3 cases are provided here as examples.

ADRENALECTOMY IN A FERRET (*MUSTELA PUTORIUS FURO*)

Hyperadrenocorticism is a common disease of ferrets, and adrenalectomy is frequently recommended either as the primary treatment or when cases are refractory to medical therapy.[6,7] Affected animals usually present with bilateral alopecia, ultrasonographic changes in one or both adrenals, and variable elevations of estradiol, androstenedione, or 17-hydroxyprogesterone.

The adrenal glands are embedded within fat and lie at the cranial poles of the kidneys. The left adrenal gland is closely associated with the aorta and lies just below the phrenicoabdominal vein. The right adrenal gland is intimately associated and generally adhered to the wall of the caudal vena cava. A large ventral midline laparotomy approach from xiphoid to caudal to the umbilicus is required to achieve sufficient exposure of the dorsal abdominal structures. A ring retractor with elastic stays (Lone-Star; Veterinary Specialty Products, Shawnee, KS, USA) facilitates retraction of the skin and linea alba and exposure of the cranial abdominal structures. The VITOM is positioned above the surgical field. Left adrenalectomy is technically easier as exposure is straightforward (**Fig. 2**A). Dissection of the left adrenal gland from surrounding fat is achieved using a combination of blunt dissection using cotton-tipped applicators and radiosurgery (4.0-MHz Surgitron; Ellman International, Oceanside, NY, USA). Dissection starts at the caudal aspect of the gland, taking care not to enter the glandular capsule (see **Fig. 2**B). As the surgeon progresses cranially, the gland is gently elevated to ensure that any adrenal tissue extending along the vessels is also removed. The only significant vessels encountered are the phrenicoabdominal vein (that lies over the ventral surface of the gland), and a small artery that enters the gland at its craniomedial border, although the aorta is in close proximity (see **Fig. 2**C). Radiosurgery and vascular clips are used to ensure hemostasis (see **Fig. 2**D–F). Right adrenalectomy is more challenging and requires incision of the hepatorenal ligament and gentle cranial retraction of the caudate liver lobe to achieve adequate exposure. In addition, the right adrenal is not only embedded within fat, but also intimately associated with the caudal vena cava. Careful dissection away from the wall of the vena cava is required and often facilitated by first placing a vascular clip between the adrenal and the vena cava. If the adrenal has invaded the wall of the vena cava, then partial resection of the vena cava is required. The affected adrenal and vessel wall is isolated using a neonatal Satinsky vascular clamp, before sharp resection, and repair of the vessel wall using 8/0 or 9/0 polydioxanone suture (PDS II; Ethicon Inc, Cornelia, GA, USA; www.ethicon.novartis.us). Partial resection is always a concern and cryosurgery,

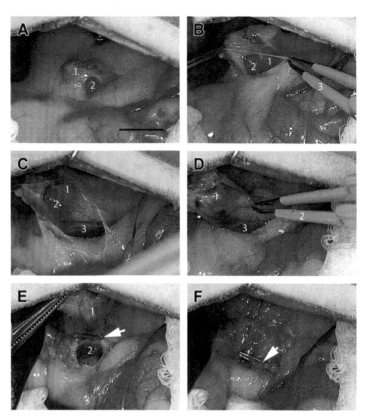

Fig. 2. Left adrenalectomy in a ferret using the VITOM system. (*A*) View of the enlarged left adrenal gland (1) and the phrenicoabdominal vein (2). Bar = 10 mm. (*B*) The left adrenal (1) and phrenicoabdominal vein (2) are preserved as radiosurgical bipolar forceps (3) are used to initiate dissection. (*C*) Following the initial fascial incision the left adrenal (1), phrenicoab-dominal vein (2) and aorta (3) can be more clearly seen. (*D*) Dissection continues around the left adrenal (1) using radiosurgery (2), taking care not to damage the aorta (3). (*E*) Once the left adrenal (1) is dissected free, a small vascular clip (*arrow*) is placed to isolate the gland from the aorta (2) and ensure hemostasis. (*F*) Following removal of the left adrenal, the vascular clip (*arrow*) and site are inspected before routine laparotomy closure.

radiosurgery, and laser have been used in an attempt to destroy any remaining neoplastic cells. On occasions, complete resection of the vena cava has proven successful if sufficient collateral blood flow has been established. Laparotomy closure is routine using techniques recommended for other small carnivores.

EXPLORATORY COELIOTOMY IN A BEARDED DRAGON (*POGONA VITTICEPS*)

Coeliotomy (laparotomy) is frequently used in reptile medicine and surgery for both diagnosis and treatment.[5,8,9] Oophorectomy, salpingotomy, salpingectomy, enterotomy, cystotomy, and the collection of visceral biopsies are just some of the reasons for performing coeliotomy. Liver disease is common in reptiles, and although changes in plasma biochemistry may be evident, hepatic biopsy is usually required for a definitive diagnosis.[10,11] Therefore, to illustrate the value of the VITOM in reptile medicine, coeliotomy and liver biopsy in a small lizard are described. The surgical approach to the lizard's coelom is complicated, not just by their diminutive size but also by the presence of a significant midline abdominal vein. With the lizard positioned in dorsal recumbency and the VITOM positioned above, a paramedian incision is made starting caudal to the umbilicus and extending cranially to the same level as the xiphoid process (**Fig. 3**A). Given the paramedian approach, sharp dissection through muscle causes hemorrhage, and therefore, blunt dissection through rectus abdominis is preferred. Retraction of the skin and muscle using a ring retractor and elastic stays helps expose the coelomic viscera (see **Fig. 3**B). Given the right paramedian approach, the gall bladder is obvious; however, biopsy from the caudal edge of the right liver lobe is still practical even in small lizards. A single loop of polydioxanone 3/0 suture is placed over the protruding margin of the right liver lobe in order to perform a guillotine biopsy procedure (see **Fig. 3**C). The suture is tightened to crush the surrounding hepatic tissue (see **Fig. 3**D), before a scalpel is used to excise the tissue distal to the suture (see **Fig. 3**E). After ensuring hemostasis, the ventral coelomic musculature is closed in a simple continuous pattern using 5/0 polydioxanone, while the skin is closed using 4/0 polydioxone using an everting horizontal mattress pattern (see **Fig. 3**F).

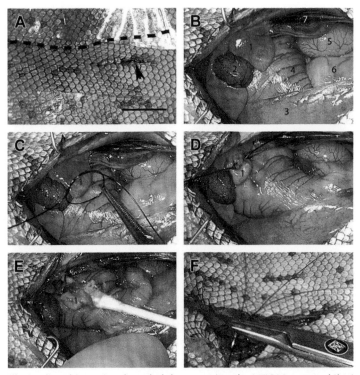

Fig. 3. Guillotine liver biopsy in a bearded dragon using the VITOM system. (*A*) View of the ventrum indicating the start of the paramedian coeliotomy incision (*arrow*), and the position of the midline and ventral abdominal vein (*dotted line*). Bar = 10 mm. (*B*) View of the exposed coelomic viscera including the liver (1), gall bladder (2), fat body (3), stomach (4), testis (5), large intestine (6), and ventral abdominal vein (7). (*C*) Placement of 3/0 polydioxanone suture around the caudal margin of the right liver lobe (1). (*D*) Tightening the suture to isolate the liver biopsy (1). (*E*) Removal of the liver biopsy (1) following sharp dissection distal to the suture. (*F*) Closing the rectus abdominis muscle using 5/0 polydioxone suture in a continuous pattern.

OVARIOHYSTERECTOMY IN A RAT (*RATTUS NORVEGICUS*)

Reproductive diseases, including cystic ovaries, pyometra, and neoplasia, remain common problems in pet rodents.[12,13] Sterilization would obviously prevent many of these diseases and has even been demonstrated to reduce the incidence of mammary neoplasia.[14] However, the practicality of performing ovariohysterectomy in small rodents necessitates magnification. With the rat positioned in dorsal recumbency and the VITOM positioned above the ventrum, a standard caudal laparotomy incision is made from umbilicus to the pelvic rim. The linea alba is incised using a scalpel or radiosurgery, taking particular care to avoid the often voluminous gastrointestinal tract below (**Fig. 4**A). Following the placement of a ring retractor and elastic stays, abdominal exposure permits the localization of the reproductive tract. The uterus is grasped and elevated and used to trace the ovaries (see **Fig. 4**B). Radiosurgery is used to first coagulate the ovarian vessels before incising the ovarian ligament (see **Fig. 4**C). The suspensory ligament of the uterus tends to be heavily infiltrated by fat that can make identification of blood vessels difficult. Therefore, radiosurgical dissection

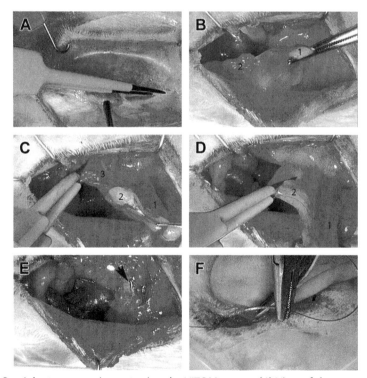

Fig. 4. Ovariohysterectomy in a rat using the VITOM system. (*A*) View of the ventrum while incisioning the linea alba using radiosurgery. (*B*) Forceps being used to grasp and elevate the uterus (1) and reveal the ovary (2). (*C*) Although elevating the uterus (1) and ovary (2), the ovarian vessels and mesovarium (3) are coagulated using radiosurgery. (*D*) The uterus (1) is elevated while radiosurgical dissection is continued through the broad ligament (2). (*E*) Once both ovaries and the entire uterus have been freed, a vascular clip (*arrow*) is placed across the cervix before radiosurgical resection and removal of the entire reproductive tract. (*F*) Following closure of the linea alba, fine absorbable monofilament is used to close the skin in a subcuticular pattern.

through this broad ligament is preferred (see **Fig.** 4D). Having freed both ovaries and the uterus to the level of the cervix, a vascular clip is used to ligate the cervix, before radiosurgical excision and removal of the reproductive tract (see **Fig.** 4E). Closure of the linea alba is accomplished using 5/0 polydioxanone in a simple continuous pattern. There is little subcutaneous tissue, and the skin is closed using antibiotic-impregnated 5/0 poliglecaprone 25 suture (Monocryl-Plus; Ethicon Inc) (see **Fig.** 4F).

SUMMARY

The VITOM system uses a practice's existing endoscopy equipment to provide a novel way for performing open microsurgical procedures in an ergonomic manner. The additional costs associated with the VITOM telescope and mechanical arm ($16,000) are 25% higher than those associated with high-quality headband or frame-mounted loupes with xenon light source and high-definition camera (eg, SurgiTel; Ann Arbor, MI, USA; www.surgitel.com). However, advantages of the VITOM system include

1. Utilization of existing endoscopy equipment, including photodocumentation for medical records, publications, client education, and practice marketing
2. Rapid positioning and ability to quickly reposition and refocus during surgery
3. Good ergonomic position with the surgeon sitting or standing and facing forward instead of down
4. Variable magnification with a good depth of field, which avoids instrument movements going in and out of focus
5. Static positioning helps:
   a. The entire operating room team to follow the procedure
   b. With taking high-quality photographs and video with less image blur and video editing
   c. Avoid obstruction of the video field by the surgeon's head (which is a common complication associated with in-light cameras)
6. The entire surgical team can observe the procedure from the monitor, which helps
   a. Teach veterinary students, interns, and residents
   b. Provide opportunities for assistants to anticipate surgeon's needs

High-quality illumination and magnification require significant capital investment, with poor-quality equipment resulting in reduced optical quality and suboptimal surgical performance. Veterinarians with existing endoscopy light source and camera equipment should consider the VITOM system as a viable alternative to traditional magnification systems.

ACKNOWLEDGMENTS

Thanks to Dr Chris Chamness and Karl Storz GmbH & Co KG for granting permission for the reproduction of the material contained in this article, which was originally submitted by the author for a Karl Storz publication (in press).

REFERENCES

1. American Veterinary Medical Association. U.S. Pet ownership & demographics sourcebook. Schaumburg (IL): American Veterinary Medical Association; 2007.
2. Bennett RA. Surgical considerations. In: Ritchie BW, Harrison GJ, Harrison LR, editors. Avian medicine: principles and application. Fort Worth (TX): Harrisons Bird Diets International Inc; 1994. p. 1081–95.

3. Divers SJ. Exotic pets. In: Tams T, Rawlings CA, editors. Small animal endoscopy. 3rd edition. St Louis (MO): Elsevier; 2011. p. 623–54.

4. Divers SJ. Endoscopy and endosurgery. Vet Clin North Am Exot Anim Pract 2010; 13(2):171–331.

5. Mader DR, Bennett RA, Funk RS, et al. Surgery. In: Mader DR, editor. Reptile medicine and surgery. 2nd edition. St. Louis (MO): Elsevier; 2006. p. 581–630.

6. Weiss CA, Scott MV. Clinical aspects and surgical treatment of hyperadrenocorticism in the domestic ferret: 94 cases (1994-1996). J Am Anim Hosp Assoc 1997; 33(6):487–93.

7. Ludwig L, Aiken S. Soft tissue surgery. In: Quesenberry KE, Carpenter JW, editors. Ferrets, rabbits and rodents - clinical medicine and surgery. St Louis (MO): Elsevier; 2004. p. 121–34.

8. Hernandez-Divers SJ. Surgery: principles and techniques. In: Raiti P, Girling S, editors. Manual of reptiles. 2nd edition. Cheltenham (United Kingdom): British Small Animal Veterinary Association; 2004. p. 147–67.

9. Hernandez-Divers SJ. Diagnostic techniques. In: Mader DR, editor. Reptile medicine and surgery. 2nd edition. St Louis (MO): Elsevier; 2006. p. 490–532.

10. Divers SJ. Reptilian liver and gastro-intestinal testing. In: Fudge AM, editor. Laboratory medicine avian and exotic pets. Philadelphia: WB Saunders; 2000. p. 205–9.

11. Hernandez-Divers SJ, Cooper JE. Hepatic lipidosis. In: Mader DR, editor. Reptile medicine and surgery. 2nd edition. St Louis (MO): Elsevier; 2006. p. 806–13.

12. O'Rourke DP. Disease problems of guinea pigs. In: Quesenberry KE, Carpenter JW, editors. Ferrets, rabbits and rodents - clinical medicine and surgery. St Louis (MO): Elsevier; 2004. p. 245–54.

13. Donnelly TM. Disease problems of small rodents. In: Quesenberry KE, Carpenter JW, editors. Ferrets, rabbits and rodents - clinical medicine and surgery. St Louis (MO): Elsevier; 2004. p. 299–315.

14. Hotchkiss CE. Effect of surgical removal of subcutaneous tumors on survival of rats. J Am Vet Med Assoc 1995;206:1575–9.

Endoscopy Practice Management, Fee Structures, and Marketing

Stephen J. Divers, BSc(Hons), BVetMed, DZooMed,
DipECZM (Herpetology, Zoo Health Management), DACZM, FRCVS

KEYWORDS

- Endoscopy • Practice management • Fee structure • Marketing

KEY POINTS

- Entry-level endoscopy equipment for the exotic animal practitioner costs around $15,000 ($300-per-month lease) and represents a significant capital investment.
- An appropriate charging mechanism and fee structure is required to offset purchase, use, maintenance, and replacement costs.
- Marketing is important to promote endoscopy services to clients.

INTRODUCTION

Although the clinical virtues of diagnostic and surgical endoscopy in exotic animal practice are obvious, appropriate management, including a fiscally responsible fee structure, seems to be more challenging. The costs of a basic rigid endoscopy system for exotic animal practice can range between $10,000 and $20,000 and is not an insignificant capital investment; therefore, a suitable fee structure is required to help recoup costs associated with purchase (or lease), use, repair, replacement, technician time, and practice facilities. From discussions with various colleagues, it became obvious that there was widespread variation in endoscopy practice management. In addition, attendees at endoscopy courses frequently raised concerns regarding fee structures. Consequently, the author designed and circulated a short survey in the summer of 2014 in an attempt to obtain basic information on endoscopy practice management in Europe and the United States.

The author has nothing to disclose.
Department of Small Animal Medicine and Surgery, College of Veterinary Medicine, University of Georgia, 2200 College Station Road, Athens, GA 30602, USA
E-mail address: sdivers@uga.edu

SURVEY

An Internet-based survey was completed by 35 veterinarians, of which 21 were from the United States or Canada, 10 from Europe, 3 from Australia or New Zealand, and one from Africa. The general demographics of their respective practices varied considerably; however, overall, the mean exotic pet caseloads were avian 31%, reptile/amphibian 21%, small mammals 23%, fish 2%, with the remainder being domesticated animals. In the following sections, the author tries to indicate the general themes and commonalities and has provided numerical mean values where appropriate.

EQUIPMENT

The total purchase costs of endoscopy equipment was, on average, $25,000; however, none of the respondents provided figures representing the recurring monthly costs associated with maintenance, repairs, and replacement. The basic 2.7-mm rigid endoscopy system can be purchased for around $15,000 (considerably less on the second-hand market) or leased for approximately $300 per month. Most survey respondents were experienced exotic animal endoscopists and had obviously expanded their endoscopy facilities from this basic starting point. Nevertheless, their continued preference for a 2.7-mm system was obvious, with most of the respondents (86%) owning this system. In addition, standard-definition cameras and monitors were twice as common (66%) compared with high-definition systems (34%), and xenon light sources were favored (60%) over cheaper halogen sources (34%). These differences probably represent a delay between new technological developments and the need to replace older items. The author expects high-definition and xenon to continue to gain in popularity in the future. Most veterinarians prefer to keep their equipment on a mobile endoscopy cart (or endoscopy tower). A complete list of endoscopy equipment and frequency of ownership can be found in **Table 1**.

EQUIPMENT CHARGES AND ANCILLARY FEES

There was considerable variation in the charging mechanism for the set up and use of endoscopy equipment. Only half of the veterinarians surveyed specifically charged for the use of an endoscopy or operating room ($150); sterilization, use, and cleaning of endoscopy equipment ($122); or standard surgical pack including traditional instruments, drape, cap, mask, and gloves ($71). Only 25% charged a specific fee for technician or nurse time ($31). No doubt, many veterinarians that do not charge the aforementioned fees separately probably incorporate them into their endoscopy procedural fees. However, there was almost universal consistency in applying separate charges for anesthesia ($184), histopathology ($210), and microbiology ($154).

ENDOSCOPY PROCEDURAL FEES

There was variation in how veterinarians actually charged for their endoscopy procedures. Approximately one-third of veterinarians used a tiered fee structure (eg, level 1–6, **Table 2**), whereas another third used an individual fee for every specific procedure (eg, reptile celioscopy, avian tracheoscopy, small mammal otoscopy, and so forth). The advantage of a tiered fee structure is that it provides flexibility to increase or decrease fees depending on difficulty, is simple and easily used by staff and doctors, and avoids numerous fee codes and individual descriptors. A major advantage of using detailed descriptors is that electronic medical record searches can be more targeted; however, this is at the expense of inputting considerably more data into a computerized accounting system.

Table 1 Endoscopy equipment ownership by exotic animal veterinarians	
Endoscopy Equipment Items	**Ownership (%)**
Separate xenon light source	60
Separate halogen light source	34
Separate standard-definition camera and monitor	66
Separate high-definition camera and monitor	34
All-in-one integrated light source, camera, and monitor system (eg, TelePak [Karl Storz Veterinary Endoscopy America Inc, Goleta, CA])	23
Carbon dioxide insufflator	40
Tilting endoscopy table	25
Integrated operating theater with endoscopy equipment on drop-down ceiling booms	3
Mobile endoscopy tower with endoscopy equipment on a mobile cart	60
<1.9-mm Rigid or semirigid endoscope	40
1.9-mm Telescope, sheath, and instruments (eg, biopsy, retrieval forceps, scissors)	40
2.7-mm Telescope, sheath, and instruments (eg, biopsy, retrieval forceps, scissors)	86
3-mm Endosurgery instruments (eg, handles, instruments, trocars/cannulae)	17
4-mm Telescope, sheath, and instruments (eg, biopsy, retrieval forceps, scissors)	20
5-mm Telescope	26
5-mm Endosurgery instruments (eg, handles, instruments, trocars/cannulae)	20
10-mm Telescope	14
10-mm Endosurgery instruments (eg, handles, instruments, trocars/ cannulae)	17
>10-mm Telescopes and instrumentation	6
Endoscopic radiosurgery or electrocautery	34
Endoscopic laser (eg, diode)	14
Flexible endoscopes <3 mm in diameter (with biopsy/retrieval instruments)	14
Flexible endoscopes 3.0–4.9 mm in diameter (with biopsy/retrieval instruments)	29
Flexible endoscopes 5–9 mm in diameter (with biopsy/retrieval instruments)	29
Flexible endoscopes >9 mm in diameter (with biopsy/retrieval instruments)	17
Separate, dedicated flexible endoscopy tower	11

Surprisingly, the final third of the survey population admitted to using no predetermined fee structure and calculated the fee to be charged on a case-by-case basis. Although this provides the greatest flexibility, general business management dogma suggests that it may result in undercharging, especially by those not directly invested in the fiscal well-being of the practice. **Table 3** lists several exotic animal endoscopy procedures and the mean fees charged. It must be appreciated that, just like any fee structure, there was considerable variation between low and high levels (approximately 50%–150% of stated means) that was probably related to geographic location and the associated costs of living. An audit of the practice caseload can be especially useful to identify likely endoscopy revenue streams (**Table 4**).

Table 2
The tiered endoscopy fee structure used at the University of Georgia by all services, including zoologic medicine

Endoscopy Fee Level	Cost ($) (January 2015)	Examples of Exotic Animal Procedures
1	81.44	Basic stomatoscopy, tracheoscopy, otoscopy
2	181.53	Complicated stomatoscopy, tracheoscopy, otoscopy Basic rhinoscopy, gastroscopy, cloacoscopy
3	264.75	Complicated rhinoscopy, gastroscopy, cloacoscopy Basic celioscopy with biopsy
4	348.38	More complicated celiotomy, bilateral entries, basic endosurgery (eg, granuloma removal)
5	431.80	More complicated endosurgery, multiple ports, surgical assistant
6	51.06	Reptile/bird sex identification fee per animal belonging to the same owner (in addition to a $500 set-up fee)

These fees only represent the procedure. Anesthesia, equipment, and laboratory tests are in addition.

MARKETING

Whenever a practice develops a new service area, appropriate marketing is essential. The ability to capture images and video for documentation makes it relatively simple to showcase the procedure to the client or referring veterinarian. It is important that the name and telephone number of the practice accompanies any image or video, as clients will frequently show their friends and family. Past materials can also be used in the examination room to demonstrate a proposed diagnostic plan to a new client (**Fig. 1**). These images should also be incorporated into letters sent to other veterinarians regarding cases that they referred for endoscopy or for referral brochures. Some practices have also discovered the benefits of holding an open day whereby the public can take behind-the-scenes tours and see demonstrations, including use of endoscopy equipment (**Fig. 2**).

When marketing endoscopy to clients, verbal delivery is critical. Take the following as an example:

> Mrs Smith your African grey seems to have respiratory disease, most likely fungal but could be bacterial. We could anesthetize for a radiograph and even perform endoscopy or we could start treatment today with both antibiotics and antifungals.

Compare the aforementioned delivery with the following and consider (1) which would be more convincing for the client and (2) more medically appropriate.

> Mrs Smith your African grey seems to have respiratory disease, but there are several possible causes and different treatments. We need to stabilize before briefly anesthetizing for radiographs and then consider endoscopy and biopsy to determine the best approach to treatment. Precise diagnosis will maximize treatment success.

The author hopes you agree that the second delivery is more convincing and avoids the inappropriate use of antimicrobials. However, it does depend on the veterinarian having confidence in his or her endoscopic abilities. To this end, it is just as important

Table 3
Mean fees charged in 2014 for specific exotic animal endoscopy procedures performed by 35 experienced clinicians. (Ranges varied between 50 and 150% of these mean values)

Procedure	Fee
Avian oculoscopy	$27
Avian tracheoscopy	$198
Avian tracheoscopy with biopsy or debridement	$280
Avian esophagus/proventriculus/ventriculus	$245
Avian esophagus/proventriculus/ventriculus with biopsy or debridement or foreign body removal	$400
Avian cloacoscopy	$173
Avian cloacoscopy with biopsy or debridement	$294
Avian celioscopy for reproductive evaluation of healthy birds (fee per bird in a group)	$194
Avian single-sided celioscopy for disease investigation	$304
Avian single-sided celioscopy with biopsy or debridement	$338
Avian multiple-entry endosurgery in a bird (eg, orchidectomy, salpingohysterectomy, mass removal)	$508
Reptile tracheoscopy	$151
Reptile tracheoscopy with biopsy or debridement	$273
Reptile esophagoscopy/gastroscopy	$195
Reptile esophagoscopy/gastroscopy with biopsy or debridement or foreign body removal	$310
Reptile celioscopy	$250
Reptile celioscopy with biopsy or debridement	$319
Reptile celioscopy and gonadectomy	$434
Reptile juvenile sex identification by celioscopy	$141
Reptile juvenile sex identification by cloacoscopy	$94
Reptile cloacoscopy for disease investigation	$172
Reptile cloacoscopy with biopsy or debridement	$228
Reptile pulmonoscopy (transcutaneous lung examination)	$253
Amphibian tracheoscopy	$135
Amphibian orograstroscopy	$55
Amphibian celioscopy	$61
Amphibian cloacoscopy	$47
Small mammal otoscopy	$129
Small mammal otoscopy with biopsy or debridement	$237
Small mammal oculoscopy	$73
Small mammal stomatoscopy for dental evaluation	$102
Small mammal stomatoscopy with biopsy, debridement, or guided dentistry	$183
Small mammal rhinoscopy	$199
Small mammal rhinoscopy with biopsy or debridement	$219
Small mammal tracheoscopy or intubation	$108
Small mammal tracheoscopy with biopsy or debridement	$213
Small mammal ovariectomy or ovariohysterectomy	$348
Small mammal laparoscopy	$308
Small mammal laparoscopy with biopsy or debridement	$361
Small mammal colonoscopy/vaginoscopy/cystoscopy	$232
Small mammal colonoscopy/vaginoscopy/cystoscopy with biopsy or debridement	$294
Fish gill endoscopy	$52
Fish orogastroscopy	$102
Fish celioscopy	$155

Table 4
An example of a case audit used to determine approximate monthly revenue using the mean fees from the survey of 35 exotic animal endoscopists

Case	Procedure	Anesthesia	Procedural Charge	Laboratory Fees	Estimated No. Per Month	Monthly Revenue
Rabbit/rodent dental	Stomatoscopy	$184	$102	Not applicable	2	$572
Small mammal otitis	Otoscopy	$184	$237	$154	1	$575
Parrot with respiratory disease	Celioscopy plus tracheoscopy	$184	$304 $280	$364	1	$1132
Anorectic lizard or turtle	Celioscopy	$184	$319	$210	1	$713
Total monthly revenue						$2992

Note: This calculation is based on only 5 exotic animal cases in a month and does not take into account any dog/cat cases; most practices could probably do more. Just one of these streams would cover the $300 monthly equipment lease.

to consider appropriate training as it is to have appropriate equipment. Fortunately, there are a variety of training opportunities within United States and Europe; short 4- to 8-hour workshops are frequently available at veterinary conferences (eg, Association of Reptilian and Amphibian Veterinarians, Association of Avian Veterinarians, Association of Exotic Mammal Veterinarians, American Association of Zoo Veterinarians, International Conference on Avian Herpetological Exotic Mammal Medicine).

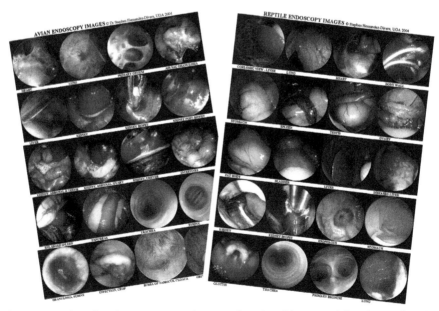

Fig. 1. Examples of endoscopy images being collated and laminated for client education and marketing.

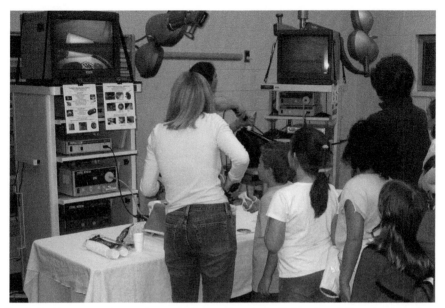

Fig. 2. Endoscopy station at the annual open day at the University of Georgia's Veterinary Teaching Hospital. Under veterinary staff supervision, children get to play various endoscopy games using old (autoclaved) disposable instruments. Such events can showcase practice facilities and staff and improve client awareness and appreciation.

More extensive 2-day courses on reptile/avian or small mammal endoscopy are regularly provided at the University of Georgia (www.vet.uga.edu/ce).

SUMMARY

The author hopes that this article, although imperfect, provides some insight into endoscopy practice management and fee structures. With a capital investment of around $15,000 (or $300-a-month lease) and basic training, a practice can offer endoscopy services to their exotic clientele and create new and exciting revenue streams.

Two-Portal Access Laparoscopic Ovariectomy Using Ligasure Atlas in Exotic Companion Mammals

Laila M. Proença, MV, DVM, MS, PhD

KEYWORDS

- Laparoscopic ovariectomy • Rabbit • Pig • Exotic mammal • Sterilization
- Endosurgery • Ligasure • Two-portal ovariectomy

KEY POINTS

- Laparoscopic sterilization techniques are becoming widely accepted because of the reported advantages of laparoscopy compared with laparotomy for sterilization in veterinary medicine.
- In human and veterinary surgery, there has been interest in reducing the number and size of portals in endosurgery, in an attempt to reduce postoperative pain.
- Novel computer-controlled bipolar electrocoagulation devices, facilitate sealing and dividing ovarian pedicles, reduce operative time and are widely used for surgical procedures in people and animals.
- The 2-portal laparoscopic ovariectomy has been proved to be safe, feasible, and effective in dogs and cats, but has not yet been described in exotic companion mammals.
- Further studies of laparoscopic ovariectomy, including 2-portal access in exotic companion mammals, are needed in order to assess safety and feasibility of the procedures.

 A video of a two-portal access laparoscopic ovariectomy accompanies this article at http://www.vetexotic.theclinics.com/

INTRODUCTION

Laparoscopic sterilization techniques are becoming widely accepted because of the reported advantages of laparoscopy compared with laparotomy for sterilization in veterinary medicine, including reduced pain and/or morbidity during the postoperative period, faster patient recovery, and better visualization of important structures during surgery.[1–5]

The author has nothing to disclose.
VCA Animals Hospitals, 12401 West Olympic Boulevard, Los Angeles, CA 90064, USA
E-mail address: laila.proenca@vca.com

Vet Clin Exot Anim 18 (2015) 587–596
http://dx.doi.org/10.1016/j.cvex.2015.04.010

Pain after laparoscopy is mostly related to abdominal distention due to pneumoperitoneum, as well as organic and chemical characteristics of the type of gas used.[6] In addition, in human and veterinary surgery, there has been interest in reducing the number and size of portals in endosurgery, in an attempt to reduce postoperative pain.[1,2,7] In a comparative study in dogs undergoing laparoscopic ovariectomy, the use of 2 cannulae significantly lower the postoperative pain score when compared with the use of 1 cannula or 3 cannulae.[1]

However, the same study showed that reducing the number of portals might prolong surgical time. The surgical time of dogs that underwent laparoscopic ovariectomy using 1 cannula was significantly longer than when using 2 or 3 cannulae. Interestingly, surgical time was not significantly different with the use of 2 or 3 cannulae (approximately 19 minutes total surgical time), and complication rates were not significantly different among the groups.[1]

Conversely, a study comparing laparoscopic ovariectomy in dogs using a single or 2-portal technique showed no significant difference in total surgical time (approximately 20 minutes) between the 2 techniques. Factors significantly affecting surgical time included body condition score, ovarian ligament fat score, ovarian bleeding, and surgeon expertize. Minor complications were similar in both groups.[2]

Novel computer-controlled bipolar electrocoagulation devices, such as the Ligasure Atlas (Covidien, Massachusetts), facilitate sealing and dividing ovarian pedicles, reduce operative time, and are widely used for surgical procedures in people and animals.[8–11] A recent study with Vietnamese Pot-bellied pigs demonstrated that open ovariectomy using the Ligasure is a faster surgical technique with less perioperative complications when compared with the ovariectomy with traditional ligatures.[9] The Ligasure Atlas with the ForceTriad generator (Covidien) was also shown to confidently promote hemostasis in arteries up to 7 mm in pigs.[12] In addition, laparoscopic-assisted 3-portal ovariectomy technique using the Ligasure device has proven to be a safe and rapid sterilization method for tigers.[13]

Elective laparoscopic ovariectomy and ovariohysterectomy, and video-assisted therapeutic ovariohysterectomy using the 2-portal techniques have been proven to be safe, feasible, and effective in dogs.[4,14–17] Moreover, ovariohysterectomy using the 2-portal technique has also been described in cats.[5] Although 3-portal laparoscopic ovariectomy has been successfully performed in rabbits,[18] the investigation of novel laparoscopic sterilization procedures, such as the use of 2-portal technique for ovariectomy, has not yet been explored in exotic companion mammals.

The purpose of this article is to describe the novel 2-portal access laparoscopic ovariectomy using the Ligasure Atlas with the ForceTriad generator in exotic companion mammals, more specifically in rabbits and Pot-bellied pigs. It is important to notice that the data presented here have not been scientifically reproduced and are based only on the author's experience.

The primary indication for 2-portal laparoscopic ovariectomy in exotic mammals is sterilization.

Contraindications for 2-portal laparoscopic ovariectomy in exotic mammals include

- Any contraindication for anesthesia and/or surgery
- Lack of appropriate equipment
- Lack of surgeon training
- Obese animals
- Any contraindication for laparoscopic ovariectomy (eg, presence of large masses on the ovaries)

LAPAROSCOPIC EQUIPMENT

For the proposed technique presented here, the dissection of the ovary is achieved with the use of the vessel sealer and divider Ligasure Atlas with the ForceTriad generator. The smallest diameter currently available for this equipment is the 5 mm, hence requiring the use of the 6 mm cannula. The Ligasure Atlas facilitates surgery and decreases surgical time, because the instrument is capable of sealing and cutting, without the need of changing instruments multiple times during the procedure. However, one should know that the use of the vessel sealer and divider is not mandatory and can be replaced by the use of bipolar endoscopic forceps and endoscopic scissors.

For the ovariectomy using a 2-portal approach in patients weighing less than 10 kg, the author prefers to use a smaller port (3.9 mm cannula) to accommodate the 2.7 mm telescope with the 3.5 mm protection sheath, and a second larger port (6 mm cannula) to accommodate the 5 mm vessel sealer and divider. For patients weighing more than 10 kg 2 6 mm cannulae can be used to house the 5 mm telescope and the 5 mm vessel sealer and divider.

Equipment for the 2-portal laparoscopic ovariectomy in exotic mammals includes

- Endovideo camera
- Xenon light source and light cable
- Imaging capture system (optional)
- Monitor—optionally 2 monitors might be connected to the camera to permit ovariectomy from either side of the table
- CO_2 insufflator with silicone tubing
- First (cranial) portal
  ○ For animals less than 10 kg: 2.7 mm, 18 cm telescope, 30° oblique view, with the 3.5 mm protection sheath and the 3.9 mm graphite and plastic cannula (with CO_2-line connection)
  ○ For animals more than 10 kg: 5 mm, 30 cm telescope, 30° oblique view, with the 6 mm threaded endotip cannula (with CO_2-line connection)
- Second (caudal) portal
  ○ 6 mm threaded endotip cannula to house the 5 mm endoscopic Babcock forceps (Karl Storz, Tuttlingen, BW, Germany) with ratchet handle and the 5 mm blunt tip (dolphin tip), 37 cm vessel sealer and divider (LigaSure Atlas).
- Energy platform for the vessel sealer and divider (ForceTriad)
- Polypropylene monofilament (150 cm), or similar, on a 5 cm, half circle curved tapper needle

PATIENT PREPARATION AND ANESTHESIA

For the 2-portal laparoscopic ovariectomy, the patient should undergo standard and routine anesthetic and surgical preparation, including physical examination, basic blood tests, and adequate fasting time for the species. In the author's experience, pigs might require a prolonged fasting time of 24 hours (food only, water should be removed 4 hours prior to the procedure) to minimize the gastrointestinal tract. Different anesthesia protocols are available, and the reader is encouraged to review the latest literature. However, one should notice that tracheal intubation and assisted ventilation are paramount due to the pneumoperitoneum.

Anesthesia should be monitored at minimum by evaluating reflexes, heart and respiratory rates, electrocardiogram (ECG), end-tidal carbon dioxide concentration, peripheral pulse, blood pressure, oxygen saturation, and body temperature. Intravenous fluid should be delivered continuously at a rate of 5 to 10 mL/kg/h during surgery.

Special attention should be taken when clipping the patient's hair, since the transabdominal suspension sutures, necessary for the technique, will be placed dorsally on each flank (**Fig. 1**).

TWO-PORTAL LAPAROSCOPIC OVARIECTOMY USING LIGASURE ATLAS
Patient Positioning

The patient should be placed in dorsal recumbency (**Fig. 2**A), or in a slight reverse Trendelenburg position, on a surgical tilting table, allowing patient rotation toward each side during surgery (see **Fig. 2**E). Alternatively, a small modified tilting table (modified after Tankersley design) can be used. The patient must be tightly tied to the table to avoid an accidental fall during rotation.

Surgical Technique

Following aseptic preparation, an approximately 1 cm long skin incision is made on the midline, 1 to 2 cm caudal to the umbilicus, exposing the linea alba. The musculature is elevated with the use of a thumb forceps to lift the body wall away from the viscera, and the linea alba is incised with the use of a No. 15 scalpel blade (see **Fig. 2**B). Then, the sheathed 30° 2.7 mm diameter telescope is inserted into the peritoneal cavity toward the right cranial quadrant. A mattress suture with 2-0 nylon is placed around the sheath to create an airtight seal (Hasson technique) (see **Fig. 2**C). CO_2 insufflation is started via the cannula port at 1 to 2 L/min to a pressure of 8 to 10 mm Hg (maximum of 12 mm Hg) (see **Fig. 2**C).

After appreciation of the abdominal cavity, a second 1 to 2-cm skin incision is made on the linea alba 2 to 3 cm cranial to the first incision. The second cannula (endotip) is inserted under direct visualization to prevent injury to the abdominal organs (see **Fig. 2**D). Then the patient is rotated 30° or more either to the right or left side to allow visualization of the left or right ovary, respectively (see **Fig. 2**E).

The kidney is visualized as a landmark, and the ovary is identified caudal to the kidney (**Fig. 3**A). The ovary is then grasped with the Babcoock forceps inserted through the cranial portal (see **Fig. 3**B). The gonad is elevated and tacked to the body wall using a transabdominal suspension suture, bypassing a 5 cm, half circle curved tapper needle through the body wall (see **Figs. 2**F and **3**C, D). A hemostat forceps is used to secure the suture on the skin surface (see **Fig. 2**G). The Babcoock forceps is retrieved

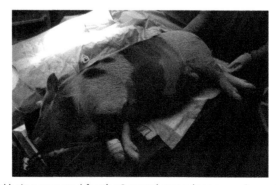

Fig. 1. Pot-bellied being prepared for the 2-portal access laparoscopic ovariectomy. Note the hair removal extended dorsally on the left flank due to the upcoming transabdominal suspension sutures. The right flank is clipped on the same manner (not seen in the picture). (Copyright © 2015 The University of Georgia. All Rights Reserved.)

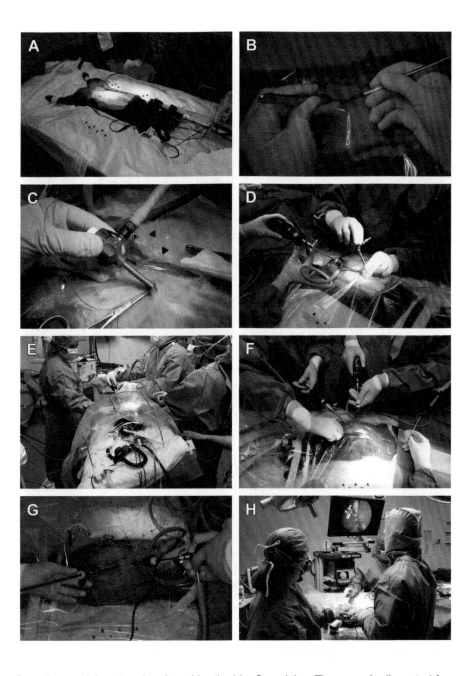

from the caudal port and replaced by the LigaSure Atlas. The ovary is dissected free by cauterizing and cutting the ovarian pedicle, proper ligament, and mesovarium (see **Figs.** 2H and **3**E). After ensuring hemostasis (see **Fig. 3**F), the ovary is left tacked to the body wall to be retrieved after contralateral ovariectomy.

The patient is rotated to the opposite side and the contralateral ovary dissected as described previously. After bilateral ovariectomy the Babcoock forceps is used to grasp the resected ovary still tacked to the body wall. Subsequently, the percutaneous

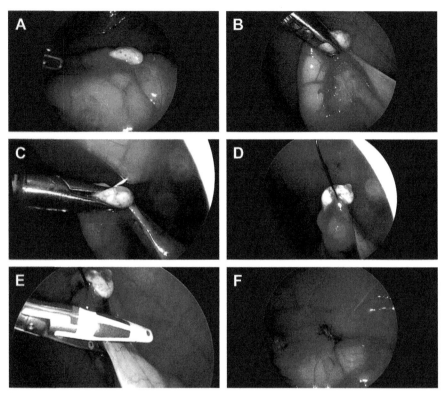

Fig. 3. Endoscopic view of the 2-portal access laparoscopic ovariectomy using Ligasure Atlas in a rabbit. (*A*) The ovary is identified. (*B*) The ovary is grasped with the Babcoock forceps and elevated to the body wall. (*C*, *D*) The gonad is tacked to the body wall using a transabdominal suspension suture, by passing a 5 cm, half circle curved tapper needle through the body wall. (*E*) The ovary is dissected free by cauterizing and cutting the ovarian pedicle, proper ligament and mesovarium. (*F*) The ovary has been removed and the surgical site observed to assure hemostasis. (Copyright © 2015 The University of Georgia. All Rights Reserved.)

Fig. 2. Two-portal access laparoscopic ovariectomy using Ligasure Atlas in a rabbit. (*A*) The patient is anesthetized and positioned on dorsal recumbency. (*B*) Following aseptic preparation and skin incision on the midline (1–2 cm caudal to the umbilicus), the musculature is elevated with the use of a thumb forceps to lift the body wall away, from the viscera and the linea alba is incised with the use of a No. 15 scalpel blade. (*C*) A 3.9 mm graphite and plastic cannula is inserted into the peritoneal cavity (first portal) toward the right cranial quadrant through the minilaparotomy incision. A mattress suture with 2-0 nylon is placed around the sheath to create an airtight seal (Hasson technique) and is secured by a hemostat. The CO_2 line is connected to the cannula, and CO_2 insufflation is started. (*D*) The 6 mm endotip cannula (second portal) is inserted on the midline cranial to the first portal under direct visualization provided by the telescope/camera. (*E*) The patient is rotated approximately 30° to the left to allow visualization of the right ovary. (*F*) Transabdominal suspension suture is applied to tack the ovary to the body wall. (*G*) A hemostat forceps is used to secure the transabdominal suspension suture on the skin surface. (*H*) The surgeon (*left*) using the LigaSure Atlas to dissect the ovary free while the assistant (*right*) holds the telescope/camera. (Copyright © 2015 The University of Georgia. All Rights Reserved.)

suture is relieved, by releasing the hemostat securing the suture to the body wall, allowing retrieval of the ovary still connected to the suture line. At this point one should not remove the suture line completely, because the line will allow retrieval of the ovary in case the grasp on the ovary is lost. The gonad is brought directly toward the cranial cannula and removed from the abdomen by gently unscrewing the cannula and pulling the forceps backwards, removing the ovary and the entire suture line tacked to it. The cannula is then replaced and the procedure repeated with the other ovary. Step-by-step two-portal laparoscopic ovariectomy using Ligasure Atlas in a rabbit can be appreciated on Video 1.

At the end of the procedure, the CO_2 previously insufflated is removed from the peritoneal cavity by manual expression. The telescope, cannulae, and mattress suture are removed, and the muscle and skin closed in 2 layers, in simple interrupted and subcuticular pattern, respectively, with 3-0 poliglecaprone 25.

COMPLICATIONS AND MANAGEMENT

Based on the author's experience, complications have occurred in 2 Pot-bellied pigs submitted to the 2-portal laparoscopic ovariectomy. Complications were attributed to the volumous gastrointestinal tract and extensive ovarian ligament fat, often hindering ovarian visualization. In the first case, bilateral ovariectomy was successfully accomplished via the 2-portal technique (**Fig. 4**A–C), but surgery time was prolonged, and the postoperatory minimally complicated due to mild ileus (possibly caused by the prolonged anesthesia time). In the second case, identification and visualization of the right ovary was not possible, and the surgery had to be converted to laparotomy. However, due to the exceptionally dorsal position of the right ovary, even the open ovariectomy was challenging but was successfully accomplished using the LigaSure Atlas. Severe postsurgical ileus occurred in this case, requiring several days of hospitalization and intensive care. The author has not experienced complications with 2-portal laparoscopic ovariectomy in rabbits.

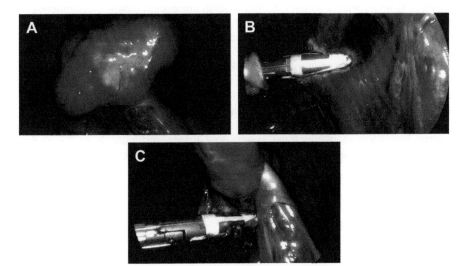

Fig. 4. Endoscopic view of the 2-portal access laparoscopic ovariectomy using Ligasure Atlas in a pot-bellied pig. (*A*) The ovary is identified and elevated. (*B, C*) The ovary is being dissected free by cauterizing and cutting the ovarian pedicle, proper ligament, and mesovarium. (Copyright © 2015 The University of Georgia. All Rights Reserved.)

In order to minimize complications, the author recommends a prolonged fasting time for pigs of 24 hours (food only, water should be removed 4 hours prior to the procedure), in an attempt to minimize the often volumous gastrointestinal tract. In addition, obese animals should be encouraged to loose weight prior to surgery. It is important to notice that the author has only performed elective laparoscopic ovariectomy in young pigs (less than 10 months) and results in older animals are unknown, but possibly more difficult, due to the tendency of pigs to become rapidly overweight.

When attempting novel techniques, such as the 2-portal laparoscopic ovariectomy, the surgeon should always be prepared to convert the procedure to traditional laparotomy and the owner should be fully informed about the risks prior to surgery (including possible emergency conversion to laparotomy and postsurgical ileus).

Postoperative Care

General postoperative care should include the use of pain medication (anti-inflammatories and opioids), gastroprotectants (for pigs), and supportive care. Usually, if no complications occur, the patient is kept hospitalized for observation for only 1 night following surgery. The author does not recommend the use of antimicrobials for routine elective laparoscopic ovariectomy. Exceptions are the use of transoperatory antibiotic in case of conversion to laparotomy (surgical time more than 1 hour) or if sterile conditions are broken. One must follow the routine standard of care regarding hospitalization, supportive, and critical care treatment based on each individual case postoperatively.

CURRENT CONTROVERSIES/FUTURE CONSIDERATIONS

Due to the small number of publications involving a selected number of species, further studies of laparoscopic ovariectomy, including 2-portal access in exotic companion mammals, are needed in order to assess safety and feasibility of the procedures. Extrapolations among species should be carefully considered.

Similar to small animal surgery, further studies comparing different approaches to laparoscopic ovariectomy (eg, 1-, 2- or 3-portal access) and different methods of ovarian dissection (eg, different vascular sealing devises and vascular clip application) are warranted.

One should expect to encounter potentially complex situations in older animals or in case of disease in the reproductive tract. It is likely that additional experiences with a wider variety of species and wider variety of endosurgical equipment will lead to more refined methods of sterilization for exotic companion mammals.

Based on the author's experience and lack of scientific comparative studies, the 2-portal laparoscopic ovariectomy seems to be safe and feasible in the rabbit. Conversely it seems that the 3-portal approach for laparoscopic ovariectomy would be preferred in pigs.

SUMMARY

Laparoscopic sterilization techniques are becoming widely accepted because of the reported advantages of laparoscopy compared with laparotomy for sterilization in veterinary medicine. In human and veterinary surgery, there has been interest in reducing the number and size of portals in endosurgery, in an attempt to reduce postoperative pain. Novel computer-controlled bipolar electrocoagulation devices, such as the Ligasure Atlas, facilitate sealing and dividing ovarian pedicles, reduce operative time, and are widely used for surgical procedures in people and animals.

The 2-portal laparoscopic ovariectomy has been proven to be safe, feasible, and effective in dogs and cats, but has not yet been described in exotic companion mammals. Based on the author's experience, the 2-portal laparoscopic ovariectomy seems to be safe and feasible in the rabbit, but complications such as emergency conversion to laparotomy and severe post-operative ileus have occurred in pigs. Further studies of laparoscopic ovariectomy, including 2-portal access in exotic companion mammals, are needed in order to assess safety and feasibility of the procedures. Extrapolations among species should be carefully considered.

ACKNOWLEDGMENTS

The author thank Supreme Pet Foods for supporting the UGA Residency in Zoologic Medicine and Dr M. Radlinsky for the support and teaching on the novel 2-portal access laparoscopic ovariectomy in exotic companion mammals. Thanks also to Dr Divers for the invitation for this VCNA issue, Dr I. Sladakovic and I. Desprez for their support, A. Schuller and C. McElhannon for their technical skills, and G. Neto for the help on editing the images.

SUPPLEMENTARY DATA

Supplementary data related to this article can be found online at http://dx.doi.org/10.1016/j.cvex.2015.04.010.

REFERENCES

1. Case JB, Marvel SJ, Boscan P, et al. Surgical time and severity of postoperative pain in dogs undergoing laparoscopic ovariectomy with one, two, or three instrument cannulas. J Am Vet Med Assoc 2011;239:203–8.
2. DuprE G, Fiorbianco V, Skalicky M, et al. Laparoscopic ovariectomy in dogs: comparison between single portal and two-portal access. Vet Surg 2009;38:818–24.
3. Davidson EB, Payton ME. Comparison of laparoscopic ovariohysterectomy and ovariohysterectomy in dogs. Vet Surg 2004;33:62–9.
4. Shariati E, Bakhtiari J, Khalaj A, et al. Comparison between two portal laparoscopy and open surgery for ovariectomy in dogs. Vet Res Forum 2014;5:219.
5. Ferreira MP, Schiochet F, Stedile R, et al. Ovário-salpingo-histerectomia videolaparoscópica em gatos domésticos: técnica com dois portais. Acta Sci Vet 2011;39:1–5.
6. Mouton W, Bessell J, Millard S, et al. A randomized controlled trial assessing the benefit of humidified insufflation gas during laparoscopic surgery. Surg Endosc 1999;13:106–8.
7. Leggett P, Churchman-Winn R, Miller G. Minimizing ports to improve laparoscopic cholecystectomy. Surg Endosc 2000;14:32–6.
8. Riegler M, Cosentini E. Update on LigaSure®/Atlas® vessel-sealing technology in general surgery. Eur Surg 2004;36:85–8.
9. Biedrzycki A, Brounts SH. A less invasive technique for spaying pet pigs. Vet Surg 2013;42:346–52.
10. Ohlund M, Hoglund O, Olsson U, et al. Laparoscopic ovariectomy in dogs: a comparison of the LigaSure (TM) and the SonoSurg (TM) systems. J Small Anim Pract 2011;52:290–4.

11. Mayhew PD, Brown DC. Comparison of three techniques for ovarian pedicle hemostasis during laparoscopic-assisted ovariohysterectomy. Vet Surg 2007;36: 541–7.

12. Katsuno G, Nagakari K, Fukunaga M. Comparison of two different energy-based vascular sealing systems for the hemostasis of various types of arteries: a porcine model—evaluation of LigaSure ForceTriad™. J Laparoendosc Adv Surg Tech A 2010;20:747–51.

13. Steeil JC, Sura PA, Ramsay EC, et al. Laparoscopic-assisted ovariectomy of tigers (*Panthera tigris*) with the use of the Ligasure™ device. J Zoo Wildl Med 2012;43:566–72.

14. Ataide MW, Brun MV, Barcellos LJ, et al. Laparoscopic-assisted or open ovariohysterectomy using Ligasure atlas™ in dogs. Ciência Rural 2010;40(9):1974–9.

15. Culp WT, Mayhew PD, Brown DC. The effect of laparoscopic versus open ovariectomy on postsurgical activity in small dogs. Vet Surg 2009;38:811–7.

16. Niranjana C, Ganesh R, Jayaprakash R, et al. Two different port placement models and ovarian pedicle hemostasis techniques in laparoscopic-assisted ovariohysterectomy-bitches. Int J Vet Sci 2013;2:155–60.

17. Guedes RL, Simeoni CP, Linhares MT, et al. Videoassisted ovariohysterectomy with two portals for pyometra's treatment in a bitch. Ciência Rural 2012;42(6): 1040–3.

18. Divers SJ. Clinical technique: endoscopic oophorectomy in the rabbit (*oryctolagus cuniculus*): the future of preventative sterilizations. Journal of Exotic Pet Medicine 2011;20:72–80.

Index

Note: Page numbers of article titles are in **boldface** type.

Printed and bound by CPI Group (UK) Ltd, Croydon, CR0 4YY

03/10/2024

01040494-0013